14TH EDITION

The Reference Manual of the

OFFICIAL
DOCUMENTS

of the American Occupational Therapy Association, Inc.

By American Occupational Therapy Association

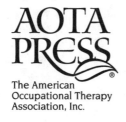

AOTA
PRESS

The American
Occupational Therapy
Association, Inc.

AOTA Vision Statement

The American Occupational Therapy Association advances occupational therapy as the pre-eminent profession in promoting the health, productivity, and quality of life of individuals and society through the therapeutic application of occupation.

AOTA Mission Statement

The American Occupational Therapy Association advances the quality, availability, use, and support of occupational therapy through standard-setting, advocacy, education, and research on behalf of its members and the public.

AOTA *Centennial Vision*

We envision that occupational therapy is a powerful, widely recognized, science-driven, and evidence-based profession with a globally connected and diverse workforce meeting society's occupational needs.

AOTA Staff

Frederick P. Somers, *Executive Director*
Christopher M. Bluhm, *Chief Operating Officer*

Chris Davis, *Director, AOTA Press*
Ashley Hofmann, *Production Editor*
Victoria Davis, *Editorial Assistant*

Beth Ledford, *Director, Marketing and Member Communications*
Emily Harlow, *Technology Marketing Specialist*
Jennifer Folden, *Marketing Specialist*

The American Occupational Therapy Association, Inc.
4720 Montgomery Lane
Bethesda, MD 20814
Phone: 301-652-AOTA (2682)
TDD: 800-377-8555
Fax: 301-652-7711
www.aota.org
To order: 1-877-404-AOTA (2682)

Disclaimers

This publication is designed to provide accurate and authoritative information in regard to the subject matter covered. It is sold or distributed with the understanding that the publisher is not engaged in rendering legal, accounting, or other professional service. If legal advice or other expert assistance is required, the services of a competent professional person should be sought.
—*From the Declaration of Principles jointly adopted by the American Bar Association and a Committee of Publishers and Associations*

It is the objective of the American Occupational Therapy Association to be a forum for free expression and interchange of ideas. The opinions expressed by the contributors to this work are their own and not necessarily those of the American Occupational Therapy Association.

ISBN 13: 978-1-56900-282-7

Design by Sarah Ely and Michael Melletz

Printing by Automated Graphic Systems, Inc., White Plains, MD.

Reference citation: American Occupational Therapy Association. (2009). *The reference manual of the official documents of the American Occupational Therapy Association, Inc.* (14th ed.). Bethesda, MD: Author.

For permissions inquiries, visit www.copyright.com.

Contents

*Articles in **bold** are new to this edition.*

---

[1]These guidelines were not adopted by the Representative Assembly.

Introduction

The Reference Manual of the Official Documents of the American Occupational Therapy Association, Inc. (AOTA) was first published in 1980 and had been fully revised biennially in even-numbered years, with an addendum produced in alternate years. In 2006, AOTA Press began publishing a fully revised edition of the *Reference Manual,* which is now produced annually. Each book purchased includes a CD for use in the classroom and in practice that provides a user-friendly search capability.

The 14th edition of this important work contains the following material:

- Part I contains AOTA's current official documents, which have been "constructed by the Association and approved by the Association for the use of the Association and its membership" (AOTA, 2007).

- Part II contains Societal Statements.

- Part III contains information about the American Occupational Therapy Foundation (AOTF).

- Part IV contains historical information on past official documents.

Types of official documents (AOTA, 2004) include the following:

- **Concept papers,** which provide a thoughtful discussion of an issue or topic, synthesizing varying perspectives to assist members to more thoroughly understand the issue or topic. These documents are developed in response to a particular issue, concern, or need and can be written for internal or external use.

- **Guidelines,** which provide descriptions, examples, or recommendations of procedures pertaining to the education and practice of occupational therapy. The *AOTA Practice Guidelines Series* has a separate development process that is part of the Evidence-Based Review Project and is not included in the official document development or adoption process.

- **Position papers,** which present the official stance of the Association on a substantive issue or subject. They are developed in response to a particular issue, concern, or need of the Association and may be written for internal or external use.

- **Roles papers,** which present a guide to the major roles common in the profession of occupational therapy. The roles listed in these documents are those frequently held by occupational therapists and occupational therapy assistants and are not all-inclusive.

- **Specialized knowledge and skills papers,** which provide a detailed outline of the specialized knowledge and skills needed for competent practice. The rationale for the development of this type of document is to provide a structure for acquiring competency in an area in which there are specialized evaluation and intervention processes.

- **Standards,** which include a general description of the topic and define the minimum requirements for performance and quality.

- **Statements,** which describe and clarify an aspect or issue related to education or practice and are linked to the fundamental concepts of occupational therapy.

Other association documents that are included in this publication are

- **Societal statements**—Written in the form of public announcements, these statements identify a societal issue of concern; state how the issue affects the participation of individuals, families, groups, or communities in society; and may offer action to be taken by individuals, groups, or communities.

- **AOTF information**—Although AOTF is separate from AOTA, this information has been included at reader request.

The documents contained in this manual have been developed by the combined efforts of many AOTA volunteers and staff. Authorship and citations for where these documents have been published in the *American Journal of Occupational Therapy* can be found at the end of each document. For additional information, visit www.aota.org.

References

American Occupational Therapy Association. (2004). *COE and COP standard operating procedures—Official documents (Attachment A).* (Available from American Occupational Therapy Association, 4720 Montgomery Lane, PO Box 31220, Bethesda, MD 20824-1220.)

American Occupational Therapy Association. (2007). *Definition of official documents.* (Adopted by the AOTA Representative Assembly during its 2006 online meeting.)

Categories of Occupational Therapy Personnel

Code: RA Motion 7/94, 4/95, 2003M54, 2006C379
Effective: 7/94
Revised: 4/95, 4/96, 4/98, 4/99, 4/01, 6/03, 4/06
BPPC Reviewed: 10/01, 1/02, 1/03, 1/06
Rescinded:

PURPOSE: To establish policy assuring that Association documents use consistent terminology when referring to individuals who provide or support the delivery of occupational therapy services.

It Shall Be the Policy of the Association That

The following terms are used as defined herein in all Association documents and publications:

1. **Occupational Therapy Personnel:** Individuals who work in an occupational therapy program/department/unit to ensure the delivery of occupational therapy services to consumers. Occupational therapy personnel may include occupational therapist (OT), occupational therapy assistant (OTA), occupational therapy student (OTS), occupational therapy assistant student (OTAS), and aide.

2. **Occupational Therapist (OT):** Any individual initially certified to practice as an OT or licensed or regulated by a state, commonwealth, district, or territory of the United States to practice as an occupational therapist and who has not had that certification, license, or regulation revoked due to disciplinary action.

3. **Occupational Therapy Assistant (OTA):** Any individual initially certified to practice as an OTA or licensed or regulated by a state, commonwealth, district, or territory of the United States to practice as an OTA and who has not had that certification, license, or regulation revoked due to disciplinary action.

4. **Occupational Therapy Student (OTS):** Any individual who is enrolled in an occupational therapy educational program that is accredited or pending accreditation by ACOTE.®

5. **Occupational Therapy Assistant Student (OTAS):** An individual who is enrolled in an occupational therapy assistant educational program that is accredited or pending accreditation by ACOTE.®

6. **Occupational Therapy Practitioner:** An individual initially certified to practice as an OT or OTA or licensed or regulated by a state, district, commonwealth, or territory of the United States to practice as an OT or OTA and who has not had that certification, license, or regulation revoked due to disciplinary action.

7. **Aide:** A person who is not licensed or regulated and who provides supportive services to OTs and OTAs. An aide shall function under the guidance and responsibility of the licensed or regulated OT and may be supervised by the OT or an OTA for specifically selected routine tasks for which the aide has been trained and has demonstrated competence. The aide is not a primary service provider of occupational therapy in a practice setting and does not provide skilled occupational therapy services.

PART I

Official Documents

Incorporation Papers and Bylaws

The

Articles of Incorporation
Of
American Occupational Therapy
Association

******

Composite Articles of Incorporation of The American Occupational Therapy Association as amended*

We, The Undersigned, All being persons of full age, and all being citizens of the United States desiring to form a corporation, pursuant to Sub-Chapter 3, of Chapter 18, of the Code of Law for the District of Columbia, do hereby make, sign and acknowledge this Certificate as follows:

FIRST: The name of the corporation is to be "The American Occupational Therapy Association."**

SECOND: The term of existence of the corporation shall be perpetual.

THIRD: The purpose or purposes which it will hereafter pursue are to *advance the therapeutic value of occupation; to research the effects of occupation upon human beings and to disseminate that research;* to promote the use of occupational therapy and to advance the standards of education and training in this field; *to educate consumers about the effect of occupation upon their well-being;* and to engage in such other activities as may be considered to be advantageous to the profession, its members, and the consumers of occupational therapy services. [Italicized portions adopted by Executive Board 1/16/76.]

FOURTH: *The corporation is to have members.*

FIFTH: *The corporation is to be divided into classes of members. The designation of each class of members, the qualifications, rights, and limitations of the members of each class and conferring, limiting, or denying the right to vote are as follows:*

a. Members: The classes of members are (1) occupational therapist, (2) occupational therapy assistant, (3) occupational therapy student, (4) organizational, and (5) associate. The bylaws may designate other classes of members.

b. Qualifications, Rights, and Limitations: The qualifications, rights, and limitations of the members of each class shall be provided in the bylaws.

c. Voting: Members are entitled to vote for Association officers and bylaw changes; members shall have such other voting rights as are provided in the bylaws. Associate members and Organizational members shall not be entitled to vote for Association Officers and bylaw changes.

SIXTH: The number of trustees, directors, or managers of the corporation shall be not less than five (5) nor more than fifty (50), and shall be known as the Board of Directors. *The manner of election or appointment of such directors shall be provided in the bylaws.*

SEVENTH: The territory in which its operations are principally to be conducted is the United States of America, the territories, possessions, and dependencies thereof and the District of Columbia, but the operations of the corporation shall not be limited to such territory.

EIGHTH: The location of the principal office of the corporation shall be fixed by the bylaws of the corporation.

NINTH: The time for holding its annual meeting shall be fixed by the bylaws of the corporation.

TENTH: *In the event this corporation shall be dissolved for any reason, any remaining assets shall be distributed for purposes within the scope of Internal Revenue code 501(c)(6) or any amendment thereto, and in accordance with the corporate statutes of the District of Columbia.*

ELEVENTH: The address, including street and number, of its registered office in the District of Columbia is 918-16th St N.W., Washington, DC 20006, and the name of its registered agent at such address is C.T. Corporation System.

TWELFTH: The names and places of residence of the persons to be its directors until its first annual meeting are as follows:
William R. Dunton, Jr., MD, of Sheppard and Enoch Pratt Hospital of Towson, Maryland; Susan C. Johnson, of 350 West 85th Street, New York City, New York; Eleanor Clarke Slagle, of the Hotel Alexandria, Chicago, Illinois; Susan E. Tracy, of Jamaica Plain, Massachusetts; and George Edward Barton, of Consolation House, Clifton Springs, New York.

IN WITNESS WHEREOF: We have made signed and acknowledged this certificate in duplicate.
Date, Clifton Springs, Ontario County, New York, this fifteenth day of March, A.D. 1917.
William R. Dunton, Jr.
Susan C. Johnson
Eleanor Clarke Slagle
George Edward Barton
Isabel G. Newton
T.B. Kidner

STATE OF NEW YORK
COUNTY OF ONTARIO: SS
On the fifteenth day of March, 1917, before me personally came William R. Dunton, Jr., Susan C. Johnson, Eleanor Clarke Slagle, George Edward Barton, Isabel G. Newton, and T.B. Kidner, to me known and known to me to be the same persons described in and who executed the foregoing certificate the same.
James A. Rolfe,
Notary Public.

(NOTARIAL SEAL)

* A resolution recommending that the corporation accept the jurisdiction of the District of Columbia Nonprofit Corporation Act (29 D.C. Code Chapter 10 then) was adopted at a meeting of the Executive Board on January 16, 1976. The formal Statement of Election to Accept was filed and certified on August 30, 1976. Italicized items were filed as part of that Statement to amend existing article number three, and to add new provisions with information required to be included in the Articles under Chapter 10 (now Chapter 5).

The 1981 amendment added the organizational category of membership without vote in Article 5, and corrected the word "The" in Article one.
The 1990 amendment added the Associate category of membership without vote in Article 5 and provides for other classes of membership to be designated in the bylaws.
This compilation represents a re-numbered composite of all official amendments or documents affecting incorporation from March 1917 through May 1990.
** Name changed from National Society for the Promotion of Occupational Therapy, Inc. Jan. 27, 1923

The

Official Bylaws
of
The American Occupational
Therapy Association, Inc.

2009

******

Table of Contents
Bylaws

The American Occupational Therapy Association, Inc.

Bylaws
Table of Contents

i

ARTICLE I.

Name

Section 1.   Name

The name of the organization shall be The American Occupational Therapy Association, Inc., hereinafter referred to as the Association.

Section 2.   Purpose

The Association is organized under the District of Columbia Nonprofit Corporation Act.

ARTICLE II.

Noninurement

Section 1.   Noninurement

No part of the net earnings of the Association shall inure to the use or benefit of any individual. The Association shall not engage in any activities that are prohibited by the Internal Revenue Code, Section 501(c)(6).

ARTICLE III.

Members

Section 1.   Membership Classes

There shall be five (5) classes of membership.

A.   Occupational Therapist (OT): Any individual initially certified to practice as an OT or licensed or regulated by a state, commonwealth, district, or territory of the United States to practice as an occupational therapist and who has not had that certification, license, or regulation revoked due to disciplinary action shall be eligible to be an Occupational Therapist Member.

B.   Occupational Therapy Assistant (OTA): Any individual initially certified to practice as an OTA or licensed or regulated by a state, commonwealth, district, or territory of the United States to practice as an occupational therapy assistant and who has not had that certification, license, or regulation revoked due to disciplinary action shall be eligible to be an Occupational Therapy Assistant Member.

1

C.   Occupational Therapy Student (OTS): Any individual enrolled in an occupational therapy educational program that is accredited, or pending accreditation by the Accreditation Council for Occupational Therapy Education (ACOTEfi) a nd that is located in the United States, or in a state, commonwealth, district, or territory of the United States, shall be eligible to be a Student Member.

D.   Organizational: An organization, institution, or agency interested in occupational therapy may be an Organizational Member.

E.   Associate: An individual interested in occupational therapy who does not satisfy the requirements of subsections A, B, C, or D of this section may be an Associate Member.

Section 2.   **Voting Rights and Privileges of Members**

A.   Occupational Therapist and Occupational Therapy Assistant Members:

1.   Shall be entitled to vote
      a.   for the officers of the Association, Board Directors, and Delegate and Alternate Delegate to the World Federation of Occupational Therapists (WFOT);
      b.   for Representative(s) and Alternate Representative(s);
      c.   for Chairpersons-Elect of the Commission on Education (COE), Commission on Practice (COP), Ethics Commission (EC), Commission on Continuing Competence and Professional Development (CCCPD), Special Interest Sections Council (SISC), and for the OTA Representative and OTA Alternate Representative to the Assembly;
      d.   at Annual Business Meetings and special meetings of the Association; and
      e.   for Association Bylaws.
2.   May submit resolutions and motions to the Agenda Committee of the Assembly.
3.   May serve on Association bodies and run for offices of the Association.
4.   Shall be eligible to receive other privileges as designated by the Board.

B.   Student Members:

1.   Shall be entitled to vote
      a.   for the officers of the Association, Board Directors, and Delegate and Alternate Delegate to the WFOT;
      b.   at Annual Business Meetings or special meetings of the

2

Association;

    c.   for Chairpersons-Elect of the COE, COP, EC, CCCPD, SISC, and for the OTA Representative and OTA Alternate Representative to the Assembly;

    d.   for the Directors of the ASD and the Student Member Representative to the Assembly; and

    e.   for Association Bylaws.

2.   May submit resolutions and motions to the Agenda Committee of the Assembly.

3.   May serve on Association bodies.

4.   Shall be eligible to be an officer or member of ASD.

5.   Shall be entitled to receive other privileges as designated by the Board.

C.   Organizational and Associate Members:

Shall be entitled to receive privileges as designated by the Board.

Section 3.   Dues and Good Standing

A.   Dues and fees, if any, for all classes of membership shall be established by the Assembly.

B.   A member shall be in good standing if he or she currently meets the qualifications for the class of membership has paid all applicable dues, and membership has not been terminated pursuant to Section 4.

Section 4.   Termination of Membership

A.   Any member whose dues are still in arrears 30 days after payment is due shall automatically be removed from membership. Membership shall automatically be reinstated by payment of dues in arrears.

B.   Members of any classification may have their membership revoked for cause. Cause may include violation of the AOTA Occupational Therapy Ethics Standards.

C.   For any cause other than nonpayment of dues, a vote for revocation shall occur only after the member has been notified of the complaint for revocation and has been given reasonable opportunity for defense pursuant to the *Enforcement Procedures for the Occupational Therapy Code of Ethics.*

ARTICLE IV.

Meetings of the Membership of the Association

3

Section 1.   **Annual Business Meeting**

A.   The Annual Business Meeting of the members shall be held within each calendar year.

B.   An official publication of the Association shall list the place, day, and hour of the Annual Business Meeting at least 90 days before the meeting date.

Section 2.   **Special Meetings**

A.   The President, a majority of voting members of the Board, two thirds of the Assembly, or 10% of the OT and OTA members of the Association may call a special meeting.

B.   Members shall be notified by mail, electronic, or telephonic transmission of the place, day, hour, and purpose of the special meeting at least 21 days before the meeting.

C.   At a special meeting, the only business conducted shall be the matters stated in the meeting notification.

Section 3.   **Quorum for Annual and Special Meetings**

A.   A quorum shall be 100 OT, OTA, and/or student members, and

B.   Representation of a majority of the election areas.

Section 4.   **Voting**

A.   Mail, electronic, or telephonic transmission may be used by OT, OTA, and student members for voting.

B.   At any annual or special meeting of the members, there shall be no voting by proxy.

C.   The Board shall determine the process for counting and recording the vote.

ARTICLE V.

Board of Directors
Section 1.   **Purpose**

The Board of Directors, herein called the Board, shall govern the affairs of the

4

Association in accordance with all duly vested statutory, corporate, and Bylaws powers.

Section 2.   **Composition**

A.   Voting Members

    1.   Officers of the Association: President, Vice President, Secretary, and Treasurer
    2.   Six Directors (at least one of whom must be an OTA and at least one of whom must be an OT)
    3.   Speaker of the Assembly

B.   Nonvoting Members

    1.   President-Elect
    2.   Public Advisor
    3.   Consumer Advisor
    4.   AOTA Executive Director

Section 3.   **Term and Qualifications of Board Directors**

A.   Term of Office

    1.   A Director shall serve a 3-year term as provided in Article XII, Section 6, or until a successor has been elected.
    2.   A Director shall only be eligible to serve another term after the expiration of 2 intervening years.

B.   Qualifications

    1.   A Director shall have been initially certified with at least 5 years of experience as an OT or OTA at the time of nomination.
    2.   A Director shall have the qualifications necessary to execute the duties of the office held as determined by the Nominating Committee.

Section 4.   **Appointment, Term, and Qualifications of Appointed Participants**

A.   Appointment

The Consumer Advisor and Public Advisor are appointed by the President.

B.   Term of Office

The Consumer Advisor and Public Advisor shall serve a 3-year term that coincides with the term of the President.

5

C.   Qualifications

          1.   Consumer Advisor
               a.   Knowledge of the profession of occupational therapy through personal experience.
               b.   Experience serving on boards, committees, or other bodies.
          2.   Public Advisor
               a.   Knowledge of the profession of occupational therapy through professional experience in the health care reimbursement, regulatory, or policy arenas.
               b.   Experience serving on boards, committees, or other bodies.

Section 5.   Functions

A.   Establish the policies and procedures of the Board.

B.   Plan, prepare, approve, and manage the Association budget for each fiscal year.

C.   Manage the Association headquarters through the appointment of the Executive Director as Chief Executive Officer of the Association headquarters.

D.   Approve and monitor grants and contracts entered into by the Association and oversee investments.

E.   Prepare and approve plans of action and the Strategic Plan of the Association.

F.   Act as, or appoint, the appeal body of the Association for matters for which such appeals are provided under these Bylaws.

G.   Determine the location of the principal office of the Association.

H.   To declare and take action during an emergency.

Section 6.   Meetings

A.   Regular Meetings

          1.   The Board shall have at least one regular meeting a year.
          2.   The time and place of the meeting shall be designated at least 30 days before the meeting date of the regular Board meeting, by mail, electronic, or telephonic transmission to the Board

6

members.

   3.   The Board may invite any person to a Board meeting to advance the business of the Board.

B.   Special Meetings

   1.   Special meetings of the Board may be called by the President or any three members to address specific issues.

   2.   Special meetings of the Board may be held by electronic means including, but not limited to, electronic or other Internet communication systems, telephone, or video conferences.

   3.   Board members shall be notified by mail, electronic, or telephonic transmission of the date, time, place, and purpose of the meeting at least 1 week before the date.

   4.   Only business as stated in the call may be transacted at the special meeting.

   5.   Urgent business may be transacted by voting members of the Board serving as an Executive Committee via conference call on a 24-hour notice.

C.   Quorum

A majority of all the voting members, including at least two officers, shall constitute a quorum.

Section 7.   Bodies of the Board

The Board shall have the authority to establish bodies as necessary to carry out the purposes of the Association provided that the Board may not delegate overall responsibility for the conduct of the business of the Association or for exercising the powers of the Board.

Section 8.   Organizational Advisors

Purpose: To provide information to the Board regarding strategic planning and budgeting with respect to matters with the expertise of the specific Organizational Advisor. The advisors include: Accreditation Council for Occupational Therapy Education (ACOTEfi) Chairperson, American Occupational Therapy Foundation (AOTF) President, American Occupational Therapy Association Political Action Committee (AOTPAC) Chairperson, Affiliated State Association Presidents (ASAP) Chairperson, Assembly of Student Delegates (ASD) Chairperson, and World Federation of Occupational Therapists (WFOT) Delegate.

Section 9.   Associated Body of the Board

ACOTEfi

Purpose: To accredit occupational therapy educational programs and occupational therapy assistant educational programs. ACOTEfi establishes, approves, and administers educational standards to evaluate occupational therapy and occupational therapy assistant educational programs. ACOTEfi shall establish its own policies and procedures.

ARTICLE VI.

Officers of the Association

Section 1.   **Officers**

The Officers shall be the President, Vice President, Secretary, and Treasurer.

Section 2.   **Officer Qualifications**

A.   Officers shall have been initially certified with at least 10 years of experience as an OT or OTA at the time of nomination.

B.   An officer shall have the qualifications necessary to execute the duties of the office held as stated in Association documents.

C.   An officer shall be a member in good standing of the Association and of a state affiliate at time of nomination and throughout the term of office.

Section 3.   **Duties**

A.   President

1.   Shall be the chief elected officer of the Association and represent the Association to the public.
2.   Shall be an ex officio member of all committees of the Association except the Nominating Committee and the EC.
3.   Shall preside at all meetings of the Association membership.
4.   Shall preside at Board meetings as Chairperson of the Board.
5.   Shall appoint ad hoc committee chairpersons.
6.   Shall appoint a member of the Board to serve as liaison to the ASD.
7.   Shall appoint liaisons to external national organizations.
8.   Shall perform all other duties incident to the office of the President.

B.   President-Elect

1.   Shall prepare for the duties of the President.

8

    2.   Shall perform assignments made by the President.

C.   Vice President

    1.   Shall fulfill presidential duties in the absence of the President.
    2.   Shall perform all other duties incident to the office of the Vice President.

D.   Secretary

    1.   Shall record the minutes of the Business Meetings of the Association and the minutes of the Board meetings and be the custodian of such records.
    2.   Shall serve as a member of the Bylaws, Policies, and Procedures Committee (BPPC) of the Assembly.
    3.   Shall call to order a Business Meeting of the Association in the absence of the President and Vice President and shall preside over an election by the members present of a chairperson pro tempore.
    4.   Shall perform all other duties incident to the office of the Secretary.

E.   Treasurer

    1.   Shall oversee the financial affairs of the Association.
    2.   Shall be bonded at the expense of the Association.
    3.   Shall have the accounts of the Association audited annually by a Certified Public Accountant.
    4.   Shall perform all other duties incident to the office of the Treasurer.

ARTICLE VII.

Representative Assembly

Section 1.   **Purpose**

The Representative Assembly, herein called the Assembly, shall be the legislative body directly responsible for the policies affecting the direction of the profession.

Section 2.   **Composition**

A.   Voting Members

    1.   Elected Representative(s), as determined by proportional representation of the election area(s), or elected Alternate

Representative(s) when seated
2. A representative of OTFC
3. Officials of the Assembly: Speaker, Vice Speaker, and Recorder
4. Officers of the Association: President, Vice President, Secretary, and Treasurer
5. Student member representative
6. OTA Representative, or Alternate OTA Representative when seated
7. The Chairpersons of the COE, COP, CCCPD, EC, and SISC
8. ASAP Representative
9. Consumer Member

B. Nonvoting Members

1. President-Elect
2. AOTA Executive Director
3. The Chairpersons-Elect of the COE, COP, CCCPD, EC, and SISC
4. Chairpersons of the Agenda, BPPC, Credentials Review and Accountability Committee (CRAC), Nominating, and Recognitions Committees

Section 3. Election, Term, and Qualifications of Elected Members

A. Election

1. Representatives and Alternate Representatives of an election area are elected by the OTs and OTAs within that election area. The election will be conducted by the Association in collaboration with the election area affiliate. An election area is defined by state, district, commonwealth, or territory boundaries and there shall be only one election area within the boundaries of each state, district, commonwealth, or territory.
2. The ASD shall conduct the election for the Student Member Representative to the RA.

B. Term of Office

1. Representatives and Alternate Representatives shall serve a 3-year term or until successors have been elected. The term of office begins July 1.
2. Representatives and Alternate Representatives shall not be eligible to serve more than two consecutive terms in the same position.
3. The Student Member Representative shall serve a 2-year term.
4. The Chairpersons of the Agenda, BPPC, CRAC, Nominating, and Recognitions Committees are elected

10

for a 3-year term and shall hold only one position in the Association at a time.

C.   Qualifications

1.   Representatives and Alternate Representatives shall be members of the Association at the time of election and throughout the term of office.

2.   Representatives and Alternate Representatives shall be members of the election area to be represented and members of an election area affiliate at the time of election and throughout the term of office.

3.   Representatives and Alternate Representatives shall maintain any election area regulatory requirements necessary to identify themselves as OTs and OTAs throughout the term of office.

4.   The OTA Representative and OTA Alternate Representative shall be members of the Association with at least 2 years of experience working in official capacities of state or national professional occupational therapy organizations at the time of election.

5.   The Student Representative shall be a voting member of the Association and may be enrolled in an accredited occupational therapy or occupational therapy assistant educational program with at least 6 months remaining in their program (coursework, fieldwork, and thesis) following induction into the office.

Section 4.   **Appointment, Term, and Qualifications of Consumer Member**

A.   Appointment

The Consumer Member is appointed by the Speaker.

B.   Term of Office

The Consumer Member shall serve a 3-year term that coincides with the term of the Speaker.

C.   Qualifications

1.   Knowledge of the profession of occupational therapy through personal experience.

2.   Experience serving on boards, committees, or other bodies.

Section 5.   **Functions**

A.   Formulate and approve Association policies and adopt Assembly procedures on, but not limited to

1.　　internal Association affairs;
2.　　external Association affairs;
3.　　budget/finance;
4.　　position statements; and
5.　　membership rights, responsibilities, and fees.

B.　　Exercise other powers and functions customary to the legislative body of an association.

C.　　Elect a Chairperson for each of the following Committees: Agenda, BPPC, CRAC, Nominating, and Recognitions. The Nominating Committee shall prepare a slate, preferably of at least two qualified candidates, and shall conduct the election.

Section 6.　　Meetings

A.　　Regular Meetings

1.　　At least one meeting of the Assembly shall be held annually.
2.　　The time and place of the meeting shall be designated by mail, electronic, or telephonic transmission to the Representatives at least 30 days before the meeting date and should be printed in an official publication before the meeting date.
3.　　The Assembly may invite any person to an Assembly meeting to advance the business of the Assembly.

B.　　Special Meetings

1.　　Special meetings may be called by one third of the Assembly members, the Speaker of the Assembly, the Board, or the President of the Association.
2.　　Special meetings of the Assembly may be held by electronic means including, but not limited to, electronic or other Internet communication systems, telephone, or video conferences.
3.　　The time, place, and purpose of the meeting shall be designated by mail, electronic, or telephonic transmission to the Representatives at least 30 days before the meeting date and should be printed in an official publication before the meeting date.
4.　　Only business stated in the notice may be transacted at the special meeting.

C.　　Conduct of the Meeting

12

All meetings are open to Association members, except when the Assembly is in Executive Session.

D.   Quorum

A majority of voting members shall constitute a quorum at any meeting of the Assembly.

Section 7.   Bodies of the Assembly

The Assembly shall have the authority to establish bodies as necessary to carry out the purposes of the Assembly. The Assembly shall establish the membership criteria for all such bodies. The Association shall have the following:

A.   COE

Purpose: To promote the quality of education for OTs and OTAs relative to educator, student, and consumer needs.

B.   COP

Purpose: To promote and guide best practice in and standards for occupational therapy relative to practitioner and consumer needs.

C.   EC

Purpose: To serve the Association members and public through the identification, development, review, interpretation, and education of the AOTA Occupational Therapy Ethics Standards and to provide the process whereby the ethics of the Association are enforced.

D.   CCCPD

Purpose: To promote continuing competence and professional development in the profession in accordance with the Association s standards for continuing competence.

E.   Agenda Committee

Purpose: To facilitate the business of the Assembly.

F.   BPPC

Purpose: To review Association governance documents and recommend changes to the appropriate body for their consideration.

G.   CRAC

13

Purpose: To ensure that Representatives and Alternate Representatives from each election area, including the OTAs and the ASD, meet the qualifications to be members of the Assembly.

H.   Nominating Committee

Purpose: To prepare slates of eligible candidates for Association elections.

I.   Recognitions Committee

Purpose: To solicit nominations and select recipients for all Association recognitions and awards.

J.   SISC

Purpose: To coordinate and facilitate the activities of the Special Interest Sections (SISs) with the bodies of the Association.

K.   Representative Assembly Coordinating Council (RACC)

Purpose: To coordinate the activities and manage integrated projects of the COE, COP, EC, CCCPD, and SISC.

L.   RA Leadership Team (RALT)

Purpose: To plan, manage, and expedite the work of the Assembly.

M.   ASD

Purpose: To provide an opportunity for student members to have input into decision making and actions of the Association, to promote well-being of students, and to enhance students knowledge and structure of the Association.

ARTICLE VIII.

Officials of the Representative Assembly

Section 1.   Officials

The officials shall be the Speaker, Vice Speaker, and Recorder.

Section 2.   Election

A.   The officials shall be elected by the voting members of the Assembly.

14

B.   The Nominating Committee shall prepare a slate, preferably of at least two qualified candidates, for each position and shall conduct the election.

C.   When a Representative or Alternate Representative is elected as an official, the person shall vacate the position of Representative or Alternate Representative.

Section 3.   **Qualifications**

A.   A candidate shall be or have been a duly elected Representative, Alternate Representative, current committee chairperson, or a current official seeking election.

B.   A candidate shall have served at least 2 full years in the Assembly within 5 years of the election.

Section 4.   **Duties**

A.   Speaker

1. Shall preside at Assembly meetings.
2. Shall have the same voting rights as other voting members of the Assembly but may abstain from voting to maintain impartiality as the presiding officer unless it would affect the outcome.
3. Shall be an ex officio member of all committees of the Assembly except the Nominating Committee and the EC.
4. Shall appoint ad hoc chairpersons and members of ad hoc committees of the Assembly.
5. Shall perform all other duties incident to the office of Speaker.
6. Shall serve as a member of the Board.

B.   Vice Speaker

1. Shall fulfill the duties of the Speaker in the absence of the Speaker.
2. Shall serve as the Chairperson to the RACC.

C.   Recorder

1. Shall take the minutes of the meetings of the Assembly.
2. Shall be the custodian of such records.

ARTICLE IX.

Nominations and Elections of the Association

15

Section 1.   Nominations

A.   Any member of the Association may submit nominations to the
            Nominating Committee for:
            1.   Officers of the Association,
            2.   Board of Directors,
            3.   Delegate and Alternate Delegate to the WFOT,
            4.   Representative or Alternate Representative of an election area in
                   which the individual member is a voting member,
            5.   OTA Representative and OTA Alternate Representative to the
                   Assembly, and
            6.   Chairpersons-Elect of the COE, COP, CCCPD, EC, and SISC.

B.   The Call for Nominations for the positions provided for in this section
            shall be placed in an official publication of the Association 45 days before
            preparation of the ballot.

Section 2.   Eligibility

An individual elected or appointed to a position may not serve in any other position at the
same time unless designated in a standard operating procedure/job description or appointed
to a smaller group of the body to which he or she was elected.

Section 3.   Slate

A.   The Nominating Committee shall prepare a slate, preferably of at least two
            qualified candidates, for all elected positions to be filled.

B.   The slate shall include all qualified individuals nominated by any -
            member of the Association.

Section 4.   Ballot for Elections of the Association

A.   Preparation

            1.   The Nominating Committee shall prepare a ballot for the election
                   of positions listed in Section 1.A of this Article.
            2.   Ballots shall be by mail, electronic, or telephonic transmission to
                   all voting members of the Association.
            3.   Ballots shall state the deadline date for the receipt of the ballot
                   and the address or location to which the ballot shall be returned.

B.   Deadline
            1.   The deadline for receipt of all marked ballots by the agent
                   authorized to receive and count ballots shall be at least 45 days
                   before the Annual Business Meeting.

16

       2.   The election shall be closed on the deadline date and no ballots received thereafter shall be counted.

C.   Vote

The election of a candidate shall be by plurality vote of those ballots that are cast and valid.

D.   Tie Vote

       1.   In the event of a tie vote the ballots shall be recounted.

       2.   In the event that the result is still tied, the election for that position shall be conducted again.

E.   Contested Vote

       1.   In the event that a vote is contested and the vote tally is separated by no more than 5% of the ballots counted, the ballots shall be recounted.

       2.   The results of the recount shall be binding.

F.   Invalid Election

The Nominating Committee shall have the authority to determine grounds for declaring an invalid election subject to the approval of the Board.

ARTICLE X.

State Affiliates

Section 1.   Boundaries

An affiliate represents members located within an individual state, commonwealth, the District of Columbia, or Puerto Rico.

Section 2.   Purpose

An affiliate is a professional organization of OTs, OTAs, and students that has been recognized by the Association. The purpose of the affiliation is to foster communication and collaboration between the Association and affiliates.

Section 3.   Recognition

An organization becomes an affiliate of the Association through the process described in the *Affiliation Principles for AOTA and State Associations.* Continued recognition is

17

dependent on compliance with the *Affiliation Principles for AOTA and State Associations.*

Section 4. Termination

Termination (disaffiliation) of an affiliate can occur for the reasons and through the process described in the *Affiliation Principles for AOTA and State Association.*

Section 5. Appeal Process

The state affiliate shall have notice and opportunity to appeal to the Board by written submission within ten days from the date of notice of termination.

Section 6. Affiliated State Association Presidents (ASAP)

The Presidents of state affiliates will be the voice and resource representing state affiliate members to the Association; advising the Board and the Assembly; and providing a forum for communicating, networking, training, and mentoring state affiliate leadership.

ARTICLE XI.

World Federation of Occupational Therapists D elegates

Section 1. Delegates

The Association shall have a Delegate and an Alternate Delegate as representatives to the World Federation of Occupational Therapists, hereinafter referred to as WFOT.

Section 2. Election and Term of Office

A. The Delegate and Alternate Delegate to the WFOT shall be elected by OT, OTA, and student members of the Association.

B. The Delegate and Alternate Delegate shall serve an initial term of 4 years or until successors are elected. The Delegate and Alternate Delegate shall be eligible for reelection to successive terms of 2 years.

C. A Delegate or Alternate Delegate may serve a maximum of 8 years in the same position.

Section 3. Qualifications

A. Shall be an OT member of the Association with a minimum of 5 years of experience.

B. Shall be an individual member of WFOT for at least 3 years prior to

18

running for office.

Section 4.   Duties

A.   Delegate

> 1.   Shall be instructed by the Board on the agenda to come before the WFOT council and shall represent the Association to WFOT.
> 2.   Shall represent international issues and WFOT to the Association.
> 3.   Shall serve as an Organizational Advisor to the Board.

B.   Alternate Delegate

> 1.   Shall serve in the Assembly with vote as Representative of the election area of Association members residing in foreign countries and territories and possessions of the United States.
> 2.   Shall assume the duties of the Delegate in the absence of the Delegate.

ARTICLE XII.

Administrative Procedures for All Elected or Appointed Positions

Section 1.   Resignation

A.   Elected or appointed officials of the Association shall submit a written resignation to the appropriate Association official as provided in the Administrative SOP.

B.   The Association shall act upon such requests, including notifying appropriate committees concerning the vacancy.

Section 2.   Censure

Motions to censure an elected or appointed official shall occur consistent with a fundamentally fair process under procedures as described in *Robert s Rules of Order* in the chapter on disciplinary procedures.

Section 3.   Removal

Motions for removal of an elected or appointed official shall occur consistent with a fundamentally fair process under procedures described in *Robert s Rules of Order* in the chapter on disciplinary procedures.

Section 4.   Appeal

The intent to appeal shall be made in accordance with due process outlined by the EC and approved by the Assembly.

Section 5.   Vacancies

In the case of vacancy in any office, except the President, the vacancy shall be filled by appointment by the presiding officer of the Board or Assembly until the next regular election.

Section 6.   Term of Office

Unless otherwise specified, a term of office shall be 3 years, or until a successor has been appointed or elected, and begins July 1. Elect positions shall serve for 1 year and assume office July 1 in the year following their election. No person will be eligible to serve consecutively in the same office for more than one term except Representatives and Alternate Representatives to the Assembly and WFOT Delegates.

Section 7.   Ballots

A.   Mail, electronic, or telephonic transmission ballots may be used to elect:

1.   Officers or Officers-Elect of the Association
2.   Board Directors
3.   Delegate or Alternate Delegate to the WFOT
4.   Representative or Alternate Representative of an election area
5.   OTA Representative and OTA Alternate Representative to the Assembly
6.   ASD Officers
7.   Chairperson-Elect of a body of the Assembly

B.   Ballots must have a method of authenticating the eligibility of each voter (e.g., a member number).

ARTICLE XIII.

Standards of the Association

Section 1.   Standards

A.   Standards of the Association shall be developed, reviewed, and promoted by the appropriate body of the Assembly.

B.   The Standards of the Association shall be approved by the Assembly and interpreted by the Board, except for educational standards, which are approved by ACOTEfi.

20

C.   All members of the Association shall be bound by the Standards of the Association.

D.   All educational programs accredited by ACOTEfi shall be bound by the ACOTEfi Standards for an Accredited Educational Program.

Section 2.   **Ethics Standards**

A.   Ethics Standards shall be developed, reviewed, and interpreted by the EC.

B.   Ethics Standards shall be approved by the Assembly.

C.   All OT, OTA, and student members of the Association shall be bound by the statements contained in the Ethics Standards.

D.   The EC shall establish and maintain the Association s procedures for enforcing the Ethics Standards.

ARTICLE XIV.

Fiscal Year

The fiscal year of the Association shall be determined by the Board.

ARTICLE XV.

Dissolution Clause

Should the corporation be dissolved for any reason, the remaining assets shall be distributed for purposes within the scope of the Internal Revenue Code, Section 501(c)(6), or any amendment thereto, and in accordance with the corporate statutes of the District of Columbia.

ARTICLE XVI.

Parliamentary Authority

The rules contained in the current edition of *Robert s Rules of Order, Newly Revised*, shall govern the Association in all cases to which they are applicable and in which they are not inconsistent with these Bylaws and any special rules of order the Association may adopt.

ARTICLE XVII.

21

Amendments to Bylaws

Section 1.   Role of Board, Assembly, and Association Members

A.   Board: Considers fiduciary responsibilities; may propose Bylaw amendments; and can recommend approval, modification, disapproval, or any other appropriate action with respect to proposed Bylaw amendments from membership or Assembly.

B.   Assembly: Considers policy and procedural implications of proposed Bylaw amendments and approves, modifies, disapproves, or takes any other appropriate action with respect to proposed Bylaw amendments, including proposing amendments.

C.   Members: Propose Bylaw amendments and vote to adopt amendments.

Section 2.   Procedure

A.   The BPPC shall announce a call for amendments in an official publication to all OT, OTA, and student members.

B.   OT, OTA, and student members shall have 60 days from the date of publication to submit suggestions to the BPPC.

C.   BPPC shall present to the Board a report containing proposed Bylaw amendments and BPPC comments on the amendments.

D.   The Board shall consider at its regular meetings any proposed Bylaws amendments. The Board shall provide a report to BPPC within 10 days of its meeting reflecting the Board s recommendations regarding proposed Bylaw amendments.

E.   The BPPC shall present to the Assembly a report containing proposed Bylaws amendments with their comments and those of the Board on the proposed amendments. This report will also be posted on the Association s Web site for consideration by the members who may offer feedback to their Representatives. The Assembly at its regular meetings shall consider, approve and recommend approval, modification, disapproval or any other appropriate action on any proposed Bylaws, including making its own proposed Bylaw amendments. The Assembly shall provide a report reflecting the Assembly s recommendations regarding proposed Bylaw amendments to BPPC within a time frame necessary to allow voting on Bylaw amendments by the membership at the Annual Business Meeting.

22

F.   Proposed Bylaw amendments within the scope of the subject matter discussed and approved by the Assembly shall be forwarded to the OT, OTA, and student members at the Annual Business Meeting for a vote.

Section 3.   Technical Corrections

The BPPC shall have authority to make technical, editorial, clerical corrections, and cross-references to other Association documents to keep the Bylaws consistent without calling for a vote of the voting members of the Association or of the Assembly.

Section 4.   Effective Date

Amendments to the Bylaws shall become effective immediately upon adoption.

ARTICLE XVIII.

Indemnification

Any present or former Board member, officer, employee, official, or agent of the Association, or other such persons so designated at the discretion of the Board, or the legal representative of such person, shall be indemnified (including advances against expenses) by the Association against all judgments, fines, settlements, and other reasonable costs, expenses, and counsel fees paid or incurred in connection with any action, suit, or proceeding to which any person or his or her legal representative may be made a party by reason of his or her being or having been such a Board member, officer, employee, official, or agent, to the greatest extent permitted by law. No indemnification or advance against expenses shall be approved by the Board or paid by the Association until after receipt from legal counsel of an opinion concerning the legality of the proposed indemnification or advance.

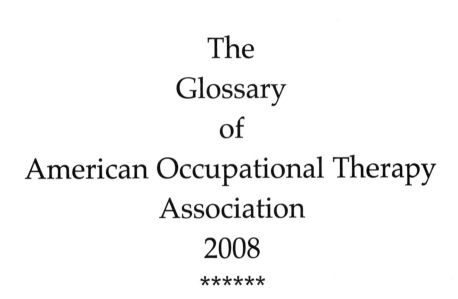

The
Glossary
of
American Occupational Therapy
Association
2008
******

Absence

Failure to attend or appear when expected; the state of being away or not present (e.g., the Treasurer is not present for the Association Annual Business Meeting).

Accreditation

The process by which an agency or organization evaluates and recognizes a program of study or an institution as meeting certain predetermined qualifications or standards. It applies only to institutions and their programs of study or their services.

ACOTE®

Accreditation Council for Occupational Therapy Education

Ad Hoc

A special body (e.g., committee, task force, task group, body) not established by the Bylaws. An ad hoc body is appointed for a specific purpose and assigned a specific task that is not an ongoing function in the Association.

Advisory

Having the function of giving advice, usually with the implication that the advice given need not be followed.

Affiliate

An Affiliate is a professional organization representing OTs, OTAs, and student members within an individual state, commonwealth, the District of Columbia, or Puerto Rico that has been recognized by the Association.

Agenda (plural for Agendum)

A list of things to be done, especially the program for a meeting (e.g., the order of business of the Assembly meeting).

Alternate Representative/Alternate Delegate

The person next in rank to the Representative/Delegate who succeeds to the position of Representative/Delegate on the resignation, removal, death, or disability of the Representative/Delegate. The alternate may act for the Representative/Delegate in the absence or on the command of the Representative/Delegate.

Amendments

Changes to the Bylaws that are neither revisions nor technical corrections.

Annual Business Meeting

The scheduled gathering of Association members that must occur at least one time per year.

Annual Conference

A meeting of persons from across the country to discuss or consult on various topics or issues (e.g., the Annual Conference of the Association).

AOTF

American Occupational Therapy Foundation

Appeal

Make an earnest request (e.g., an officer pleads against removal from office).

BPPC Reviewed: 9/7/03, 1/05, 1/07, 1/08
Adopted RA: 11/03, 5/05, 4/07 2

Approval Articles of Incorporation
This is synonymous with ratification. The original statements that provided the framework for the development and organization of the Association.

ASAP
Affiliated State Association Presidents

Assembly
A group of people meeting as a deliberative or lawmaking body.

ASD
Assembly of Student Delegates

Associated Body of the Board
A body that operates at "arm's length" according to specific legal or regulatory requirements to achieve its stated purpose.

Association
An organized body of people who have some interest, activity, or purpose in common (e.g., The American Occupational Therapy Association, Inc.).

Association headquarters
The headquarters of the Association, which houses the staff who are responsible for carrying out activities as assigned by the Board or Assembly.

Award
An honor that is conferred on designated individuals (e.g., Slagle Lectureship, Award of Merit).

Ballot
A written or printed paper used to cast or register a vote (e.g., a printed piece of paper containing the names of candidates and instructions for voting).

Board
A group of people chosen to make executive or managerial decisions for an organization.

Board
The Board of Directors

Body
An organized group of individuals that has an official function.

Boundaries
A border or limit (e.g., the border that defines an election area or state association).

Budget
An estimate of expected income and expenses, an itemized allotment of funds for a given year (e.g., a yearly allotment of Association funds for a committee).

Bylaw
A rule adopted by an organization for the governance of its members and the regulation of its affairs (e.g., the Bylaws of The American Occupational Therapy Association, Inc.).

BPPC
Bylaws, Policies, and Procedures Committee

BPPC Reviewed: 9/7/03, 1/05, 1/07, 1/08
Adopted RA: 11/03, 5/05, 4/07 3

Censure
A formal expression of strong disapproval that is public.

Certification
The process by which a nongovernmental agency or association grants recognition to an individual who has met certain predetermined qualifications specified by that agency or association.

Chairperson
The presiding officer

Commission
A group of people authorized or directed to carry out a duty or task. A commission is responsible for a broad area of information relevant to the Association.

CCCPD
Commission on Continuing Competence and Professional Development

COE
Commission on Education

COP
Commission on Practice

Committee
A body of one or more persons, elected or appointed by the Board or Assembly, to consider, investigate, or take action on certain matters or subjects.

Communication
The means of sending or giving messages, orders, and so forth, including telephone, telegraph, radio, books, films, and e-mail.

Component
An element or part of something larger in structure and organization (e.g., a subcommittee is a component of a committee).

Council
An appointed or elected body of people with an administrative, advisory, or representative function.

Credentials
Evidence of authority, status, rights, entitlement, or privileges, usually in written form (e.g., written notice of election of a person as a representative from an election area).

CRAC
Credentials Review and Accountability Committee

Delegate
Somebody chosen to represent or given the authority to act on behalf of another person, group, or organization (e.g., at a meeting or conference).

Dissolution
The breaking up or undoing of an Assembly or organization (e.g., the dissolution of The American Occupational Therapy Association, Inc.).

Duty
Something that one is expected or required to do by moral or legal obligation (e.g., conduct the meeting).

BPPC Reviewed: 9/7/03, 1/05, 1/07, 1/08
Adopted RA: 11/03, 5/05, 4/07 4

Editorial
To alter, adapt, or refine, especially to bring about conformity to a standard or to suit a particular purpose.

Education
The act or process of importing or acquiring general knowledge and of developing the powers of reasoning and judgment.

Election
The selection of a person or persons for office by vote (e.g., choosing a President, Secretary, etc.).

Election-Area
A geographic area or class of persons that is defined as eligible for Representation in the Assembly.

Election-Area Affiliate
A professional Association in a particular state, commonwealth, district, territory, or possession that has been recognized by the Association.

Emblem
A sign, design, or figure that identifies or represents (e.g., the "practice patch," which identifies the person as an OT or OTA).

Emergency, Association
An emergency that would alter the Association's ability to effectively conduct business may be declared by the Executive Director, President, or Vice President.

Emergency, National
Declared by the President of the United States or Congress that results in restriction of travel, expenditures or collections, or personal activity, and a temporary policy or procedure is required to meet the situation.

Ethics
A body of moral principles or values.

EC
Ethics Commission

Ethics Standards
A term that includes three documents: the *Occupational Therapy Code of Ethics, Core Values and Attitudes,* and *Guidelines to the Occupational Therapy Code of Ethics.*

Executive Director
The person having administrative or managerial authority (e.g., of the headquarters of the Association).

Executive Session
A meeting or portion of a meeting at which the proceedings are secret and only members, special invitees, and designated staff may be present. In the Association, Executive Session is used primarily to discuss information and issues that involve privileged data affecting individual member and personnel matters of the Association, or matters that may be the subject of litigation and/or are subject to attorney–client privilege. The purpose is to protect confidentiality, not to deprive members of their right to know (e.g., the Assembly is in Executive Session to hear the case of a member charged with unethical behavior).

BPPC Reviewed: 9/7/03, 1/05, 1/07, 1/08
Adopted RA: 11/03, 5/05, 4/07 5

Fee
A sum paid or charged for a privilege (e.g., the fee for membership in the Association).

Fiscal
Pertaining to financial matters in general.

Formation
How the group is organized to do business (e.g., Assembly business is conducted in formal session).

Function
What the group is charged to do (e.g., the Assembly is charged to make policy for the Association).

Good Standing
A statement that identifies that a member has met and maintained the qualifications to belong to the Association.

Job Description
Regular procedures or actions that are taken by an individual to accomplish an activity, charge, or item of business. Job descriptions are recorded in written form.

Legislative
Involved in writing and passing laws or regulations.

Liaison
The contact maintained between bodies to ensure concerted action. An individual serving in this position is not an official member of the body to which he or she is serving as a liaison.

Logo (short for logotype)
A trademark or company name or device (e.g., the name, "The American Occupational Therapy Association, Inc.").

Meetings
The sequence of events an Association body experiences to conduct business, from the initial call to order to adjournment. Meeting agendas generally include approval of prior minutes, reports, and old and new business. A meeting may be made up of several sessions.

Members
Persons or organizations that meet and maintain the qualifications to belong to and compose the Association.

Motion
A formal proposal by a member in an official meeting for a certain action. The proposed action may be of a substantive nature, or it may express a certain view or direct that a particular investigation be conducted and the findings be reported for possible further action.

NBCOT
National Board for Certification in Occupational Therapy®

Nominate
To propose someone as a proper or suitable person for appointment or election to an office.

Noninurement
Not to accrue to the advantage or benefit of an individual(s); specifically, monies earned by or for the Association cannot be given or taken by individuals for their own use.

BPPC Reviewed: 9/7/03, 1/05, 1/07, 1/08
Adopted RA: 11/03, 5/05, 4/07 5

Occupational Therapist

Any individual initially certified to practice as an OT or licensed or regulated by a state, commonwealth, district, or territory of the United States to practice as an occupational therapist and who has not had that certification, license, or regulation revoked due to disciplinary action shall be eligible to be an Occupational Therapist Member.

OT

Occupational Therapist

Occupational Therapy Assistant

Any individual initially certified to practice as an OTA or licensed or regulated by a state, commonwealth, district, or territory of the United States to practice as an occupational therapy assistant and who has not had that certification, license, or regulation revoked due to disciplinary action shall be eligible to be an Occupational Therapy Assistant Member.

OTA

Occupational Therapy Assistant

Officer

One who holds a position of authority or command and serves in a designated capacity in the Association and Board (e.g., President, Treasurer).

Official Document

Those documents constructed by the Association and approved by the Association for the use of the Association and its members.

Organizational Advisors

Critical governance bodies within the organization that advise the Board and promote active collaboration and effective dialogue among the Board, appropriate bodies of the Board, the Assembly, and AOTA.

Organizational Member

Institutions or agencies that are interested in the profession or practice of occupational therapy (e.g., another professional health care organization).

OTFC Parliamentary

OTs in Foreign Countries. In accordance with the rules governing deliberative bodies.

Personnel

A body of persons employed in any work, undertaking, or service (e.g., the Association staff).

Policy

A definite course or method of action selected to guide and determine present and future decisions.

Postprofessional Program

An educational curriculum in occupational therapy that offers courses designed to enhance knowledge and skills beyond the basic entry level for persons who are already OTs.

Practice

Action or process of performing or doing something, the exercise or pursuit of a profession or occupation (e.g., delivering occupational therapy services to a client).

BPPC Reviewed: 9/7/03, 1/05, 1/07, 1/08

Adopted RA: 11/03, 5/05, 4/07 5

President
The highest executive officer elected to preside over an organized body.

President-Elect
A person who has been duly elected to the presidency but whose term of office as President has not begun.

Principal Office
The main or central place of business.

Privileges
Those things or activities that a member is permitted to do by virtue of being a member of the Association (e.g., seek services that are provided).

Procedure
A particular way or series of steps followed to accomplish something or a way of acting; an established way of doing things.

Professional Education
An educational curriculum in occupational therapy that offers courses designed to provide education for entry-level performance of the OT.

Proportional Representation
The means of determining the number of representatives on the basis of percentage.

Pro Tem (Pro Tempore)
Temporarily; for the time being (e.g., a person who acts as a Chairperson for a group for this meeting).

Publications
Those publications that are designated as belonging to or representing the views of The American Occupational Therapy Association, Inc.

Purpose
A summary statement of the goals and/or objectives of the group.

Qualifications
An accomplishment, experience, or skill that fits a person for some function, office, or the like (e.g., has served on a committee).

Quorum
A quorum is the number of voting members who must be present in order that business can be legally transacted. The quorum refers to the number of such members present, not to the number actually voting on a particular question.

RA
Representative Assembly

RACC
Representative Assembly Coordinating Council

Recognition
The act of showing appreciation, achievement, service, merit, and so forth, as by some reward, public honor, or the like (e.g., Award of Merit, Slagle Lectureship).

BPPC Reviewed: 9/7/03, 1/05, 1/07, 1/08
Adopted RA: 11/03, 5/05, 4/07 5

Recorder
A person who sets down something in writing or other permanent form (e.g., the person who prepares and keeps the minutes of the Assembly).

Removal
The act of taking away the title and duties of a position.

Representative
An individual who votes or speaks on behalf of others.

Representative Assembly
The body composed of representatives from identified constituencies (election areas) whose function is to legislate and establish policy for the Association.

Reprimand
Formal expression of disapproval that is privately communicated.

Resignation
The act of giving up or renouncing one's office or position (e.g., the Secretary notifies the President that he or she will no longer perform the duties of Secretary).

Resolution
A complex motion that is a formal statement of an expression of opinion put before an Assembly or decision adopted by an Assembly (e.g., a resolution submitted to and passed by the Assembly).

Revision
Changes of the Bylaws that are so extensive and general that they are scattered throughout the Bylaws and should be effected through the substitution of an entirely new set of Bylaws (*Robert's Rules of Order,* p. 575). Revisions include roles and responsibilities of individuals, functions of the bodies, relationships between bodies, election of individuals to bodies, and number of voting members.

Rights
Those things to which a member has just claim by virtue of being a member of the Association (e.g., access Member pages on the Web site).

Robert's Rules
The rules contained in the current edition of *Robert's Rules of Order, Newly Revised,* shall govern the Association in all cases in which they are applicable and in which they are not inconsistent with the Bylaws and any special rules of order the Association may adopt.

SCB
Specialty Certification Board

Seated
A position from which authority is exercised; also, the approval a person receives from the group authorizing participation in the conduct of business.

Secretary
An officer who is in charge of the records, correspondence, minutes of Board meetings and Annual Business Meetings, and related affairs of an organization, company, or Association.

Session
A portion of a meeting, from the Call to Order to a Recess.

BPPC Reviewed: 9/7/03, 1/05, 1/07, 1/08
Adopted RA: 11/03, 5/05, 4/07 5

Slate
A list of candidates, officers, and so forth to be considered for nomination, appointment, election, and the like.

Speaker
The presiding officer of a legislative assembly (e.g., Speaker of the Assembly).

Special Interest Section
A group of members recognized by the Assembly as having a mutual interest in a practical area of practice in occupational therapy.

SISs
Special Interest Sections

SISC
Special Interest Sections Council

Standard
Something considered by an authority as a basis of comparison, as an approved model.

Standard Operating Procedure
Regular procedures or actions that are taken by a group to accomplish an activity, charge, or item of business. Standard operating procedures are recorded in written form and are referred to as SOPS.

Standing Committee
A permanent committee established in the Bylaws dealing with a designated subject (e.g., fees, personnel, recognitions). A committee is responsible for a specific area of information relevant to the Association.

State Association
A group of persons living in a state, commonwealth, the District of Columbia, or Puerto Rico who are interested in and concerned with occupational therapy who have formed an organization for mutual benefit and sharing of information.

Steering Committee
A selected group of persons charged to function as an organizing unit to conduct certain business for a larger group. The function of the Steering Committee is to expedite the work of a larger group.

Strategic Plan
A document outlining the goals and activities that the Association members have agreed to strive to achieve and to which resources will be assigned.

Student
Any person who is enrolled in an occupational therapy education program that is accredited or approved by the Association for the first technical or professional degree.

Substantive Change
A change of an essential part, or constituent, or relating to what is essential.

Technical Education
An educational curriculum in occupational therapy that offers courses designed to provide education for entry-level performance of the OTA.

Term (of Office)
A period of time to which limits have been set (e.g., selected for a term of 2 years).

BPPC Reviewed: 9/7/03, 1/05, 1/07, 1/08
Adopted RA: 11/03, 5/05, 4/07 5

Tracking
Following the course or progress of or keeping informed about (e.g., the secretary is charged to monitor the progress of motions and charges so that tasks are assigned and completed and reports are filed).

Treasurer
An officer who is charged with the receipt, care, and disbursement of money.

Treasurer-Elect
A person who has been duly elected to the treasury, but whose term of office as Treasurer has not begun.

Vacancy
An unoccupied position or office (e.g., the Presidency is vacant due to the resignation of the President).

Vice President
The officer next in rank to the President who succeeds to the Presidency on the resignation, removal, death, or disability of the President. The Vice President may act for the President in the absence or on the command of the President.

Vice Speaker
The officer who is next in rank to the Speaker and succeeds to the position of Speaker on the resignation, removal, death, or disability of the Speaker. The Vice Speaker may act for the Speaker in the absence or on the command of the Speaker.

Vote
A formal expression of preference for a candidate for office, proposed resolution, motion of an issue, or Bylaws change.

WFOT
World Federation of Occupational Therapists

BPPC Reviewed: 9/7/03, 1/05, 1/07, 1/08
Adopted RA: 11/03, 5/05, 4/07 12

Accreditation

Accreditation Standards for a Doctoral-Degree-Level Educational Program for the Occupational Therapist

Adopted December 2006. Effective January 1, 2008.

The Accreditation Council for Occupational Therapy Education (ACOTE®) of the American Occupational Therapy Association (AOTA) accredits educational programs for the occupational therapist. The Standards comply with the United States Department of Education (USDE) criteria for recognition of accrediting agencies.

These Standards are the requirements used in accrediting educational programs that prepare individuals to enter the occupational therapy profession. The extent to which a program complies with these Standards determines its accreditation status.

Preamble

The rapidly changing and dynamic nature of contemporary health and human services delivery systems provides challenging opportunities for the occupational therapist to use knowledge and skills in a practice area as a direct care provider, consultant, educator, manager, leader, researcher, and advocate for the profession and the consumer.

A graduate from an ACOTE-accredited doctoral-degree-level occupational therapy program must

- Have acquired, as a foundation for professional study, a breadth and depth of knowledge in the liberal arts and sciences and an understanding of issues related to diversity.

- Be educated as a generalist with a broad exposure to the delivery models and systems used in settings where occupational therapy is currently practiced and where it is emerging as a service.

- Have achieved entry-level competence through a combination of academic and fieldwork education.

- Be prepared to articulate and apply occupational therapy theory and evidence-based evaluations and interventions to achieve expected outcomes as related to occupation.

- Be prepared to be a lifelong learner and keep current with evidence-based professional practice.

- Uphold the ethical standards, values, and attitudes of the occupational therapy profession.

- Understand the distinct roles and responsibilities of the occupational therapist and occupational therapy assistant in the supervisory process.

- Be prepared to advocate as a professional for the occupational therapy services offered and for the recipients of those services.

- Be prepared to be an effective consumer of the latest research and knowledge bases that support practice and contribute to the growth and dissemination of research and knowledge.

- Demonstrate in-depth knowledge of delivery models, policies, and systems related to the area of practice in settings where occupational therapy is currently practiced and where it is emerging as a service.

- Demonstrate thorough knowledge of evidence-based practice.

- Demonstrate active involvement in professional development, leadership, and advocacy.

- Relate theory to practice and demonstrate synthesis of advanced knowledge in a practice area through completion of a culminating project.

- Develop in-depth experience in one or more of the following areas through completion of a doctoral experiential component: clinical practice skills, research skills, administration, leadership, program and policy development, advocacy, education, and theory development.

Section A:
General Requirements for Accreditation

A.1.0. Sponsorship and Accreditation

A.1.1.   The sponsoring institution(s) and affiliates, if any, must be accredited by recognized national, regional, or state agencies with accrediting authority. For programs in countries other than the United States, ACOTE will determine an alternative and equivalent external review process.

A.1.2.   Sponsoring institutions must be authorized under applicable law or other acceptable authority to provide a program of post-secondary education and have appropriate doctoral-degree-granting authority.

A.1.3.   Accredited occupational therapy educational programs may be established only in senior colleges, universities, or medical schools.

A.1.4.   The sponsoring institution must assume primary responsibility for appointment of faculty, admission of students, and curriculum planning. This would include course content, satisfactory completion of the educational program, and granting of the degree. The sponsoring institution must also be responsible for the coordination of classroom teaching and supervised fieldwork practice and for providing assurance that the practice activities assigned to students in a fieldwork setting are appropriate to the program.

A.1.5.   The sponsoring institution or program must

- Inform ACOTE of the transfer of program sponsorship or change of the institution's name within 30 days of the transfer or change.

- Inform ACOTE within 30 days of the date of notification of any adverse accreditation action taken to change the sponsoring institution's accreditation status to probation or withdrawal of accreditation.

- Submit a Letter of Intent to add or change a program degree level at least 1 year prior to the planned admission of students into that level.

- Inform ACOTE within 30 days of the resignation of the program director or appointment of a new or interim program director.

- Pay accreditation fees within 90 days of the invoice date.

- Submit a Report of Self-Study and other required reports (e.g., Biennial Report, Plan of Correction, Progress Report) within the period of time designated by ACOTE. All reports must be complete and contain all requested information.

- Agree to a site visit date before the end of the period for which accreditation was previously awarded.

- Demonstrate honesty and integrity in all interactions with ACOTE.

A.2.0. Academic Resources

A.2.1.   The program must have a director who is assigned to the occupational therapy educational program on a full-time basis. The director may be assigned other institutional duties that do not interfere with the management and administration of the program. The institution must ensure that the needs of the program are being met.

A.2.2.   The program director must be an initially certified occupational therapist who is licensed or credentialed according to regulations in the state or jurisdiction in which the program is located. The director must hold a doctoral degree.

A.2.3.   The program director must have a minimum of 8 years of documented experience in the field of occupational therapy. This experience must include clinical practice as an occupational therapist, administrative or supervisory experience, clinical research, and at least 3 years of experience in a full-time academic appointment with teaching responsibilities at the postbaccalaureate level.

A.2.4.   The program director must be responsible for the management and administration of the program, including planning, evaluation, budgeting, selection of faculty and staff, maintenance of accreditation, and commitment to strategies for professional development.

A.2.5.   The program director and faculty must possess the academic and experiential qualifications and backgrounds (identified in documented descriptions of roles and responsibilities) that are necessary to meet program objectives and the mission of the institution.

A.2.6.   The program must document policies and procedures to ensure that the program director and faculty are aware of and abide by the current code of ethics of the profession of occupational therapy.

A.2.7.   The program must identify an individual responsible for the experiential component of the program and ensure the program's compliance with the requirements of Standards Section B.10.0 and B.11.0. This individual must be a licensed or credentialed occupational therapist. Coordinators who hold a faculty position must meet the requirements of Standard A.2.9.

A.2.8.   The faculty must include currently licensed or credentialed occupational therapists.

A.2.9.   All full-time faculty teaching in the program must hold a doctoral degree.

A.2.10. The faculty must have documented expertise in their area(s) of teaching responsibility and knowledge of the content delivery method (e.g., distance learning).

A.2.11. The occupational therapy faculty at each accredited location where the program is offered must be sufficient in number and must possess the expertise necessary to ensure appropriate curriculum design, content delivery, and program evaluation.

A.2.12. Faculty responsibilities must be consistent with and supportive of the mission of the institution.

A.2.13. The faculty–student ratio must permit the achievement of the purpose and stated objectives for laboratory and lecture courses, be compatible with accepted practices of the institution for similar programs, and ensure student and consumer safety.

A.2.14. Clerical and support staff must be provided to the program, consistent with institutional practice, to meet programmatic and administrative requirements, including support for any portion of the program offered by distance education.

A.2.15. The program must be allocated a budget of regular institutional funds, not including grants, gifts, and other restricted sources, sufficient to implement and maintain the objectives of the program and to fulfill the program's obligation to matriculated and entering students.

A.2.16. Classrooms and laboratories must be provided that are consistent with the program's educational objectives, teaching methods, number of students, and safety and health standards of the institution, and must allow for efficient operation of the program. If any portion of the program is offered by distance education, technology and resources must be adequate to support a distance-learning environment.

A.2.17. Laboratory space provided by the institution must be assigned to the occupational therapy program on a priority basis. If laboratory space is provided by another institution or agency, there must be a written and signed agreement to ensure assignment of space for program use.

A.2.18. Adequate space must be provided to store and secure equipment and supplies.

A.2.19. The program director and faculty must have office space consistent with institutional practice.

A.2.20. Adequate space must be provided for the private advising of students.

A.2.21. Appropriate and sufficient equipment and supplies must be provided by the institution for student use and for the didactic, supervised fieldwork, and experiential components of the curriculum.

A.2.22. Students must be given access to and have the opportunity to use the evaluative and treatment methodologies that reflect both current practice and practice in the geographic area served by the program.

A.2.23. Students must have ready access to a supply of current and relevant books, journals, periodicals, computers, software, and other reference materials needed for the practice areas and to meet the requirements of the curriculum. This may include, but is not limited to, libraries, online services, interlibrary loan, and resource centers.

A.2.24. Instructional aids and technology must be available in sufficient quantity and quality to be consistent with the program objectives and teaching methods.

A.3.0. Students

A.3.1. Admission of students to the occupational therapy program must be made in accordance with the practices of the institution and the program design. There must be stated admission criteria that are clearly defined and published and reflective of the demands of the program.

A.3.2. By July 1, 2010, institutions must require that program applicants hold a baccalaureate degree or higher prior to admission to the program.

A.3.3. Policies pertaining to standards for admission, advanced placement, transfer of credit, credit for experiential learning (if applicable), residency requirements, and prerequisite educational or work experience requirements must be readily accessible to prospective students and the public.

A.3.4. Programs must document implementation of a mechanism to ensure that students receiving credit for previous courses and/or work experience have met the content requirements of the appropriate doctoral Standards.

A.3.5. Criteria for successful completion of each segment of the educational program and for graduation must be given in advance to each student.

A.3.6. Evaluation content and methods must be consistent with the curriculum design; objectives; and competencies of the didactic, fieldwork, and experiential components of the program.

A.3.7. Evaluation must be conducted on a regular basis to provide students and program officials with timely indications of the students' progress and academic standing.

A.3.8.   Students must be informed of and have access to the student support services that are provided to other students in the institution.

A.3.9.   Advising related to professional coursework, fieldwork education, and the experiential component of the program must be the responsibility of the occupational therapy faculty.

A.4.0. Operational Policies

A.4.1.   All program publications and advertising—including, but not limited to, academic calendars, announcements, catalogs, handbooks, and Web sites—must accurately reflect the program offered.

A.4.2.   Accurate and current information regarding student outcomes must be readily available to the public in at least one publication or Web page. The following data must be reported as an aggregate for the 3 most recent calendar years and specify the

- 3-year time period being reported,

- total number of program graduates during that period,

- total number of eligible first-time test takers of the national certification examination during that period,

- total number of eligible first-time test takers who passed the exam during that period, and

- percentage of the total number of eligible first-time test takers who passed the exam during that period.

A.4.3.   The program's accreditation status and the name, address, and telephone number of ACOTE must be published in all of the following used by the institution: catalog, Web site, and program-related brochures or flyers available to prospective students.

A.4.4.   Faculty recruitment and employment practices, as well as student recruitment and admission procedures, must be nondiscriminatory.

A.4.5.   Graduation requirements, tuition, and fees must be accurately stated, published, and made known to all applicants. When published fees are subject to change, a statement to that effect must be included.

A.4.6.   The program or sponsoring institution must have a defined and published policy and procedure for processing student and faculty grievances.

A.4.7.   Policies and procedures for handling complaints against the program must be published and made known. The program must maintain a record of student complaints that includes the nature and disposition of each complaint.

A.4.8.   Policies and processes for student withdrawal and for refunds of tuition and fees must be published and made known to all applicants.

A.4.9.   Policies and procedures for student probation, suspension, and dismissal must be published and made known.

A.4.10. Policies and procedures must be published and made known for human-subject research protocol.

A.4.11. Written policies and procedures must be made available to students regarding appropriate use of equipment and supplies and for all educational activities that have implications for the health and safety of clients, students, and faculty (including infection control and evacuation procedures).

A.4.12. A program admitting students on the basis of ability to benefit (defined by the U.S. Department of Education as admitting students who do not have either a high school diploma or its equivalent) must publicize its objectives, assessment measures, and means of evaluating the student's ability to benefit.

A.4.13. Documentation of all progression, retention, residency, graduation, certification, and credentialing requirements must be published and made known to applicants. If applicable, this must include a statement about the potential impact of a felony conviction on a graduate's eligibility for certification and credentialing.

A.4.14. The program must have a documented and published policy to ensure students complete all graduation, fieldwork, and experiential component requirements in a timely manner. This must include a statement that all Level II fieldwork and the experiential component of the program must be completed within a time frame established by the program.

A.4.15. Records regarding student admission, enrollment, and achievement must be maintained and kept in a secure setting. Grades and credits for courses must be recorded on students' transcripts and permanently maintained by the sponsoring institution.

A.5.0. *Strategic Plan and Program Assessment*

A.5.1. The program must document a current strategic plan that articulates the program's future vision and guides the program development (e.g., faculty recruitment and professional growth, scholarship, changes in the curriculum design, priorities in academic resources, procurement of fieldwork and experiential component sites). A program strategic plan must include, but need not be limited to

- Evidence that the plan is based on program evaluation and an analysis of external and internal environments.

- Long-term goals that address the vision and mission of both the institution and program, as well as specific needs of the program.

- Specific measurable action steps with expected timelines by which the program will reach its long-term goals.

- Persons(s) responsible for action steps.

- Evidence of periodic updating of action steps and long-term goals as they are met or as circumstances change.

A.5.2. The program director and each faculty member who teaches two or more courses must have a current written professional growth and development plan. Each plan must contain the signature of the faculty member and supervisor. At a minimum the plan must include, but need not be limited to

- Goals to enhance the faculty member's ability to fulfill designated responsibilities (e.g., goals related to currency in areas of teaching responsibility, teaching effectiveness, research, scholarly activity).

- Specific measurable action steps with expected timelines by which the faculty member will achieve the goals.

- Evidence of annual updates of action steps and goals as they are met or as circumstances change.

- Identification of the ways in which the faculty member's professional development plan will contribute to attaining the program's strategic goals.

A.5.3. Programs must routinely secure and document sufficient qualitative and quantitative information to allow for meaningful analysis about the extent to which the program is meeting its stated goals and objectives. This must include, but need not be limited to

- Faculty effectiveness in their assigned teaching responsibilities.

- Students' progression through the program.

- Fieldwork and experiential component performance evaluation.

- Student evaluation of fieldwork and the experiential component experience.

- Student satisfaction with the program.

- Graduates' performance on the NBCOT certification exam, if applicable.

- Graduates' job placement and performance based on employer satisfaction.

- Graduates' scholarly activity (e.g., presentations, publications, grants obtained, state and national leadership positions, awards).

A.5.4. The average total pass rate of OT doctoral program graduates taking the national certification exam for the first time over the 3 most recent calendar years must be 70% or higher.

A.5.5. Programs must routinely and systematically analyze data to determine the extent to which the program is meeting its stated goals and objectives. An annual report summarizing analysis of data and planned action responses must be maintained.

A.5.6. The results of ongoing evaluation must be appropriately reflected in the program's strategic plan, curriculum, and other dimensions of the program.

A.6.0. Curriculum Framework

The curriculum framework is a description of the program that includes the program's mission, philosophy, and curriculum design.

A.6.1. The curriculum must ensure preparation to practice as a generalist with a broad exposure to current practice settings (e.g., school, hospital, community, long-term care) and emerging practice areas (as defined by the program). The curriculum must prepare students to work with a variety of populations including, but not limited to, children, adolescents, adults, and elderly persons in areas of physical and mental health.

A.6.2. The curriculum must include course objectives and learning activities demonstrating preparation beyond a generalist level in, but not limited to, practice skills, research skills, administration, leadership, and theory.

A.6.3. The OT doctoral degree must be awarded after a period of study such that the total time to the degree, including both pre-professional and professional preparation, equals at least 6 full-time equivalent academic years. The program must document a system and rationale for ensuring that the length of study of the program is appropriate to the expected learning and competence of the graduate.

A.6.4. The curriculum must include application of knowledge to practice through a combination of experiential activities and a culminating project.

A.6.5. The statement of philosophy of the occupational therapy program must reflect the current published philosophy of the profession and must include a statement of the program's fundamental beliefs about human beings and how they learn.

A.6.6. The statement of the mission of the occupational therapy program must be consistent with and supportive of the mission of the sponsoring institution.

A.6.7. The curriculum design must reflect the mission and philosophy of both the occupational therapy program and the institution and must provide the basis for program planning, implementation, and evaluation. The design must identify educational goals and describe the selection of the content, scope, and sequencing of coursework.

A.6.8. The program must have clearly documented assessment measures by which students are regularly evaluated on their acquisition of knowledge, skills, attitudes, and competencies required for graduation.

A.6.9. The program must have written syllabi for each course that include course objectives and learning activities that, in total, reflect all course content required by the Standards. Instructional methods (e.g., presentations, demonstrations, discussion) and materials used to accomplish course objectives must be documented. Programs must also demonstrate the consistency between course syllabi and the curriculum design.

Section B:
Specific Requirements for Accreditation

The specific requirements for accreditation contain the content that a program must include. The content requirements are written as expected student outcomes. Faculty are responsible for developing learning activities and evaluation methods to document that students meet these outcomes.

B.1.0. Foundational Content Requirements

Program content must be based on a broad foundation in the liberal arts and sciences. A strong foundation in the biological, physical, social, and behavioral sciences supports an understanding of occupation across the life span. Coursework in these areas may be prerequisite to or concurrent with professional education and must facilitate development of the performance criteria listed below. The student will be able to

B.1.1. Demonstrate oral and written communication skills.

B.1.2. Employ logical thinking, critical analysis, problem solving, and creativity.

B.1.3. Demonstrate competence in basic computer use, including the ability to use databases and search engines to access information, word processing for writing, and presentation software (e.g., PowerPoint™).

B.1.4. Demonstrate knowledge and understanding of the structure and function of the human body to include the biological and physical sciences. Course content must include, but is not limited to, biology, anatomy, physiology, neuroscience, and kinesiology or biomechanics.

B.1.5. Demonstrate knowledge and understanding of human development throughout the life span (infants, children, adolescents, adults, and elderly persons). Course content must include, but is not limited to, developmental psychology.

B.1.6. Demonstrate knowledge and understanding of the concepts of human behavior to include the behavioral and social sciences. Course content must include, but is not limited to, introductory psychology, abnormal psychology, and introductory sociology or introductory anthropology.

B.1.7.   Demonstrate knowledge and appreciation of the role of sociocultural, socioeconomic, and diversity factors and lifestyle choices in contemporary society. Course content must include, but is not limited to, introductory psychology, abnormal psychology, and introductory sociology or introductory anthropology.

B.1.8.   Articulate the influence of social conditions and the ethical context in which humans choose and engage in occupations.

B.1.9.   Demonstrate knowledge of global social issues and prevailing health and welfare needs.

B.1.10.   Apply quantitative statistics and qualitative analysis to interpret tests, measurements, and other data.

B.1.11.   Demonstrate the ability to use technology in screening, evaluation, intervention, and data analysis as appropriate for the area of practice.

B.2.0. *Basic Tenets of Occupational Therapy*

Coursework must facilitate development of the performance criteria listed below. The student will be able to

B.2.1.   Explain the history and philosophical base of the profession of occupational therapy and its importance.

B.2.2.   Explain the meaning and dynamics of occupation and activity, including the interaction of areas of occupation, performance skills, performance patterns, activity demands, context(s), and client factors.

B.2.3.   Articulate to consumers, potential employers, colleagues, third-party payers, regulatory boards, policymakers, other audiences, and the general public both the unique nature of occupation as viewed by the profession of occupational therapy and the value of occupation to support participation in context(s) for the client.

B.2.4.   Articulate the importance of balancing areas of occupation with the achievement of health and wellness.

B.2.5.   Explain the role of occupation in the promotion of health and the prevention of disease and disability for the individual, family, and society.

B.2.6.   Analyze the effects of physical and mental health, heritable diseases and predisposing genetic conditions, disability, disease processes, and traumatic injury to the individual within the cultural context of family and society on occupational performance.

B.2.7.   Exhibit the ability to analyze tasks relative to areas of occupation, performance skills, performance patterns, activity demands, context(s), and client factors to formulate an intervention plan.

B.2.8.   Use sound judgment in regard to safety of self and others, and adhere to safety regulations throughout the occupational therapy process.

B.2.9.   Express support for the quality of life, well-being, and occupation of the individual, group, or population to promote physical and mental health and prevention of injury and disease considering the context (e.g., cultural, physical, social, personal, spiritual, temporal, virtual).

B.2.10.   Use clinical reasoning to explain the rationale for and use of compensatory strategies when desired life tasks cannot be performed.

B.2.11.   Analyze, synthesize, evaluate, and apply models of occupational performance and theories of occupation.

B.3.0. Occupational Therapy Theoretical Perspectives

The program must facilitate the development of the performance criteria listed below. The student will be able to

B.3.1.   Apply theories that underlie the practice of occupational therapy.

B.3.2.   Compare, contrast, and integrate a variety of models of practice and frames of reference that are used in occupational therapy.

B.3.3.   Use theories, models of practice, and frames of reference to guide and inform evaluation and intervention.

B.3.4.   Analyze and discuss how history, theory, and the sociopolitical climate influence and are influenced by practice.

B.3.5.   Apply theoretical constructs to evaluation and intervention with various types of clients and practice contexts, including population-based approaches, to analyze and effect meaningful occupation.

B.3.6.   Articulate the process of theory development in occupational therapy and its desired impact and influence on society.

B.4.0. Screening, Evaluation, and Referral

The process of screening, evaluation, referral, and diagnosis as related to occupational performance and participation must be culturally relevant and based on theoretical perspectives, models of practice, frames of reference, and available evidence. In addition, this process must consider the continuum of need from individuals to populations. The program must facilitate development of the performance criteria listed below. The student will be able to

B.4.1.   Use standardized and nonstandardized screening and assessment tools to determine the need for occupational therapy intervention. These include, but are not limited to, specified screening tools; assessments; skilled observations; checklists; histories; consultations with other professionals; and interviews with the client, family, significant others, and community.

B.4.2.   Select appropriate assessment tools based on client needs, contextual factors, and psychometric properties of tests. These must be relevant to a variety of populations across the life span, culturally relevant, based on available evidence, and incorporate use of occupation in the assessment process.

B.4.3.   Use appropriate procedures and protocols (including standardized formats) when administering assessments.

B.4.4.   Evaluate client(s)' occupational performance in activities of daily living (ADL), instrumental activities of daily living (IADL), education, work, play, leisure, and social participation. Evaluation of occupational performance using standardized and nonstandardized assessment tools includes

• The occupational profile, including participation in activities that are meaningful and necessary for the client to carry out roles in home, work, and community environments.

• Client factors, including body functions (e.g., neuromuscular, sensory, visual, perceptual, cognitive, mental) and body structures (e.g., cardiovascular, digestive, integumentary systems).

• Performance patterns (e.g., habits, routines, roles) and behavior patterns.

- Cultural, physical, social, personal, spiritual, temporal, and virtual contexts and activity demands that affect performance.

- Performance skills, including motor (e.g., posture, mobility, coordination, strength, energy), process (e.g., energy, knowledge, temporal organization, organizing space and objects, adaptation), and communication and interaction skills (e.g., physicality, information exchange, relations).

B.4.5. Compare and contrast the role of the occupational therapist and occupational therapy assistant in the screening and evaluation process along with the importance of and rationale for supervision and collaborative work between the occupational therapist and occupational therapy assistant in that process.

B.4.6. Interpret criterion-referenced and norm-referenced standardized test scores based on an understanding of sampling, normative data, standard and criterion scores, reliability, and validity.

B.4.7. Consider factors that might bias assessment results, such as culture, disability status, and situational variables related to the individual and context.

B.4.8. Interpret the evaluation data in relation to accepted terminology of the profession, relevant theoretical frameworks, and interdisciplinary knowledge.

B.4.9. Evaluate appropriateness and discuss mechanisms for referring clients for additional evaluation to specialists who are internal and external to the profession.

B.4.10. Document occupational therapy services to ensure accountability of service provision and to meet standards for reimbursement of services, adhering to applicable facility, local, state, federal, and reimbursement agencies. Documentation must effectively communicate the need and rationale for occupational therapy services.

B.4.11. Articulate screening and evaluation processes for a practice area. Use evidence-based reasoning to analyze, synthesize, evaluate, and diagnose problems related to occupational performance and participation.

B.5.0. *Intervention Plan: Formulation and Implementation*

The process of formulation and implementation of the therapeutic intervention plan to facilitate occupational performance and participation must be culturally relevant; reflective of current occupational therapy practice; based on available evidence; and based on theoretical perspectives, models of practice, and frames of reference. In addition, this process must consider the continuum of need from individuals to populations. The program must facilitate development of the performance criteria listed below. The student will be able to

B.5.1. Use evaluation findings to diagnose occupational performance and participation based on appropriate theoretical approaches, models of practice, frames of reference, and interdisciplinary knowledge. Develop occupation-based intervention plans and strategies (including goals and methods to achieve them) based on the stated needs of the client as well as data gathered during the evaluation process in collaboration with the client and others. Intervention plans and strategies must be culturally relevant, reflective of current occupational therapy practice, and based on available evidence. Interventions address the following components:

- The occupational profile, including participation in activities that are meaningful and necessary for the client to carry out roles in home, work, and community environments.

- Client factors, including body functions (e.g., neuromuscular, sensory, visual, perceptual, cognitive, mental) and body structures (e.g., cardiovascular, digestive, integumentary systems).

- Performance patterns (e.g., habits, routines, roles) and behavior patterns.

- Cultural, physical, social, personal, spiritual, temporal, and virtual contexts and activity demands that affect performance.

- Performance skills, including motor (e.g., posture, mobility, coordination, strength, energy), process (e.g., energy, knowledge, temporal organization, organizing space and objects, adaptation), and communication and interaction skills (e.g., physicality, information exchange, relations).

B.5.2. Select and provide direct occupational therapy interventions and procedures to enhance safety, wellness, and performance in activities of daily living (ADL), instrumental activities of daily living (IADL), education, work, play, leisure, and social participation.

B.5.3. Provide therapeutic use of occupation and activities (e.g., occupation-based activity, practice skills, preparatory methods).

B.5.4. Provide training in self-care, self-management, home management, and community and work integration.

B.5.5. Provide development, remediation, and compensation for physical, cognitive, perceptual, sensory (e.g., vision, tactile, auditory, gustatory, olfactory, pain, temperature, pressure, vestibular, proprioception), neuromuscular, and behavioral skills.

B.5.6. Provide therapeutic use of self, including one's personality, insights, perceptions, and judgments as part of the therapeutic process in both individual and group interaction.

B.5.7. Demonstrate care coordination, case management, and transition services in traditional and emerging practice environments.

B.5.8. Modify environments (e.g., home, work, school, community) and adapt processes, including the application of ergonomic principles.

B.5.9. Design, fabricate, apply, fit, and train in assistive technologies and devices (e.g., electronic aids to daily living, seating systems) used to enhance occupational performance.

B.5.10. Provide design, fabrication, application, fitting, and training in orthotic devices used to enhance occupational performance and training in the use of prosthetic devices, based on scientific principles of kinesiology, biomechanics, and physics.

B.5.11. Provide recommendations and training in techniques to enhance mobility, including physical transfers, wheelchair management, and community mobility, and address issues related to driver rehabilitation.

B.5.12. Provide management of feeding and eating to enable performance (including the process of bringing food or fluids from the plate or cup to the mouth, the ability to keep and manipulate food or fluid in the mouth, and the initiation of swallowing) and train others in precautions and techniques while considering client and contextual factors.

B.5.13. Explain the use of superficial thermal and mechanical modalities as a preparatory measure to improve occupational performance, including foundational knowledge, underlying principles, indications, contraindications, and precautions. Demonstrate safe and effective application of superficial thermal and mechanical modalities.

B.5.14. Explain the use of deep thermal and electrotherapeutic modalities as a preparatory measure to improve occupational performance, including indications, contraindications, and precautions.

B.5.15. Develop and promote the use of appropriate home and community programming to support performance in the client's natural environment and participation in all contexts relevant to the client.

B.5.16. Demonstrate the ability to educate the client, caregiver, family, significant others, and communities to facilitate skills in areas of occupation as well as prevention, health maintenance, and safety.

B.5.17. Apply the principles of the teaching–learning process using educational methods to design educational experiences to address the needs of the client, family, significant others, communities, colleagues, other health providers, and the public.

B.5.18. Effectively interact through written, oral, and nonverbal communication with the client, family, significant others, communities, colleagues, other health providers, and the public in a professionally acceptable manner.

B.5.19. Grade and adapt the environment, tools, materials, occupations, and interventions to reflect the changing needs of the client, sociocultural context, and technological advances.

B.5.20. Select and teach compensatory strategies, such as use of technology, adaptations to the environment, and involvement of humans and nonhumans in the completion of tasks.

B.5.21. Identify and demonstrate techniques in skills of supervision and collaboration with occupational therapy assistants and other professionals on therapeutic interventions.

B.5.22. Understand when and how to use the consultative process with groups, programs, organizations, or communities.

B.5.23. Refer to specialists (both internal and external to the profession) for consultation and intervention.

B.5.24. Monitor and reassess, in collaboration with the client, caregiver, family, and significant others, the effect of occupational therapy intervention and the need for continued or modified intervention.

B.5.25. Plan for discharge, in collaboration with the client, by reviewing the needs of the client, caregiver, family, and significant others; resources; and discharge environment. This includes, but is not limited to, identification of client's current status within the continuum of care and the identification of community, human, and fiscal resources; recommendations for environmental adaptations; and home programming to facilitate the client's progression along the continuum toward outcome goals.

B.5.26. Organize, collect, and analyze data in a systematic manner for evaluation of practice outcomes. Report evaluation results and modify practice as needed to improve outcomes.

B.5.27. Terminate occupational therapy services when stated outcomes have been achieved or it has been determined that they cannot be achieved. This includes developing a summary of occupational therapy outcomes, appropriate recommendations and referrals, and discussion with the client and with appropriate others of post-discharge needs.

B.5.28. Document occupational therapy services to ensure accountability of service provision and to meet standards for reimbursement of services. Documentation must effectively communicate the need and rationale for occupational therapy services and must be appropriate to the context in which the service is delivered.

B.5.29. Provide population-based occupational therapy intervention that addresses occupational needs as identified by a community.

B.6.0. Context of Service Delivery

Context of service delivery includes the knowledge and understanding of the various contexts, such as professional, social, cultural, political, economic, and ecological, in which occupational therapy services are provided. The program must facilitate development of the performance criteria listed below. The student will be able to

B.6.1.   Critically evaluate and address the various contexts of health care, education, community, political, and social systems as they relate to the practice of occupational therapy.

B.6.2.   Critically analyze the current policy issues and the social, economic, political, geographic, and demographic factors that influence the various contexts for practice of occupational therapy.

B.6.3.   Integrate the current social, economic, political, geographic, and demographic factors to promote policy development and the provision of occupational therapy services.

B.6.4.   Advocate for changes in service delivery policies, effect changes in the system, and identify opportunities to address societal needs.

B.6.5.   Critically analyze the trends in models of service delivery and their potential effect on the practice of occupational therapy, including, but not limited to, medical, educational, community, and social models.

B.6.6.   Use national and international resources in making assessment or intervention choices, and appreciate the influence of international occupational therapy contributions to education, research, and practice.

B.7.0. Leadership and Management

Leadership and management skills include principles and applications of leadership and management theory. The program must facilitate development of the performance criteria listed below. The student will be able to

B.7.1.   Identify and critically evaluate how the various practice settings (e.g., medical institutions, community practice, school systems) affect the delivery of occupational therapy services for individuals and populations.

B.7.2.   Identify and critically evaluate the impact of contextual factors on the management and delivery of occupational therapy services for individuals and populations.

B.7.3.   Identify and critically evaluate the systems and structures that create federal and state legislation and regulation and their implications and effects on practice and policy.

B.7.4.   Demonstrate knowledge of applicable national requirements for credentialing and requirements for licensure, certification, or registration under state laws.

B.7.5.   Demonstrate knowledge of various reimbursement systems (e.g., federal, state, third-party, private-payer), appeals mechanisms, and documentation requirements that affect society and the practice of occupational therapy.

B.7.6.   Describe the mechanisms, systems, and techniques needed to properly maintain, organize, and prioritize workloads and intervention settings including inventories.

B.7.7.   Demonstrate leadership skills in the ability to plan, develop, organize, and market the delivery of services to include the determination of programmatic needs, service delivery options, and formulation and management of staffing for effective service provision.

B.7.8.   Demonstrate leadership skills in the ability to design ongoing processes for quality improvement (e.g., outcome studies analysis) and develop program changes as needed to ensure quality of services and to direct administrative changes.

B.7.9.   Develop strategies for effective, competency-based legal and ethical supervision of occupational therapy and non–occupational therapy personnel.

B.7.10. Describe the ongoing professional responsibility for providing fieldwork education and the criteria for becoming a fieldwork educator.

B.7.11. Demonstrate knowledge of and the ability to write program development plans for provision of occupational therapy services to individuals and populations.

B.7.12. Identify and adapt existing models or develop new service provision models to respond to policy, regulatory agencies, and reimbursement and compliance standards.

B.7.13. Identify and develop strategies to enable occupational therapy to respond to society's changing needs.

B.7.14. Identify and implement strategies to promote staff development based on evaluation of the personal and professional abilities and competencies of supervised staff as they relate to job responsibilities.

B.8.0. Research

Application of research includes the ability to read, understand, and conduct research that affects practice and the provision of occupational therapy services. The program must facilitate development of the performance criteria listed below. The student will be able to

B.8.1.   Articulate the importance of research, scholarly activities, and the continued development of a body of knowledge relevant to the profession of occupational therapy.

B.8.2.   Effectively locate, understand, and evaluate information, including the quality of research evidence.

B.8.3.   Use research literature to make evidence-based decisions.

B.8.4.   Select, apply, and interpret basic descriptive, correlational, and inferential quantitative statistics and code, analyze, and synthesize qualitative data.

B.8.5.   Understand and critique the validity of research studies, including designs (both quantitative and qualitative) and methodologies.

B.8.6.   Demonstrate the skills necessary to design a research proposal that includes the research question, relevant literature, sample, design, measurement, and data analysis.

B.8.7.   Design and implement a research study that evaluates clinical practice, service delivery, and/or professional issues.

B.8.8.   Write scholarly reports appropriate for presentation or for publication in a peer-reviewed journal.

B.8.9.   Demonstrate an understanding of the process of locating and securing grants and how grants can serve as a fiscal resource for research and practice.

B.8.10. Complete a culminating project that relates theory to practice and demonstrates synthesis of advanced knowledge in a practice area.

B.9.0. Professional Ethics, Values, and Responsibilities

Professional ethics, values, and responsibilities include an understanding and appreciation of ethics and values of the profession of occupational therapy. The program must facilitate development of the performance criteria listed below. The student will be able to

B.9.1.   Demonstrate a knowledge and understanding of the American Occupational Therapy Association (AOTA) *Occupational Therapy Code of Ethics, Core Values and Attitudes of Occupational Therapy Practice,* and AOTA Standards of Practice and use them as a guide for ethical decision making in professional interactions, client interventions, and employment settings.

B.9.2.   Discuss and justify how the role of a professional is enhanced by knowledge of and involvement in international, national, state, and local occupational therapy associations and related professional associations.

B.9.3.   Promote occupational therapy by educating other professionals, service providers, consumers, third-party payers, regulatory bodies, and the public.

B.9.4.   Identify and develop strategies for ongoing professional development to ensure that practice is consistent with current and accepted standards.

B.9.5.   Discuss professional responsibilities related to liability issues under current models of service provision.

B.9.6.   Discuss and evaluate personal and professional abilities and competencies as they relate to job responsibilities.

B.9.7.   Discuss and justify the varied roles of the occupational therapist as a practitioner, educator, researcher, policy developer, program developer, advocate, administrator, consultant, and entrepreneur.

B.9.8.   Explain and justify the importance of supervisory roles, responsibilities, and collaborative professional relationships between the occupational therapist and the occupational therapy assistant.

B.9.9.   Describe and discuss professional responsibilities and issues when providing service on a contractual basis.

B.9.10.   Demonstrate strategies for analyzing issues and making decisions to resolve personal and organizational ethical conflicts.

B.9.11.   Demonstrate a variety of informal and formal ethical dispute–resolution strategies.

B.9.12.   Describe and implement strategies to assist the consumer in gaining access to occupational therapy and other health and social services.

B.9.13.   Demonstrate advocacy by participating in and exploring leadership positions in organizations or agencies promoting the profession (e.g., American Occupational Therapy Association, state occupational therapy associations, World Federation of Occupational Therapists, advocacy organizations), consumer access and services, and the welfare of the community.

B.10.0. Fieldwork Education

Fieldwork education is a crucial part of professional preparation and is best integrated as a component of the curriculum design. Fieldwork experiences should be implemented and evaluated for their effectiveness by the educational institution. The experience should provide the student with the opportunity to carry out professional responsibilities under supervision and for professional role

modeling. The academic fieldwork coordinator is responsible for the program's compliance with fieldwork education requirements. The academic fieldwork coordinator will

B.10.1. Document the criteria and process for selecting fieldwork sites. Ensure that the fieldwork program reflects the sequence, depth, focus, and scope of content in the curriculum design.

B.10.2. Ensure that the academic fieldwork coordinator and faculty collaborate to design fieldwork experiences that strengthen the ties between didactic and fieldwork education.

B.10.3. Provide fieldwork education in settings that are equipped to meet the curriculum goals, provide educational experiences applicable to the academic program, and have fieldwork educators who are able to effectively meet the learning needs of the students.

B.10.4. Ensure that the academic fieldwork coordinator is responsible for advocating the development of links between the fieldwork and didactic aspects of the curriculum, for communicating about the curriculum to fieldwork educators, and for maintaining contracts and site data related to fieldwork placements.

B.10.5. Demonstrate that academic and fieldwork educators collaborate in establishing fieldwork objectives, identifying site requirements, and communicating with the student and fieldwork educator about progress and performance during fieldwork.

B.10.6. Document a policy and procedure for complying with fieldwork site health requirements and maintaining student health records in a secure setting.

B.10.7. Ensure that the ratio of fieldwork educators to student(s) enables proper supervision and the ability to provide frequent assessment of student progress in achieving stated fieldwork objectives.

B.10.8. Ensure that fieldwork agreements are sufficient in scope and number to allow completion of graduation requirements in a timely manner in accordance with the policy adopted by the program.

B.10.9. For programs in which the academic and fieldwork components of the curriculum are provided by two or more institutions, responsibilities of each sponsoring institution and fieldwork site must be clearly documented in a memorandum of understanding. For active Level I and Level II fieldwork sites, programs must have current fieldwork agreements or memoranda of understanding that are signed by both parties. (Electronic contracts and signatures are acceptable.)

B.10.10. Documentation must be provided that each memorandum of understanding between institutions and active fieldwork sites is reviewed at least every 5 years by both parties. Programs must provide documentation that both parties have reviewed the contract.

The goal of Level I fieldwork is to introduce students to the fieldwork experience, to apply knowledge to practice, and to develop understanding of the needs of clients. The program will

B.10.11. Ensure that Level I fieldwork is integral to the program's curriculum design and include experiences designed to enrich didactic coursework through directed observation and participation in selected aspects of the occupational therapy process.

B.10.12. Ensure that qualified personnel supervise Level I fieldwork. Examples may include, but are not limited to, currently licensed or credentialed occupational therapists and occupational therapy assistants, psychologists, physician assistants, teachers, social workers, nurses, and physical therapists.

B.10.13. Document all Level I fieldwork experiences that are provided to students, including mechanisms for formal evaluation of student performance. Ensure that Level I fieldwork is not substituted for any part of Level II fieldwork.

The goal of Level II fieldwork is to develop competent, entry-level, generalist occupational therapists. Level II fieldwork must be integral to the program's curriculum design and must include an in-depth experience in delivering occupational therapy services to clients, focusing on the application of purposeful and meaningful occupation and research, administration, and management of occupational therapy services. It is recommended that the student be exposed to a variety of clients across the life span and to a variety of settings. The program will

B.10.14. Ensure that the fieldwork experience is designed to promote clinical reasoning and reflective practice, to transmit the values and beliefs that enable ethical practice, and to develop professionalism and competence in career responsibilities.

B.10.15. Provide Level II fieldwork in traditional and/or emerging settings, consistent with the curriculum design. In all settings, psychosocial factors influencing engagement in occupation must be understood and integrated for the development of client-centered, meaningful, occupation-based outcomes. The student can complete Level II fieldwork in a minimum of one setting if it is reflective of more than one practice area, or in a maximum of four different settings.

B.10.16. Require a minimum of 24 weeks' full-time Level II fieldwork. This may be completed on a part-time basis as defined by the fieldwork placement in accordance with the fieldwork placement's usual and customary personnel policies as long as it is at least 50% of a full-time equivalent at that site.

B.10.17. Ensure that the student is supervised by a currently licensed or credentialed occupational therapist who has a minimum of 1 year of practice experience subsequent to initial certification, and is adequately prepared to serve as a fieldwork educator. The supervising therapist may be engaged by the fieldwork site or by the educational program.

B.10.18. Document a mechanism for evaluating the effectiveness of supervision (e.g., student evaluation of fieldwork) and for providing resources for enhancing supervision (e.g., materials on supervisory skills, continuing education opportunities, articles on theory and practice).

B.10.19. Ensure that supervision provides protection of consumers and opportunities for appropriate role modeling of occupational therapy practice. Initially, supervision should be direct and then decrease to less direct supervision as is appropriate for the setting, the severity of the client's condition, and the ability of the student.

B.10.20. Ensure that supervision provided in a setting where no occupational therapy services exist includes a documented plan for provision of occupational therapy services and supervision by a currently licensed or credentialed occupational therapist with at least 3 years of professional experience. Supervision must include a minimum of 8 hours per week. Supervision must be initially direct and then may be decreased to less direct supervision as is appropriate for the setting, the client's needs, and the ability of the student. An occupational therapy supervisor must be available, via a variety of contact measures, to the student during all working hours. An on-site supervisor designee of another profession must be assigned while the occupational therapy supervisor is off site.

B.10.21. Document mechanisms for requiring formal evaluation of student performance on Level II fieldwork (e.g., the American Occupational Therapy Association *Fieldwork Performance Evaluation for the Occupational Therapy Student* or equivalent).

B.10.22. Ensure that students attending Level II fieldwork outside the United States are supervised by an occupational therapist who graduated from a program approved by the World Federation of Occupational Therapists and has 1 year of experience in practice. Such fieldwork must not exceed 12 weeks.

B.11.0. Doctoral-Level Experiential Component

The student must successfully complete all coursework and Level II fieldwork and pass a competency requirement prior to commencement of the doctoral experiential component. The goal of the doctoral experiential component is to develop occupational therapists with advanced skills (those that are beyond a generalist level). The doctoral experiential component shall be an integral part of the program's curriculum design and shall include an in-depth experience in one or more of the following: clinical practice skills, research skills, administration, leadership, program and policy development, advocacy, education, or theory development. The program will

B.11.1.   Ensure that the doctoral experiential component is provided in a setting consistent with the program's curriculum design, including individualized specific objectives and plans for supervision.

B.11.2.   Require that the length of this doctoral experiential component be a minimum of 16 weeks (640 hours). This may be completed on a part-time basis and must be consistent with the individualized specific objectives and culminating project.

B.11.3.   Ensure that the student is mentored by an individual with expertise consistent with the student's area of focus.

B.11.4.   Document a formal evaluation mechanism for objective assessment of the student's performance during and at the completion of the doctoral experiential component.

Accreditation Standards for a Master's-Degree-Level Educational Program for the Occupational Therapist

Adopted August 2006. Effective January 1, 2008.

The Accreditation Council for Occupational Therapy Education (ACOTE®) of the American Occupational Therapy Association (AOTA) accredits educational programs for the occupational therapist. The Standards comply with the United States Department of Education (USDE) criteria for recognition of accrediting agencies.

These Standards are the requirements used in accrediting educational programs that prepare individuals to enter the occupational therapy profession. The extent to which a program complies with these Standards determines its accreditation status.

Preamble

The rapidly changing and dynamic nature of contemporary health and human services delivery systems requires the occupational therapist to possess basic skills as a direct care provider, consultant, educator, manager, researcher, and advocate for the profession and the consumer.

A graduate from an ACOTE-accredited master's-degree-level occupational therapy program must

- Have acquired, as a foundation for professional study, a breadth and depth of knowledge in the liberal arts and sciences and an understanding of issues related to diversity.

- Be educated as a generalist with a broad exposure to the delivery models and systems used in settings where occupational therapy is currently practiced and where it is emerging as a service.

- Have achieved entry-level competence through a combination of academic and fieldwork education.

- Be prepared to articulate and apply occupational therapy theory and evidence-based evaluations and interventions to achieve expected outcomes as related to occupation.

- Be prepared to be a lifelong learner and keep current with evidence-based professional practice.

- Uphold the ethical standards, values, and attitudes of the occupational therapy profession.

- Understand the distinct roles and responsibilities of the occupational therapist and occupational therapy assistant in the supervisory process.

- Be prepared to advocate as a professional for the occupational therapy services offered and for the recipients of those services.

- Be prepared to be an effective consumer of the latest research and knowledge bases that support practice and contribute to the growth and dissemination of research and knowledge.

Section A:
General Requirements for Accreditation

A.1.0. Sponsorship and Accreditation

A.1.1. The sponsoring institution(s) and affiliates, if any, must be accredited by recognized national, regional, or state agencies with accrediting authority. For programs in countries other than the United States, ACOTE will determine an alternative and equivalent external review process.

A.1.2. Sponsoring institutions must be authorized under applicable law or other acceptable authority to provide a program of post-secondary education and have appropriate degree-granting authority.

A.1.3. Accredited occupational therapy educational programs may be established only in senior colleges, universities, or medical schools.

A.1.4. The sponsoring institution must assume primary responsibility for appointment of faculty, admission of students, and curriculum planning. This would include course content, satisfactory completion of the educational program, and granting of the degree. The sponsoring institution must also be responsible for the coordination of classroom teaching and supervised fieldwork practice and for providing assurance that the practice activities assigned to students in a fieldwork setting are appropriate to the program.

A.1.5. The sponsoring institution or program must

- Inform ACOTE of the transfer of program sponsorship or change of the institution's name within 30 days of the transfer or change.

- Inform ACOTE within 30 days of the date of notification of any adverse accreditation action taken to change the sponsoring institution's accreditation status to probation or withdrawal of accreditation.

- Submit a Letter of Intent to add or change a program degree level at least 1 year prior to the planned admission of students into that level.

- Inform ACOTE within 30 days of the resignation of the program director or appointment of a new or interim program director.

- Pay accreditation fees within 90 days of the invoice date.

- Submit a Report of Self-Study and other required reports (e.g., Biennial Report, Plan of Correction, Progress Report) within the period of time designated by ACOTE. All reports must be complete and contain all requested information.

- Agree to a site visit date before the end of the period for which accreditation was previously awarded.

- Demonstrate honesty and integrity in all interactions with ACOTE.

A.2.0. Academic Resources

A.2.1. The program must have a director who is assigned to the occupational therapy educational program on a full-time basis. The director may be assigned other institutional duties that do not interfere with the management and administration of the program. The institution must ensure that the needs of the program are being met.

A.2.2. The program director must be an initially certified occupational therapist who is licensed or credentialed according to regulations in the state or jurisdiction in which the program is located.

The director must hold academic qualifications comparable to the majority of other program directors within the institutional unit (e.g., division, college, school) to which the program is assigned. By July 1, 2012, the program director must hold a doctoral degree.

A.2.3.   The program director must have a minimum of 6 years of experience in the field of occupational therapy, including practice as an occupational therapist, administrative or supervisory experience, and at least 2 years of experience in a full-time academic appointment with teaching responsibilities.

A.2.4.   The program director must be responsible for the management and administration of the program, including planning, evaluation, budgeting, selection of faculty and staff, maintenance of accreditation, and commitment to strategies for professional development.

A.2.5.   The program director and faculty must possess the academic and experiential qualifications and backgrounds (identified in documented descriptions of roles and responsibilities) that are necessary to meet program objectives and the mission of the institution.

A.2.6.   The program must document policies and procedures to ensure that the program director and faculty are aware of and abide by the current code of ethics of the profession of occupational therapy.

A.2.7.   The program must identify an individual as academic fieldwork coordinator who is specifically responsible for the program's compliance with the fieldwork requirements of Standards Section B.10.0. This individual must be a licensed or credentialed occupational therapist. Academic fieldwork coordinators who hold a faculty position must meet the requirements of Standard A.2.9.

A.2.8.   The faculty must include currently licensed or credentialed occupational therapists.

A.2.9.   All full-time faculty must hold a minimum of a master's degree. By July 1, 2012, the majority of full-time faculty who are occupational therapists must hold a doctoral degree.

A.2.10. The faculty must have documented expertise in their area(s) of teaching responsibility and knowledge of the content delivery method (e.g., distance learning).

A.2.11. The occupational therapy faculty at each accredited location where the program is offered must be sufficient in number and must possess the expertise necessary to ensure appropriate curriculum design, content delivery, and program evaluation.

A.2.12. Faculty responsibilities must be consistent with and supportive of the mission of the institution.

A.2.13. The faculty–student ratio must permit the achievement of the purpose and stated objectives for laboratory and lecture courses, be compatible with accepted practices of the institution for similar programs, and ensure student and consumer safety.

A.2.14. Clerical and support staff must be provided to the program, consistent with institutional practice, to meet programmatic and administrative requirements, including support for any portion of the program offered by distance education.

A.2.15. The program must be allocated a budget of regular institutional funds, not including grants, gifts, and other restricted sources, sufficient to implement and maintain the objectives of the program and to fulfill the program's obligation to matriculated and entering students.

A.2.16. Classrooms and laboratories must be provided that are consistent with the program's educational objectives, teaching methods, number of students, and safety and health standards of the institution, and must allow for efficient operation of the program. If any portion of the program is offered by distance education, technology and resources must be adequate to support a distance-learning environment.

A.2.17. Laboratory space provided by the institution must be assigned to the occupational therapy program on a priority basis. If laboratory space is provided by another institution or agency, there must be a written and signed agreement to ensure assignment of space for program use.

A.2.18. Adequate space must be provided to store and secure equipment and supplies.

A.2.19. The program director and faculty must have office space consistent with institutional practice.

A.2.20. Adequate space must be provided for the private advising of students.

A.2.21. Appropriate and sufficient equipment and supplies must be provided by the institution for student use and for the didactic and supervised fieldwork components of the curriculum.

A.2.22. Students must be given access to and have the opportunity to use the evaluative and treatment methodologies that reflect both current practice and practice in the geographic area served by the program.

A.2.23. Students must have ready access to a supply of current and relevant books, journals, periodicals, computers, software, and other reference materials needed to meet the requirements of the curriculum. This may include, but is not limited to, libraries, online services, interlibrary loan, and resource centers.

A.2.24. Instructional aids and technology must be available in sufficient quantity and quality to be consistent with the program objectives and teaching methods.

A.3.0. Students

A.3.1. Admission of students to the occupational therapy program must be made in accordance with the practices of the institution. There must be stated admission criteria that are clearly defined and published and reflective of the demands of the program.

A.3.2. Policies pertaining to standards for admission, advanced placement, transfer of credit, credit for experiential learning (if applicable), and prerequisite educational or work experience requirements must be readily accessible to prospective students and the public.

A.3.3. Programs must document implementation of a mechanism to ensure that students receiving credit for previous courses and/or work experience have met the content requirements of the appropriate master's Standards.

A.3.4. Criteria for successful completion of each segment of the educational program and for graduation must be given in advance to each student.

A.3.5. Evaluation content and methods must be consistent with the curriculum design, objectives, and competencies of the didactic and fieldwork components of the program.

A.3.6. Evaluation must be conducted on a regular basis to provide students and program officials with timely indications of the students' progress and academic standing.

A.3.7. Students must be informed of and have access to the student support services that are provided to other students in the institution.

A.3.8. Advising related to professional coursework and fieldwork education must be the responsibility of the occupational therapy faculty.

A.4.0. Operational Policies

A.4.1. All program publications and advertising—including, but not limited to, academic calendars, announcements, catalogs, handbooks, and Web sites—must accurately reflect the program offered.

A.4.2. Accurate and current information regarding student outcomes must be readily available to the public in at least one publication or Web page. The following data must be reported as an aggregate for the 3 most recent calendar years and specify the

- 3-year time period being reported,

- total number of program graduates during that period,

- total number of first-time test takers of the national certification examination during that period,

- total number of first-time test takers who passed the exam during that period, and

- percentage of the total number of first-time test takers who passed the exam during that period.

A.4.3. The program's accreditation status and the name, address, and telephone number of ACOTE must be published in all of the following used by the institution: catalog, Web site, and program-related brochures or flyers available to prospective students.

A.4.4. Faculty recruitment and employment practices, as well as student recruitment and admission procedures, must be nondiscriminatory.

A.4.5. Graduation requirements, tuition, and fees must be accurately stated, published, and made known to all applicants. When published fees are subject to change, a statement to that effect must be included.

A.4.6. The program or sponsoring institution must have a defined and published policy and procedure for processing student and faculty grievances.

A.4.7. Policies and procedures for handling complaints against the program must be published and made known. The program must maintain a record of student complaints that includes the nature and disposition of each complaint.

A.4.8. Policies and processes for student withdrawal and for refunds of tuition and fees must be published and made known to all applicants.

A.4.9. Policies and procedures for student probation, suspension, and dismissal must be published and made known.

A.4.10. Policies and procedures must be published and made known for human-subject research protocol.

A.4.11. Written policies and procedures must be made available to students regarding appropriate use of equipment and supplies and for all educational activities that have implications for the health and safety of clients, students, and faculty (including infection control and evacuation procedures).

A.4.12. A program admitting students on the basis of ability to benefit (defined by the U.S. Department of Education as admitting students who do not have either a high school diploma or its equivalent) must publicize its objectives, assessment measures, and means of evaluating the student's ability to benefit.

A.4.13. Documentation of all progression, retention, graduation, certification, and credentialing requirements must be published and made known to applicants. This must include a statement about the potential impact of a felony conviction on a graduate's eligibility for certification and credentialing.

A.4.14. The program must have a documented and published policy to ensure students complete all graduation and fieldwork requirements in a timely manner. This must include a statement that all Level II fieldwork be completed within a time frame established by the program.

A.4.15. Records regarding student admission, enrollment, and achievement must be maintained and kept in a secure setting. Grades and credits for courses must be recorded on students' transcripts and permanently maintained by the sponsoring institution.

A.5.0. Strategic Plan and Program Assessment

A.5.1.   The program must document a current strategic plan that articulates the program's future vision and guides the program development (e.g., faculty recruitment and professional growth, changes in the curriculum design, priorities in academic resources, procurement of fieldwork sites). A program strategic plan must include, but need not be limited to

- Evidence that the plan is based on program evaluation and an analysis of external and internal environments.

- Long-term goals that address the vision and mission of both the institution and program, as well as specific needs of the program.

- Specific measurable action steps with expected timelines by which the program will reach its long-term goals.

- Persons(s) responsible for action steps.

- Evidence of periodic updating of action steps and long-term goals as they are met or as circumstances change.

A.5.2.   The program director and each faculty member who teaches two or more courses must have a current written professional growth and development plan. Each plan must contain the signature of the faculty member and supervisor. At a minimum the plan must include, but need not be limited to

- Goals to enhance the faculty member's ability to fulfill designated responsibilities (e.g., goals related to currency in areas of teaching responsibility, teaching effectiveness, research, scholarly activity).

- Specific measurable action steps with expected timelines by which the faculty member will achieve the goals.

- Evidence of annual updates of action steps and goals as they are met or as circumstances change.

- Identification of the ways in which the faculty member's professional development plan will contribute to attaining the program's strategic goals.

A.5.3.   Programs must routinely secure and document sufficient qualitative and quantitative information to allow for meaningful analysis about the extent to which the program is meeting its stated goals and objectives. This must include, but need not be limited to

- Faculty effectiveness in their assigned teaching responsibilities.

- Students' progression through the program.

- Fieldwork performance evaluation.

- Student evaluation of fieldwork experience.

- Student satisfaction with the program.

- Graduates' performance on the NBCOT certification exam.

- Graduates' job placement and performance based on employer satisfaction.

A.5.4.   The average total pass rate of OT master's program graduates taking the national certification exam for the first time over the 3 most recent calendar years must be 70% or higher.

A.5.5.   Programs must routinely and systematically analyze data to determine the extent to which the program is meeting its stated goals and objectives. An annual report summarizing analysis of data and planned action responses must be maintained.

A.5.6.   The results of ongoing evaluation must be appropriately reflected in the program's strategic plan, curriculum, and other dimensions of the program.

A.6.0. Curriculum Framework

The curriculum framework is a description of the program that includes the program's mission, philosophy, and curriculum design.

A.6.1.   The curriculum must include preparation for practice as a generalist with a broad exposure to current practice settings (e.g., school, hospital, community, long-term care) and emerging practice areas (as defined by the program). The curriculum must prepare students to work with a variety of populations including, but not limited to, children, adolescents, adults, and elderly persons in areas of physical and mental health.

A.6.2.   The program must document a system and rationale for ensuring that the length of study of the program is appropriate to the expected learning and competence of the graduate.

A.6.3.   The statement of philosophy of the occupational therapy program must reflect the current published philosophy of the profession and must include a statement of the program's fundamental beliefs about human beings and how they learn.

A.6.4.   The statement of the mission of the occupational therapy program must be consistent with and supportive of the mission of the sponsoring institution.

A.6.5.   The curriculum design must reflect the mission and philosophy of both the occupational therapy program and the institution and must provide the basis for program planning, implementation, and evaluation. The design must identify educational goals and describe the selection of the content, scope, and sequencing of coursework.

A.6.6.   The program must have clearly documented assessment measures by which students are regularly evaluated on their acquisition of knowledge, skills, attitudes, and competencies required for graduation.

A.6.7.   The program must have written syllabi for each course that include course objectives and learning activities that, in total, reflect all course content required by the Standards. Instructional methods (e.g., presentations, demonstrations, discussion) and materials used to accomplish course objectives must be documented. Programs must also demonstrate the consistency between course syllabi and the curriculum design.

Section B:
Specific Requirements for Accreditation

The specific requirements for accreditation contain the content that a program must include. The content requirements are written as expected student outcomes. Faculty are responsible for developing learning activities and evaluation methods to document that students meet these outcomes.

B.1.0. Foundational Content Requirements

Program content must be based on a broad foundation in the liberal arts and sciences. A strong foundation in the biological, physical, social, and behavioral sciences supports an understanding of occupation across the life span. Coursework in these areas may be prerequisite to or concurrent with professional education and must facilitate development of the performance criteria listed below. The student will be able to

B.1.1.   Demonstrate oral and written communication skills.

B.1.2.   Employ logical thinking, critical analysis, problem solving, and creativity.

B.1.3. Demonstrate competence in basic computer use, including the ability to use databases and search engines to access information, word processing for writing, and presentation software (e.g., PowerPoint™).

B.1.4. Demonstrate knowledge and understanding of the structure and function of the human body to include the biological and physical sciences. Course content must include, but is not limited to, biology, anatomy, physiology, neuroscience, and kinesiology or biomechanics.

B.1.5. Demonstrate knowledge and understanding of human development throughout the life span (infants, children, adolescents, adults, and elderly persons). Course content must include, but is not limited to, developmental psychology.

B.1.6. Demonstrate knowledge and understanding of the concepts of human behavior to include the behavioral and social sciences. Course content must include, but is not limited to, introductory psychology, abnormal psychology, and introductory sociology or introductory anthropology.

B.1.7. Demonstrate knowledge and appreciation of the role of sociocultural, socioeconomic, and diversity factors and lifestyle choices in contemporary society. Course content must include, but is not limited to, introductory psychology, abnormal psychology, and introductory sociology or introductory anthropology.

B.1.8. Articulate the influence of social conditions and the ethical context in which humans choose and engage in occupations.

B.1.9. Demonstrate knowledge of global social issues and prevailing health and welfare needs.

B.1.10. Demonstrate the ability to use statistics to interpret tests and measurements.

B.2.0. Basic Tenets of Occupational Therapy

Coursework must facilitate development of the performance criteria listed below. The student will be able to

B.2.1. Articulate an understanding of the importance of the history and philosophical base of the profession of occupational therapy.

B.2.2. Explain the meaning and dynamics of occupation and activity, including the interaction of areas of occupation, performance skills, performance patterns, activity demands, context(s), and client factors.

B.2.3. Articulate to consumers, potential employers, colleagues, third-party payers, regulatory boards, policymakers, other audiences, and the general public both the unique nature of occupation as viewed by the profession of occupational therapy and the value of occupation to support participation in context(s) for the client.

B.2.4. Articulate the importance of balancing areas of occupation with the achievement of health and wellness.

B.2.5. Explain the role of occupation in the promotion of health and the prevention of disease and disability for the individual, family, and society.

B.2.6. Analyze the effects of physical and mental health, heritable diseases and predisposing genetic conditions, disability, disease processes, and traumatic injury to the individual within the cultural context of family and society on occupational performance.

B.2.7. Exhibit the ability to analyze tasks relative to areas of occupation, performance skills, performance patterns, activity demands, context(s), and client factors to formulate an intervention plan.

B.2.8.   Use sound judgment in regard to safety of self and others, and adhere to safety regulations throughout the occupational therapy process.

B.2.9.   Express support for the quality of life, well-being, and occupation of the individual, group, or population to promote physical and mental health and prevention of injury and disease considering the context (e.g., cultural, physical, social, personal, spiritual, temporal, virtual).

B.2.10. Use clinical reasoning to explain the rationale for and use of compensatory strategies when desired life tasks cannot be performed.

B.2.11. Analyze, synthesize, and apply models of occupational performance and theories of occupation.

B.3.0. Occupational Therapy Theoretical Perspectives

The program must facilitate the development of the performance criteria listed below. The student will be able to

B.3.1.   Describe theories that underlie the practice of occupational therapy.

B.3.2.   Compare and contrast models of practice and frames of reference that are used in occupational therapy.

B.3.3.   Discuss how theories, models of practice, and frames of reference are used in occupational therapy evaluation and intervention.

B.3.4.   Analyze and discuss how history, theory, and the sociopolitical climate influence practice.

B.3.5.   Apply theoretical constructs to evaluation and intervention with various types of clients and practice contexts to analyze and effect meaningful occupation.

B.3.6.   Discuss the process of theory development and its importance to occupational therapy.

B.4.0. Screening, Evaluation, and Referral

The process of screening, evaluation, and referral as related to occupational performance and participation must be culturally relevant and based on theoretical perspectives, models of practice, frames of reference, and available evidence. The program must facilitate development of the performance criteria listed below. The student will be able to

B.4.1.   Use standardized and nonstandardized screening and assessment tools to determine the need for occupational therapy intervention. These include, but are not limited to, specified screening tools; assessments; skilled observations; checklists; histories; consultations with other professionals; and interviews with the client, family, and significant others.

B.4.2.   Select appropriate assessment tools based on client needs, contextual factors, and psychometric properties of tests. These must be relevant to a variety of populations across the life span, culturally relevant, based on available evidence, and incorporate use of occupation in the assessment process.

B.4.3.   Use appropriate procedures and protocols (including standardized formats) when administering assessments.

B.4.4.   Evaluate client(s)' occupational performance in activities of daily living (ADL), instrumental activities of daily living (IADL), education, work, play, leisure, and social participation. Evaluation of occupational performance using standardized and nonstandardized assessment tools includes

- The occupational profile, including participation in activities that are meaningful and necessary for the client to carry out roles in home, work, and community environments.

- Client factors, including body functions (e.g., neuromuscular, sensory, visual, perceptual, cognitive, mental) and body structures (e.g., cardiovascular, digestive, integumentary systems).

- Performance patterns (e.g., habits, routines, roles) and behavior patterns.

- Cultural, physical, social, personal, spiritual, temporal, and virtual contexts and activity demands that affect performance.

- Performance skills, including motor (e.g., posture, mobility, coordination, strength, energy), process (e.g., energy, knowledge, temporal organization, organizing space and objects, adaptation), and communication and interaction skills (e.g., physicality, information exchange, relations).

B.4.5.   Compare and contrast the role of the occupational therapist and occupational therapy assistant in the screening and evaluation process along with the importance of and rationale for supervision and collaborative work between the occupational therapist and occupational therapy assistant in that process.

B.4.6.   Interpret criterion-referenced and norm-referenced standardized test scores based on an understanding of sampling, normative data, standard and criterion scores, reliability, and validity.

B.4.7.   Consider factors that might bias assessment results, such as culture, disability status, and situational variables related to the individual and context.

B.4.8.   Interpret the evaluation data in relation to accepted terminology of the profession and relevant theoretical frameworks.

B.4.9.   Evaluate appropriateness and discuss mechanisms for referring clients for additional evaluation to specialists who are internal and external to the profession.

B.4.10. Document occupational therapy services to ensure accountability of service provision and to meet standards for reimbursement of services, adhering to applicable facility, local, state, federal, and reimbursement agencies. Documentation must effectively communicate the need and rationale for occupational therapy services.

B.5.0. Intervention Plan: Formulation and Implementation

The process of formulation and implementation of the therapeutic intervention plan to facilitate occupational performance and participation must be culturally relevant; reflective of current occupational therapy practice; based on available evidence; and based on theoretical perspectives, models of practice, and frames of reference. The program must facilitate development of the performance criteria listed below. The student will be able to

B.5.1.   Use evaluation findings based on appropriate theoretical approaches, models of practice, and frames of reference to develop occupation-based intervention plans and strategies (including goals and methods to achieve them) based on the stated needs of the client as well as data gathered during the evaluation process in collaboration with the client and others. Intervention plans and strategies must be culturally relevant, reflective of current occupational therapy practice, and based on available evidence. Interventions address the following components:

- The occupational profile, including participation in activities that are meaningful and necessary for the client to carry out roles in home, work, and community environments.

- Client factors, including body functions (e.g., neuromuscular, sensory, visual, perceptual, cognitive, mental) and body structures (e.g., cardiovascular, digestive, integumentary systems).

- Performance patterns (e.g., habits, routines, roles) and behavior patterns.

- Cultural, physical, social, personal, spiritual, temporal, and virtual contexts and activity demands that affect performance.

- Performance skills, including motor (e.g., posture, mobility, coordination, strength, energy), process (e.g., energy, knowledge, temporal organization, organizing space and objects, adaptation), and communication and interaction skills (e.g., physicality, information exchange, relations).

B.5.2. Select and provide direct occupational therapy interventions and procedures to enhance safety, wellness, and performance in activities of daily living (ADL), instrumental activities of daily living (IADL), education, work, play, leisure, and social participation.

B.5.3. Provide therapeutic use of occupation and activities (e.g., occupation-based activity, practice skills, preparatory methods).

B.5.4. Provide training in self-care, self-management, home management, and community and work integration.

B.5.5. Provide development, remediation, and compensation for physical, cognitive, perceptual, sensory (e.g., vision, tactile, auditory, gustatory, olfactory, pain, temperature, pressure, vestibular, proprioception), neuromuscular, and behavioral skills.

B.5.6. Provide therapeutic use of self, including one's personality, insights, perceptions, and judgments as part of the therapeutic process in both individual and group interaction.

B.5.7. Describe the role of the occupational therapist in care coordination, case management, and transition services in traditional and emerging practice environments.

B.5.8. Modify environments (e.g., home, work, school, community) and adapt processes, including the application of ergonomic principles.

B.5.9. Articulate principles of and be able to design, fabricate, apply, fit, and train in assistive technologies and devices (e.g., electronic aids to daily living, seating systems) used to enhance occupational performance.

B.5.10. Provide design, fabrication, application, fitting, and training in orthotic devices used to enhance occupational performance and training in the use of prosthetic devices, based on scientific principles of kinesiology, biomechanics, and physics.

B.5.11. Provide recommendations and training in techniques to enhance mobility, including physical transfers, wheelchair management, and community mobility, and address issues related to driver rehabilitation.

B.5.12. Provide management of feeding and eating to enable performance (including the process of bringing food or fluids from the plate or cup to the mouth, the ability to keep and manipulate food or fluid in the mouth, and the initiation of swallowing) and train others in precautions and techniques while considering client and contextual factors.

B.5.13. Explain the use of superficial thermal and mechanical modalities as a preparatory measure to improve occupational performance, including foundational knowledge, underlying principles, indications, contraindications, and precautions. Demonstrate safe and effective application of superficial thermal and mechanical modalities.

B.5.14. Explain the use of deep thermal and electrotherapeutic modalities as a preparatory measure to improve occupational performance, including indications, contraindications, and precautions.

B.5.15. Develop and promote the use of appropriate home and community programming to support performance in the client's natural environment and participation in all contexts relevant to the client.

B.5.16. Demonstrate the ability to educate the client, caregiver, family, and significant others to facilitate skills in areas of occupation as well as prevention, health maintenance, and safety.

B.5.17. Apply the principles of the teaching–learning process using educational methods to design educational experiences to address the needs of the client, family, significant others, colleagues, other health providers, and the public.

B.5.18. Effectively interact through written, oral, and nonverbal communication with the client, family, significant others, colleagues, other health providers, and the public in a professionally acceptable manner.

B.5.19. Grade and adapt the environment, tools, materials, occupations, and interventions to reflect the changing needs of the client and the sociocultural context.

B.5.20. Select and teach compensatory strategies, such as use of technology, adaptations to the environment, and involvement of humans and nonhumans in the completion of tasks.

B.5.21. Identify and demonstrate techniques in skills of supervision and collaboration with occupational therapy assistants on therapeutic interventions.

B.5.22. Understand when and how to use the consultative process with groups, programs, organizations, or communities.

B.5.23. Refer to specialists (both internal and external to the profession) for consultation and intervention.

B.5.24. Monitor and reassess, in collaboration with the client, caregiver, family, and significant others, the effect of occupational therapy intervention and the need for continued or modified intervention.

B.5.25. Plan for discharge, in collaboration with the client, by reviewing the needs of the client, caregiver, family, and significant others; resources; and discharge environment. This includes, but is not limited to, identification of client's current status within the continuum of care and the identification of community, human, and fiscal resources; recommendations for environmental adaptations; and home programming to facilitate the client's progression along the continuum toward outcome goals.

B.5.26. Organize, collect, and analyze data in a systematic manner for evaluation of practice outcomes. Report evaluation results and modify practice as needed to improve outcomes.

B.5.27. Terminate occupational therapy services when stated outcomes have been achieved or it has been determined that they cannot be achieved. This includes developing a summary of occupational therapy outcomes, appropriate recommendations and referrals, and discussion with the client and with appropriate others of post-discharge needs.

B.5.28. Document occupational therapy services to ensure accountability of service provision and to meet standards for reimbursement of services. Documentation must effectively communicate the need and rationale for occupational therapy services and must be appropriate to the context in which the service is delivered.

B.6.0. *Context of Service Delivery*

Context of service delivery includes the knowledge and understanding of the various contexts in which occupational therapy services are provided. The program must facilitate development of the performance criteria listed below. The student will be able to

B.6.1.   Differentiate among the contexts of health care, education, community, and social systems as they relate to the practice of occupational therapy.

B.6.2.   Discuss the current policy issues and the social, economic, political, geographic, and demographic factors that influence the various contexts for practice of occupational therapy.

B.6.3.   Describe the current social, economic, political, geographic, and demographic factors to promote policy development and the provision of occupational therapy services.

B.6.4.   Articulate the role and responsibility of the practitioner to address changes in service delivery policies to effect changes in the system, and to identify opportunities in emerging practice areas.

B.6.5.   Articulate the trends in models of service delivery and their potential effect on the practice of occupational therapy, including, but not limited to, medical, educational, community, and social models.

B.6.6.   Use national and international resources in making assessment or intervention choices, and appreciate the influence of international occupational therapy contributions to education, research, and practice.

B.7.0. *Management of Occupational Therapy Services*

Management of occupational therapy services includes the application of principles of management and systems in the provision of occupational therapy services to individuals and organizations. The program must facilitate development of the performance criteria listed below. The student will be able to

B.7.1.   Explain how the various practice settings (e.g., medical institutions, community practice, school systems) affect the delivery of occupational therapy services.

B.7.2.   Describe and discuss the impact of contextual factors on the management and delivery of occupational therapy services.

B.7.3.   Describe the systems and structures that create federal and state legislation and regulation and their implications and effects on practice.

B.7.4.   Demonstrate knowledge of applicable national requirements for credentialing and requirements for licensure, certification, or registration under state laws.

B.7.5.   Demonstrate knowledge of various reimbursement systems (e.g., federal, state, third-party, private-payer), appeals mechanisms, and documentation requirements that affect the practice of occupational therapy.

B.7.6.   Describe the mechanisms, systems, and techniques needed to properly maintain, organize, and prioritize workloads and intervention settings, including inventories.

B.7.7.   Demonstrate the ability to plan, develop, organize, and market the delivery of services to include the determination of programmatic needs, service delivery options, and formulation and management of staffing for effective service provision.

B.7.8.   Demonstrate the ability to design ongoing processes for quality improvement (e.g., outcome studies analysis) and develop program changes as needed to ensure quality of services and to direct administrative changes.

B.7.9.   Develop strategies for effective, competency-based legal and ethical supervision of occupational therapy and non–occupational therapy personnel.

B.7.10.   Describe the ongoing professional responsibility for providing fieldwork education and the criteria for becoming a fieldwork educator.

B.8.0. Research

Application of research includes the ability to read and understand current research that affects practice and the provision of occupational therapy services. The program must facilitate development of the performance criteria listed below. The student will be able to

B.8.1.   Articulate the importance of research, scholarly activities, and the continued development of a body of knowledge relevant to the profession of occupational therapy.

B.8.2.   Effectively locate, understand, and evaluate information, including the quality of research evidence.

B.8.3.   Use research literature to make evidence-based decisions.

B.8.4.   Understand and use basic descriptive, correlational, and inferential quantitative statistics and code, analyze, and synthesize qualitative data.

B.8.5.   Understand and critique the validity of research studies, including designs (both quantitative and qualitative) and methodologies.

B.8.6.   Demonstrate the skills necessary to design a research proposal that includes the research question, relevant literature, sample, design, measurement, and data analysis.

B.8.7.   Implement one or more aspects of research methodology. These may be simulated or actual and may include, but are not limited to, designing research instruments, collecting data, and analyzing or synthesizing data. These research activities may be completed individually, with a group, or with a faculty member.

B.8.8.   Demonstrate basic skills necessary to write a research report in a format for presentation or publication.

B.8.9.   Demonstrate an understanding of the process of locating and securing grants and how grants can serve as a fiscal resource for research and practice.

B.9.0. Professional Ethics, Values, and Responsibilities

Professional ethics, values, and responsibilities include an understanding and appreciation of ethics and values of the profession of occupational therapy. The program must facilitate development of the performance criteria listed below. The student will be able to

B.9.1.   Demonstrate a knowledge and understanding of the American Occupational Therapy Association (AOTA) *Occupational Therapy Code of Ethics, Core Values and Attitudes of Occupational Therapy Practice*, and AOTA *Standards of Practice* and use them as a guide for ethical decision making in professional interactions, client interventions, and employment settings.

B.9.2.   Discuss and justify how the role of a professional is enhanced by knowledge of and involvement in international, national, state, and local occupational therapy associations and related professional associations.

B.9.3.   Promote occupational therapy by educating other professionals, service providers, consumers, third-party payers, regulatory bodies, and the public.

B.9.4.   Discuss strategies for ongoing professional development to ensure that practice is consistent with current and accepted standards.

B.9.5.   Discuss professional responsibilities related to liability issues under current models of service provision.

B.9.6.   Discuss and evaluate personal and professional abilities and competencies as they relate to job responsibilities.

B.9.7.   Discuss and justify the varied roles of the occupational therapist as a practitioner, educator, researcher, consultant, and entrepreneur.

B.9.8.   Explain and justify the importance of supervisory roles, responsibilities, and collaborative professional relationships between the occupational therapist and the occupational therapy assistant.

B.9.9.   Describe and discuss professional responsibilities and issues when providing service on a contractual basis.

B.9.10.   Explain strategies for analyzing issues and making decisions to resolve personal and organizational ethical conflicts.

B.9.11.   Explain the variety of informal and formal ethical dispute–resolution systems that have jurisdiction over occupational therapy practice.

B.9.12.   Describe and discuss strategies to assist the consumer in gaining access to occupational therapy services.

B.9.13.   Demonstrate professional advocacy by participating in organizations or agencies promoting the profession (e.g., American Occupational Therapy Association, state occupational therapy associations, advocacy organizations).

B.10.0. *Fieldwork Education*

Fieldwork education is a crucial part of professional preparation and is best integrated as a component of the curriculum design. Fieldwork experiences should be implemented and evaluated for their effectiveness by the educational institution. The experience should provide the student with the opportunity to carry out professional responsibilities under supervision and for professional role modeling. The academic fieldwork coordinator is responsible for the program's compliance with fieldwork education requirements. The academic fieldwork coordinator will

B.10.1.   Document the criteria and process for selecting fieldwork sites. Ensure that the fieldwork program reflects the sequence, depth, focus, and scope of content in the curriculum design.

B.10.2.   Ensure that the academic fieldwork coordinator and faculty collaborate to design fieldwork experiences that strengthen the ties between didactic and fieldwork education.

B.10.3.   Provide fieldwork education in settings that are equipped to meet the curriculum goals, provide educational experiences applicable to the academic program, and have fieldwork educators who are able to effectively meet the learning needs of the students.

B.10.4.   Ensure that the academic fieldwork coordinator is responsible for advocating the development of links between the fieldwork and didactic aspects of the curriculum, for communicating about the curriculum to fieldwork educators, and for maintaining contracts and site data related to fieldwork placements.

B.10.5. Demonstrate that academic and fieldwork educators collaborate in establishing fieldwork objectives, identifying site requirements, and communicating with the student and fieldwork educator about progress and performance during fieldwork.

B.10.6. Document a policy and procedure for complying with fieldwork site health requirements and maintaining student health records in a secure setting.

B.10.7. Ensure that the ratio of fieldwork educators to student(s) enables proper supervision and the ability to provide frequent assessment of student progress in achieving stated fieldwork objectives.

B.10.8. Ensure that fieldwork agreements are sufficient in scope and number to allow completion of graduation requirements in a timely manner in accordance with the policy adopted by the program.

B.10.9. For programs in which the academic and fieldwork components of the curriculum are provided by two or more institutions, responsibilities of each sponsoring institution and fieldwork site must be clearly documented in a memorandum of understanding. For active Level I and Level II fieldwork sites, programs must have current fieldwork agreements or memoranda of understanding that are signed by both parties. (Electronic contracts and signatures are acceptable.)

B.10.10. Documentation must be provided that each memorandum of understanding between institutions and active fieldwork sites is reviewed at least every 5 years by both parties. Programs must provide documentation that both parties have reviewed the contract.

The goal of Level I fieldwork is to introduce students to the fieldwork experience, to apply knowledge to practice, and to develop understanding of the needs of clients. The program will

B.10.11. Ensure that Level I fieldwork is integral to the program's curriculum design and include experiences designed to enrich didactic coursework through directed observation and participation in selected aspects of the occupational therapy process.

B.10.12. Ensure that qualified personnel supervise Level I fieldwork. Examples may include, but are not limited to, currently licensed or credentialed occupational therapists and occupational therapy assistants, psychologists, physician assistants, teachers, social workers, nurses, and physical therapists.

B.10.13. Document all Level I fieldwork experiences that are provided to students, including mechanisms for formal evaluation of student performance. Ensure that Level I fieldwork is not substituted for any part of Level II fieldwork.

The goal of Level II fieldwork is to develop competent, entry-level, generalist occupational therapists. Level II fieldwork must be integral to the program's curriculum design and must include an in-depth experience in delivering occupational therapy services to clients, focusing on the application of purposeful and meaningful occupation and research, administration, and management of occupational therapy services. It is recommended that the student be exposed to a variety of clients across the life span and to a variety of settings. The program will

B.10.14. Ensure that the fieldwork experience is designed to promote clinical reasoning and reflective practice, to transmit the values and beliefs that enable ethical practice, and to develop professionalism and competence in career responsibilities.

B.10.15. Provide Level II fieldwork in traditional and/or emerging settings, consistent with the curriculum design. In all settings, psychosocial factors influencing engagement in occupation must be understood and integrated for the development of client-centered, meaningful, occupation-based outcomes. The student can complete Level II fieldwork in a minimum of one setting if it is reflective of more than one practice area, or in a maximum of four different settings.

B.10.16. Require a minimum of 24 weeks' full-time Level II fieldwork. This may be completed on a part-time basis as defined by the fieldwork placement in accordance with the fieldwork placement's usual and customary personnel policies as long as it is at least 50% of a full-time equivalent at that site.

B.10.17. Ensure that the student is supervised by a currently licensed or credentialed occupational therapist who has a minimum of 1 year of practice experience subsequent to initial certification, and is adequately prepared to serve as a fieldwork educator. The supervising therapist may be engaged by the fieldwork site or by the educational program.

B.10.18. Document a mechanism for evaluating the effectiveness of supervision (e.g., student evaluation of fieldwork) and for providing resources for enhancing supervision (e.g., materials on supervisory skills, continuing education opportunities, articles on theory and practice).

B.10.19. Ensure that supervision provides protection of consumers and opportunities for appropriate role modeling of occupational therapy practice. Initially, supervision should be direct and then decrease to less direct supervision as is appropriate for the setting, the severity of the client's condition, and the ability of the student.

B.10.20. Ensure that supervision provided in a setting where no occupational therapy services exist includes a documented plan for provision of occupational therapy services and supervision by a currently licensed or credentialed occupational therapist with at least 3 years of professional experience. Supervision must include a minimum of 8 hours per week. Supervision must be initially direct and then may be decreased to less direct supervision as is appropriate for the setting, the client's needs, and the ability of the student. An occupational therapy supervisor must be available, via a variety of contact measures, to the student during all working hours. An on-site supervisor designee of another profession must be assigned while the occupational therapy supervisor is off site.

B.10.21. Document mechanisms for requiring formal evaluation of student performance on Level II fieldwork (e.g., the American Occupational Therapy Association *Fieldwork Performance Evaluation for the Occupational Therapy Student* or equivalent).

B.10.22. Ensure that students attending Level II fieldwork outside the United States are supervised by an occupational therapist who graduated from a program approved by the World Federation of Occupational Therapists and has 1 year of experience in practice. Such fieldwork must not exceed 12 weeks.

Accreditation Standards for an Educational Program for the Occupational Therapy Assistant

Adopted August 2006. Effective January 1, 2008.

The Accreditation Council for Occupational Therapy Education (ACOTE®) of the American Occupational Therapy Association (AOTA) accredits educational programs for the occupational therapy assistant. The Standards comply with the United States Department of Education (USDE) criteria for recognition of accrediting agencies.

These Standards are the requirements used in accrediting educational programs that prepare individuals to become occupational therapy assistants. The extent to which a program complies with these Standards determines its accreditation status.

Preamble

The rapidly changing and dynamic nature of contemporary health and human services delivery systems requires the occupational therapy assistant to possess basic skills as a direct care provider, educator, and advocate for the profession and the consumer.

A graduate from an ACOTE-accredited occupational therapy assistant program must

- Have acquired an educational foundation in the liberal arts and sciences, including a focus on issues related to diversity.

- Be educated as a generalist with a broad exposure to the delivery models and systems used in settings where occupational therapy is currently practiced and where it is emerging as a service.

- Have achieved entry-level competence through a combination of academic and fieldwork education.

- Be prepared to articulate and apply occupational therapy principles and intervention tools to achieve expected outcomes as related to occupation.

- Be prepared to be a lifelong learner and keep current with the best practice.

- Uphold the ethical standards, values, and attitudes of the occupational therapy profession.

- Understand the distinct roles and responsibilities of the occupational therapist and occupational therapy assistant in the supervisory process.

- Be prepared to advocate as a professional for the occupational therapy services offered and for the recipients of those services.

Section A:
General Requirements for Accreditation

A.1.0. Sponsorship and Accreditation

A.1.1.   The sponsoring institution(s) and affiliates, if any, must be accredited by recognized national, regional, or state agencies with accrediting authority.

A.1.2.   Sponsoring institutions must be authorized under applicable law or other acceptable authority to provide a program of post-secondary education, have appropriate degree-granting authority, or be a program offered within the military services.

A.1.3.   Accredited occupational therapy assistant educational programs may be established only in community, technical, junior and senior colleges, universities, medical schools, vocational schools or institutions, or military services.

A.1.4.   The sponsoring institution must assume primary responsibility for appointment of faculty, admission of students, and curriculum planning. This would include course content, satisfactory completion of the educational program, and granting of the degree. The sponsoring institution must also be responsible for the coordination of classroom teaching and supervised fieldwork practice and for providing assurance that the practice activities assigned to students in a fieldwork setting are appropriate to the program.

A.1.5.   The sponsoring institution or program must

- Inform ACOTE of the transfer of program sponsorship or change of the institution's name within 30 days of the transfer or change.

- Inform ACOTE within 30 days of the date of notification of any adverse accreditation action taken to change the sponsoring institution's accreditation status to probation or withdrawal of accreditation.

- Submit a Letter of Intent to add or change a program degree level at least 1 year prior to the planned admission of students into that level.

- Inform ACOTE within 30 days of the resignation of the program director or appointment of a new or interim program director.

- Pay accreditation fees within 90 days of the invoice date.

- Submit a Report of Self-Study and other required reports (e.g., Biennial Report, Plan of Correction, Progress Report) within the period of time designated by ACOTE. All reports must be complete and contain all requested information.

- Agree to a site visit date before the end of the period for which accreditation was previously awarded.

- Demonstrate honesty and integrity in all interactions with ACOTE.

A.2.0. Academic Resources

A.2.1.   The program must have a director who is assigned to the occupational therapy educational program on a full-time basis. The director may be assigned other institutional duties that do not interfere with the management and administration of the program. The institution must ensure that the needs of the program are being met.

A.2.2.   The program director must be an initially certified occupational therapist or occupational therapy assistant who is licensed or credentialed according to regulations in the state or jurisdiction in which the program is located. The director must hold academic qualifications comparable to the majority of other program directors within the institutional unit (e.g., division, college, school) to which the program is assigned. By July 1, 2012, the program director must hold a minimum of a master's degree.

A.2.3. The program director must have a minimum of 5 years of experience in the field of occupational therapy, including practice as an occupational therapist or occupational therapy assistant, administrative or supervisory experience, and at least 1 year of experience in a full-time academic appointment with teaching responsibilities.

A.2.4. The program director must have an understanding of and experience with occupational therapy assistants.

A.2.5. The program director must be responsible for the management and administration of the program, including planning, evaluation, budgeting, selection of faculty and staff, maintenance of accreditation, and commitment to strategies for professional development.

A.2.6. In addition to the program director, the program must have at least one full-time equivalent (FTE) faculty position at each accredited location where the program is offered. This position may be shared by several individuals who teach as adjunct faculty and have one or more additional responsibilities related to student advisement, fieldwork administration or supervision, committee work, program planning, evaluation, recruitment, and marketing activities.

A.2.7. The program director and faculty must possess the academic and experiential qualifications and backgrounds (identified in documented descriptions of roles and responsibilities) that are necessary to meet program objectives and the mission of the institution.

A.2.8. The program must document policies and procedures to ensure that the program director and faculty are aware of and abide by the current code of ethics of the profession of occupational therapy.

A.2.9. The program must identify an individual as academic fieldwork coordinator who is specifically responsible for the program's compliance with the fieldwork requirements of Standards Section B.10.0. This individual must be a licensed or credentialed occupational therapist or occupational therapy assistant. Academic fieldwork coordinators who hold a faculty position must meet the requirements of Standard A.2.11.

A.2.10. The faculty must include currently licensed or credentialed occupational therapists and occupational therapy assistants.

A.2.11. By July 1, 2012, all occupational therapy assistant faculty who are either full-time or who comprise the second FTE faculty position must hold a minimum of a baccalaureate degree.

A.2.12. The faculty must have documented expertise in their area(s) of teaching responsibility and knowledge of the content delivery method (e.g., distance learning).

A.2.13. The occupational therapy assistant faculty at each accredited location where the program is offered must be sufficient in number and possess the expertise necessary to ensure appropriate curriculum design, content delivery, and program evaluation.

A.2.14. Faculty responsibilities must be consistent with and supportive of the mission of the institution.

A.2.15. The faculty–student ratio must permit the achievement of the purpose and stated objectives for laboratory and lecture courses, be compatible with accepted practices of the institution for similar programs, and ensure student and consumer safety.

A.2.16. Clerical and support staff must be provided to the program, consistent with institutional practice, to meet programmatic and administrative requirements including support for any portion of the program offered by distance education.

A.2.17. The program must be allocated a budget of regular institutional funds, not including grants, gifts, and other restricted sources, sufficient to implement and maintain the objectives of the program and to fulfill the program's obligation to matriculated and entering students.

A.2.18. Classrooms and laboratories must be provided that are consistent with the program's educational objectives, teaching methods, number of students, and safety and health standards of the institution, and must allow for efficient operation of the program. If any portion of the program is offered by distance education, technology and resources must be adequate to support a distance-learning environment.

A.2.19. Laboratory space provided by the institution must be assigned to the occupational therapy assistant program on a priority basis. If laboratory space is provided by another institution or agency, there must be a written and signed agreement to ensure assignment of space for program use.

A.2.20. Adequate space must be provided to store and secure equipment and supplies.

A.2.21. The program director and faculty must have office space consistent with institutional practice.

A.2.22. Adequate space must be provided for the private advising of students.

A.2.23. Appropriate and sufficient equipment and supplies must be provided by the institution for student use and for the didactic and supervised fieldwork components of the curriculum.

A.2.24. Students must be given access to and have the opportunity to use the evaluative and treatment methodologies that reflect both current practice and practice in the geographic area served by the program.

A.2.25. Students must have ready access to a supply of current and relevant books, journals, periodicals, computers, software, and other reference materials needed to meet the requirements of the curriculum. This may include, but is not limited to, libraries, online services, interlibrary loan, and resource centers.

A.2.26. Instructional aids and technology must be available in sufficient quantity and quality to be consistent with the program objectives and teaching methods.

A.3.0. Students

A.3.1. Admission of students to the occupational therapy assistant program must be made in accordance with the practices of the institution. There must be stated admission criteria that are clearly defined and published and reflective of the demands of the program.

A.3.2. Policies pertaining to standards for admission, advanced placement, transfer of credit, credit for experiential learning (if applicable), and prerequisite educational or work experience requirements must be readily accessible to prospective students and the public.

A.3.3. Programs must document implementation of a mechanism to ensure that students receiving credit for previous courses and/or work experience have met the content requirements of the appropriate OTA Standards.

A.3.4. Criteria for successful completion of each segment of the educational program and for graduation must be given in advance to each student.

A.3.5.   Evaluation content and methods must be consistent with the curriculum design, objectives, and competencies of the didactic and fieldwork components of the program.

A.3.6.   Evaluation must be conducted on a regular basis to provide students and program officials with timely indications of the students' progress and academic standing.

A.3.7.   Students must be informed of and have access to the student support services that are provided to other students in the institution.

A.3.8.   Advising related to coursework in the occupational therapy assistant program and fieldwork education must be the responsibility of the occupational therapy assistant faculty.

A.4.0. Operational Policies

A.4.1.   All program publications and advertising—including, but not limited to, academic calendars, announcements, catalogs, handbooks, and Web sites—must accurately reflect the program offered.

A.4.2.   Accurate and current information regarding student outcomes must be readily available to the public in at least one publication or Web page. The following data must be reported as an aggregate for the 3 most recent calendar years and specify the

- 3-year time period being reported,

- total number of program graduates during that period,

- total number of first-time test takers of the national certification examination during that period,

- total number of first-time test takers who passed the exam during that period, and

- percentage of the total number of first-time test takers who passed the exam during that period.

A.4.3.   The program's accreditation status and the name, address, and telephone number of ACOTE must be published in all of the following used by the institution: catalog, Web site, and program-related brochures or flyers available to prospective students.

A.4.4.   Faculty recruitment and employment practices, as well as student recruitment and admission procedures, must be nondiscriminatory.

A.4.5.   Graduation requirements, tuition, and fees must be accurately stated, published, and made known to all applicants. When published fees are subject to change, a statement to that effect must be included.

A.4.6.   The program or sponsoring institution must have a defined and published policy and procedure for processing student and faculty grievances.

A.4.7.   Policies and procedures for handling complaints against the program must be published and made known. The program must maintain a record of student complaints that includes the nature and disposition of each complaint.

A.4.8.   Policies and processes for student withdrawal and for refunds of tuition and fees must be published and made known to all applicants.

A.4.9.   Policies and procedures for student probation, suspension, and dismissal must be published and made known.

A.4.10. Policies and procedures must be published and made known for human-subject research protocol (if applicable to the program).

A.4.11. Written policies and procedures must be made available to students regarding appropriate use of equipment and supplies and for all educational activities that have implications for the health and safety of clients, students, and faculty (including infection control and evacuation procedures).

A.4.12. A program admitting students on the basis of ability to benefit (defined by U.S. Department of Education as admitting students who do not have either a high school diploma or its equivalent) must publicize its objectives, assessment measures, and means of evaluating the student's ability to benefit.

A.4.13. Documentation of all progression, retention, graduation, certification, and credentialing requirements must be published and made known to applicants. This must include a statement about the potential impact of a felony conviction on a graduate's eligibility for certification and credentialing.

A.4.14. The program must have a documented and published policy to ensure students complete all graduation and fieldwork requirements in a timely manner. This must include a statement that all Level II fieldwork be completed within a time frame established by the program.

A.4.15. Records regarding student admission, enrollment, and achievement must be maintained and kept in a secure setting. Grades and credits for courses must be recorded on students' transcripts and permanently maintained by the sponsoring institution.

A.5.0. Strategic Plan and Program Assessment

A.5.1. The program must document a current strategic plan that articulates the program's future vision and guides the program development (e.g., faculty recruitment and professional growth, changes in the curriculum design, priorities in academic resources, procurement of fieldwork sites). A program strategic plan must include, but need not be limited to

- Evidence that the plan is based on program evaluation and an analysis of external and internal environments.

- Long-term goals that address the vision and mission of both the institution and program, as well as specific needs of the program.

- Specific measurable action steps with expected timelines by which the program will reach its long-term goals.

- Persons(s) responsible for action steps.

- Evidence of periodic updating of action steps and long-term goals as they are met or as circumstances change.

A.5.2. The program director and each faculty member who teach two or more courses must have a current written professional growth and development plan. Each plan must contain the signature of the faculty member and supervisor. At a minimum the plan must include, but need not be limited to

- Goals to enhance the faculty member's ability to fulfill designated responsibilities (e.g., goals related to currency in areas of teaching responsibility, teaching effectiveness, research, scholarly activity).

- Specific measurable action steps with expected timelines by which the faculty member will achieve the goals.

- Evidence of annual updates of action steps and goals as they are met or as circumstances change.

- Identification of the ways in which the faculty member's professional development plan will contribute to attaining the program's strategic goals.

A.5.3.   Programs must routinely secure and document sufficient qualitative and quantitative information to allow for meaningful analysis about the extent to which the program is meeting its stated goals and objectives. This must include, but need not be limited to

- Faculty effectiveness in their assigned teaching responsibilities.

- Students' progression through the program.

- Fieldwork performance evaluation.

- Student evaluation of fieldwork experience.

- Student satisfaction with the program.

- Graduates' performance on the NBCOT certification exam.

- Graduates' job placement and performance based on employer satisfaction.

A.5.4.   The average total pass rate of OTA program graduates taking the national certification exam for the first time over the 3 most recent calendar years must be 70% or higher.

A.5.5.   Programs must routinely and systematically analyze data to determine the extent to which the program is meeting its stated goals and objectives. An annual report summarizing analysis of data and planned action responses must be maintained.

A.5.6.   The results of ongoing evaluation must be appropriately reflected in the program's strategic plan, curriculum, and other dimensions of the program.

A.6.0. Curriculum Framework

The curriculum framework is a description of the program that includes the program's mission, philosophy, and curriculum design.

A.6.1.   The curriculum must include preparation for practice as a generalist with a broad exposure to current practice settings (e.g., school, hospital, community, long-term care) and emerging practice areas (as defined by the program). The curriculum must prepare students to work with a variety of populations including, but not limited to, children, adolescents, adults, and elderly persons in areas of physical and mental health.

A.6.2.   The program must document a system and rationale for ensuring that the length of study of the program is appropriate to the expected learning and competence of the graduate.

A.6.3.   The statement of philosophy of the occupational therapy assistant program must reflect the current published philosophy of the profession and must include a statement of the program's fundamental beliefs about human beings and how they learn.

A.6.4.   The statement of the mission of the occupational therapy assistant program must be consistent with and supportive of the mission of the sponsoring institution.

A.6.5.   The curriculum design must reflect the mission and philosophy of both the occupational therapy assistant program and the institution and must provide the basis for program planning, implementation, and evaluation. The design must identify educational goals and describe the selection of the content, scope, and sequencing of coursework.

A.6.6.   The program must have clearly documented assessment measures by which students are regularly evaluated on their acquisition of knowledge, skills, attitudes, and competencies required for graduation.

A.6.7.   The program must have written syllabi for each course that include course objectives and learning activities that, in total, reflect all course content required by the Standards. Instructional methods (e.g., presentations, demonstrations, discussion) and materials used to accomplish course objectives must be documented. Programs must also demonstrate the consistency between course syllabi and the curriculum design.

Section B:
Specific Requirements for Accreditation

The specific requirements for accreditation contain the content that a program must include. The content requirements are written as expected student outcomes. Faculty are responsible for developing learning activities and evaluation methods to document that students meet these outcomes.

B.1.0. Foundational Content Requirements

Program content must be based on a foundation of the liberal arts and sciences. A foundation in the biological, physical, social, and behavioral sciences supports an understanding of occupation across the life span. Coursework in these areas may be prerequisite to or concurrent with occupational therapy assistant education and must facilitate development of the performance criteria listed below. The student will be able to

B.1.1.   Demonstrate oral and written communication skills.

B.1.2.   Employ logical thinking, critical analysis, problem solving, and creativity.

B.1.3.   Demonstrate competence in basic computer use, including the ability to use databases and search engines to access information, word processing for writing, and presentation software (e.g., PowerPoint™).

B.1.4.   Demonstrate knowledge and understanding of the structure and function of the human body to include the biological and physical sciences. Course content must include, but is not limited to, anatomy, physiology, and biomechanics.

B.1.5.   Demonstrate knowledge and understanding of human development throughout the life span (infants, children, adolescents, adults, and elderly persons). Course content must include, but is not limited to, developmental psychology.

B.1.6.   Demonstrate knowledge and understanding of the concepts of human behavior to include the behavioral and social sciences (e.g., principles of psychology, sociology, abnormal psychology).

B.1.7.   Demonstrate knowledge and appreciation of the role of sociocultural, socioeconomic, and diversity factors and lifestyle choices in contemporary society (e.g., principles of psychology, sociology, and abnormal psychology).

B.1.8.   Articulate the influence of social conditions and the ethical context in which humans choose and engage in occupations.

B.1.9.   Demonstrate knowledge of global social issues and prevailing health and welfare needs.

B.1.10.   Articulate the importance of using statistics, tests, and measurements.

B.2.0. Basic Tenets of Occupational Therapy

Coursework must facilitate development of the performance criteria listed below. The student will be able to

B.2.1. Articulate an understanding of the importance of the history and philosophical base of the profession of occupational therapy.

B.2.2. Describe the meaning and dynamics of occupation and activity, including the interaction of areas of occupation, performance skills, performance patterns, activity demands, context(s), and client factors.

B.2.3. Articulate to consumers, potential employers, colleagues, third-party payers, regulatory boards, policymakers, other audiences, and the general public both the unique nature of occupation as viewed by the profession of occupational therapy and the value of occupation to support participation in context(s) for the client.

B.2.4. Articulate the importance of balancing areas of occupation with the achievement of health and wellness.

B.2.5. Explain the role of occupation in the promotion of health and the prevention of disease and disability for the individual, family, and society.

B.2.6. Understand the effects of physical and mental health, heritable diseases and predisposing genetic conditions, disability, disease processes, and traumatic injury to the individual within the cultural context of family and society on occupational performance.

B.2.7. Exhibit the ability to analyze tasks relative to areas of occupation, performance skills, performance patterns, activity demands, context(s), and client factors to implement the intervention plan.

B.2.8. Use sound judgment in regard to safety of self and others, and adhere to safety regulations throughout the occupational therapy process.

B.2.9. Express support for the quality of life, well-being, and occupation of the individual, group, or population to promote physical and mental health and prevention of injury and disease considering the context (e.g., cultural, physical, social, personal, spiritual, temporal, virtual).

B.2.10. Explain the need for and use of compensatory strategies when desired life tasks cannot be performed.

B.2.11. Apply models of occupational performance and theories of occupation.

B.3.0. Occupational Therapy Theoretical Perspectives

The program must facilitate the development of the performance criteria listed below. The student will be able to

B.3.1. Describe basic features of the theories that underlie the practice of occupational therapy.

B.3.2. Describe models of practice and frames of reference that are used in occupational therapy.

B.3.3. Analyze and discuss how history, theory, and the sociopolitical climate influence practice.

B.4.0. Screening and Evaluation

The process of screening and evaluation as related to occupational performance and participation must be conducted under the supervision of and in cooperation with the occupational therapist and must be culturally relevant and based on theoretical perspectives, models of practice, frames of reference,

and available evidence. The program must facilitate development of the performance criteria listed below. The student will be able to

B.4.1. Gather and share data for the purpose of screening and evaluation including, but not limited to, specified screening tools; assessments; skilled observations; checklists; histories; consultations with other professionals; and interviews with the client, family, and significant others.

B.4.2. Administer selected assessments using appropriate procedures and protocols (including standardized formats) and use occupation for the purpose of assessment.

B.4.3. Gather and share data for the purpose of evaluating client(s)' occupational performance in activities of daily living (ADL), instrumental activities of daily living (IADL), education, work, play, leisure, and social participation. Evaluation of occupational performance includes

* The occupational profile, including participation in activities that are meaningful and necessary for the client to carry out roles in home, work, and community environments.

* Client factors, including body functions (e.g., neuromuscular, sensory, visual, perceptual, cognitive, mental) and body structures (e.g., cardiovascular, digestive, integumentary systems).

* Performance patterns (e.g., habits, routines, roles) and behavior patterns.

* Cultural, physical, social, personal, spiritual, temporal, and virtual contexts and activity demands that affect performance.

* Performance skills, including motor (e.g., posture, mobility, coordination, strength, energy), process (e.g., energy, knowledge, temporal organization, organizing space and objects, adaptation), and communication and interaction skills (e.g., physicality, information exchange, relations).

B.4.4. Articulate the role of the occupational therapy assistant and occupational therapist in the screening and evaluation process along with the importance of and rationale for supervision and collaborative work between the occupational therapy assistant and occupational therapist in that process.

B.4.5. Identify when to recommend to the occupational therapist the need for referring clients for additional evaluation.

B.4.6. Document occupational therapy services to ensure accountability of service provision and to meet standards for reimbursement of services, adhering to applicable facility, local, state, federal, and reimbursement agencies. Documentation must effectively communicate the need and rationale for occupational therapy services.

B.5.0. Intervention and Implementation

The process of intervention to facilitate occupational performance and participation must be done under the supervision of and in cooperation with the occupational therapist and must be culturally relevant, reflective of current occupational therapy practice, and based on available evidence. The program must facilitate development of the performance criteria listed below. The student will be able to

B.5.1. Assist with the development of occupation-based intervention plans and strategies (including goals and methods to achieve them) based on the stated needs of the client as well as data gathered during the evaluation process in collaboration with the client and others. Intervention plans and strategies must be culturally relevant, reflective of current occupational therapy practice, and based on available evidence. Interventions address the following components:

* The occupational profile, including participation in activities that are meaningful and necessary for the client to carry out roles in home, work, and community environments.

- Client factors, including body functions (e.g., neuromuscular, sensory, visual, perceptual, cognitive, mental) and body structures (e.g., cardiovascular, digestive, integumentary systems).

- Performance patterns (e.g., habits, routines, roles) and behavior patterns.

- Cultural, physical, social, personal, spiritual, temporal, and virtual contexts and activity demands that affect performance.

- Performance skills, including motor (e.g., posture, mobility, coordination, strength, energy), process (e.g., energy, knowledge, temporal organization, organizing space and objects, adaptation), and communication and interaction skills (e.g., physicality, information exchange, relations).

B.5.2.   Select and provide direct occupational therapy interventions and procedures to enhance safety, wellness, and performance in activities of daily living (ADL), instrumental activities of daily living (IADL), education, work, play, leisure, and social participation.

B.5.3.   Provide therapeutic use of occupation and activities (e.g., occupation-based activity, practice skills, preparatory methods).

B.5.4.   Provide training in self-care, self-management, home management, and community and work integration.

B.5.5.   Provide development, remediation, and compensation for physical, cognitive, perceptual, sensory (e.g., vision, tactile, auditory, gustatory, olfactory, pain, temperature, pressure, vestibular, proprioception), neuromuscular, and behavioral skills.

B.5.6.   Provide therapeutic use of self, including one's personality, insights, perceptions, and judgments as part of the therapeutic process in both individual and group interaction.

B.5.7.   Describe the role of the occupational therapy assistant in care coordination, case management, and transition services in traditional and emerging practice environments.

B.5.8.   Modify environments (e.g., home, work, school, community) and adapt processes, including the application of ergonomic principles.

B.5.9.   Articulate principles of and demonstrate strategies with assistive technologies and devices (e.g., electronic aids to daily living, seating systems) used to enhance occupational performance.

B.5.10. Provide fabrication, application, fitting, and training in orthotic devices used to enhance occupational performance and training in the use of prosthetic devices.

B.5.11. Provide training in techniques to enhance mobility, including physical transfers, wheelchair management, and community mobility, and participate in addressing issues related to driving.

B.5.12. Enable feeding and eating performance (including the process of bringing food or fluids from the plate or cup to the mouth, the ability to keep and manipulate food or fluid in the mouth, and the initiation of swallowing) and train others in precautions and techniques while considering client and contextual factors.

B.5.13. Recognize the use of superficial thermal and mechanical modalities as a preparatory measure to improve occupational performance. Based on the intervention plan, demonstrate safe and effective administration of superficial thermal and mechanical modalities to achieve established goals while adhering to contraindications and precautions.

B.5.14. Promote the use of appropriate home and community programming to support performance in the client's natural environment and participation in all contexts relevant to the client.

B.5.15. Demonstrate the ability to educate the client, caregiver, family, and significant others to facilitate skills in areas of occupation as well as prevention, health maintenance, and safety.

B.5.16. Use the teaching–learning process with the client, family, significant others, colleagues, other health providers, and the public. Collaborate with the occupational therapist and learner to identify appropriate educational methods.

B.5.17. Effectively interact through written, oral, and nonverbal communication with the client, family, significant others, colleagues, other health providers, and the public in a professionally acceptable manner.

B.5.18. Grade and adapt the environment, tools, materials, occupations, and interventions to reflect the changing needs of the client and the sociocultural context.

B.5.19. Teach compensatory strategies, such as use of technology, adaptations to the environment, and involvement of humans and nonhumans in the completion of tasks.

B.5.20. Demonstrate skills of collaboration with occupational therapists on therapeutic interventions.

B.5.21. Understand when and how to use the consultative process where appropriate with specific consumers or consumer groups as directed by an occupational therapist.

B.5.22. Recognize and communicate the need to refer to specialists (both internal and external to the profession) for consultation and intervention.

B.5.23. Monitor and reassess, in collaboration with the client, caregiver, family, and significant others, the effect of occupational therapy intervention and the need for continued or modified intervention, and communicate the identified needs to the occupational therapist.

B.5.24. Facilitate discharge planning by reviewing the needs of the client, caregiver, family, and significant others; resources; and discharge environment, and identify those needs to the occupational therapist, client, and others involved in discharge planning. This includes, but is not limited to, identification of community, human, and fiscal resources; recommendations for environmental adaptations; and home programming.

B.5.25. Under the direction of an administrator, manager, or occupational therapist, collect, organize, and report on data for evaluation of practice outcomes.

B.5.26. Recommend to the occupational therapist the need for termination of occupational therapy services when stated outcomes have been achieved or it has been determined that they cannot be achieved. Assist with developing a summary of occupational therapy outcomes, recommendations, and referrals.

B.5.27. Document occupational therapy services to ensure accountability of service provision and to meet standards for reimbursement of services. Documentation must effectively communicate the need and rationale for occupational therapy services and must be appropriate to the context in which the service is delivered.

B.6.0. Context of Service Delivery

Context of service delivery includes the knowledge and understanding of the various contexts in which occupational therapy services are provided. The program must facilitate development of the performance criteria listed below. The student will be able to

B.6.1. Describe the contexts of health care, education, community, and social models or systems as they relate to the practice of occupational therapy.

B.6.2. Identify potential impacts of social, economic, political, geographic, or demographic factors on the practice of occupational therapy.

B.6.3. Identify the role and responsibility of the practitioner to address changes in service delivery policies, to effect changes in the system, and to recognize opportunities in emerging practice areas.

B.7.0. Assistance with Management of Occupational Therapy Services

Assistance with management of occupational therapy services includes the application of principles of management and systems in the provision of occupational therapy services to individuals and organizations. The program must facilitate development of the performance criteria listed below. The student will be able to

B.7.1.   Identify how the various practice settings (e.g., medical institutions, community practice, school systems) affect the delivery of occupational therapy services.

B.7.2.   Identify the impact of contextual factors on the management and delivery of occupational therapy services.

B.7.3.   Identify the systems and structures that create federal and state legislation and regulation and their implications and effects on practice.

B.7.4.   Demonstrate knowledge of applicable national requirements for credentialing and requirements for licensure, certification, or registration under state laws.

B.7.5.   Demonstrate knowledge of various reimbursement systems (e.g., federal, state, third-party, private-payer) and documentation requirements that affect the practice of occupational therapy.

B.7.6.   Identify the mechanisms, systems, and techniques needed to properly maintain, organize, and prioritize workloads and intervention settings including inventories.

B.7.7.   Demonstrate the ability to participate in the development, marketing, and management of service delivery options.

B.7.8.   Participate in the documentation of ongoing processes for quality improvement and implement program changes as needed to ensure quality of services.

B.7.9.   Identify strategies for effective, competency-based legal and ethical supervision of non–professional personnel.

B.7.10. Describe the ongoing professional responsibility for providing fieldwork education and the criteria for becoming a fieldwork educator.

B.8.0. Professional Literature

Application of professional literature includes the ability to read and understand professional literature and recognize its implications for practice and the provision of occupational therapy services. The program must facilitate development of the performance criteria listed below. The student will be able to

B.8.1.   Articulate the importance of professional research and literature and the continued development of the profession.

B.8.2.   Use professional literature to make evidence-based practice decisions in collaboration with the occupational therapist that are supported by research.

B.8.3.   Identify the skills necessary to follow a research protocol including accurate and confidential collection of data and related documentation.

B.9.0. Professional Ethics, Values, and Responsibilities

Professional ethics, values, and responsibilities include an understanding and appreciation of ethics and values of the profession of occupational therapy. The program must facilitate development of the performance criteria listed below. The student will be able to

B.9.1.   Demonstrate a knowledge and understanding of the American Occupational Therapy Association (AOTA) *Occupational Therapy Code of Ethics, Core Values and Attitudes of Occupational Therapy Practice,* and AOTA *Standards of Practice* and use them as a guide for ethical decision making in professional interactions, client interventions, and employment settings.

B.9.2.   Explain and give examples of how the role of a professional is enhanced by knowledge of and involvement in international, national, state, and local occupational therapy associations and related professional associations.

B.9.3.   Promote occupational therapy by educating other professionals, service providers, consumers, and the public.

B.9.4.   Discuss strategies for ongoing professional development to ensure that practice is consistent with current and accepted standards.

B.9.5.   Identify professional responsibilities related to liability issues under current models of service provision.

B.9.6.   Identify personal and professional abilities and competencies as they relate to job responsibilities.

B.9.7.   Identify and appreciate the varied roles of the occupational therapy assistant as a practitioner, educator, and research assistant.

B.9.8.   Identify and explain the need for supervisory roles, responsibilities, and collaborative professional relationships between the occupational therapist and the occupational therapy assistant.

B.9.9.   Identify professional responsibilities and issues when providing service on a contractual basis.

B.9.10. Identify strategies for analyzing issues and making decisions to resolve personal and organizational ethical conflicts.

B.9.11. Identify the variety of informal and formal ethical dispute–resolution systems that have jurisdiction over occupational therapy practice.

B.9.12. Identify strategies to assist the consumer in gaining access to occupational therapy services.

B.9.13. Demonstrate professional advocacy by participating in organizations or agencies promoting the profession (e.g., American Occupational Therapy Association, state occupational therapy associations, advocacy organizations).

B.10.0. Fieldwork Education

Fieldwork education is a crucial part of the preparation of the occupational therapy assistant and is best integrated as a component of the curriculum design. Fieldwork experiences should be implemented and evaluated for their effectiveness by the educational institution. The experience should provide the student with the opportunity to carry out professional responsibilities under supervision and for role modeling. The academic fieldwork coordinator is responsible for the program's compliance with fieldwork education requirements. The academic fieldwork coordinator will

B.10.1. Document the criteria and process for selecting fieldwork sites. Ensure that the fieldwork program reflects the sequence, depth, focus, and scope of content in the curriculum design.

B.10.2. Ensure that the academic fieldwork coordinator and faculty collaborate to design fieldwork experiences that strengthen the ties between didactic and fieldwork education.

B.10.3. Provide fieldwork education in settings that are equipped to meet the curriculum goals, provide educational experiences applicable to the academic program, and have fieldwork educators who are able to effectively meet the learning needs of the students.

B.10.4.   Ensure that the academic fieldwork coordinator is responsible for advocating the development of links between the fieldwork and didactic aspects of the curriculum, for communicating about the curriculum to fieldwork educators, and for maintaining contracts and site data related to fieldwork placements.

B.10.5.   Demonstrate that academic and fieldwork educators collaborate in establishing fieldwork objectives, identifying site requirements, and communicating with the student and fieldwork educator about progress and performance during fieldwork.

B.10.6.   Document a policy and procedure for complying with fieldwork site health requirements and maintaining student health records in a secure setting.

B.10.7.   Ensure that the ratio of fieldwork educators to student(s) enables proper supervision and the ability to provide frequent assessment of student progress in achieving stated fieldwork objectives.

B.10.8.   Ensure that fieldwork agreements are sufficient in scope and number to allow completion of graduation requirements in a timely manner in accordance with the policy adopted by the program.

B.10.9.   For programs in which the academic and fieldwork components of the curriculum are provided by two or more institutions, responsibilities of each sponsoring institution and fieldwork site must be clearly documented in a memorandum of understanding. For active Level I and Level II fieldwork sites, programs must have current fieldwork agreements or memoranda of understanding that are signed by both parties. (Electronic contracts and signatures are acceptable.)

B.10.10. Documentation must be provided that each memorandum of understanding between institutions and active fieldwork sites is reviewed at least every 5 years by both parties. Programs must provide documentation that both parties have reviewed the contract.

The goal of Level I fieldwork is to introduce students to the fieldwork experience, to apply knowledge to practice, and to develop understanding of the needs of clients. The program will

B.10.11. Ensure that Level I fieldwork is integral to the program's curriculum design and include experiences designed to enrich didactic coursework through directed observation and participation in selected aspects of the occupational therapy process.

B.10.12. Ensure that qualified personnel supervise Level I fieldwork. Examples may include, but are not limited to, currently licensed or credentialed occupational therapists and occupational therapy assistants, psychologists, physician assistants, teachers, social workers, nurses, and physical therapists.

B.10.13. Document all Level I fieldwork experiences that are provided to students, including mechanisms for formal evaluation of student performance. Ensure that Level I fieldwork is not substituted for any part of Level II fieldwork.

The goal of Level II fieldwork is to develop competent, entry-level, generalist occupational therapy assistants. Level II fieldwork must be integral to the program's curriculum design and must include an in-depth experience in delivering occupational therapy services to clients, focusing on the application of purposeful and meaningful occupation. It is recommended that the student be exposed to a variety of clients across the life span and to a variety of settings. The program will:

B.10.14. Ensure that the fieldwork experience is designed to promote clinical reasoning appropriate to the occupational therapy assistant role, to transmit the values and beliefs that enable ethical practice, and to develop professionalism and competence in career responsibilities.

B.10.15. Provide Level II fieldwork in traditional and/or emerging settings, consistent with the curriculum design. In all settings, psychosocial factors influencing engagement in occupation must be understood and integrated for the development of client-centered, meaningful, occupation-based outcomes. The student can complete Level II fieldwork in a minimum of one setting if it is reflective of more than one practice area, or in a maximum of three different settings.

B.10.16. Require a minimum of 16 weeks' full-time Level II fieldwork. This may be completed on a part-time basis as defined by the fieldwork placement in accordance with the fieldwork placement's usual and customary personnel policies as long as it is at least 50% of a full-time equivalent at that site.

B.10.17. Ensure that the student is supervised by a currently licensed or credentialed occupational therapist or occupational therapy assistant who has a minimum of 1 year of practice experience subsequent to initial certification, and is adequately prepared to serve as a fieldwork educator. The supervising therapist may be engaged by the fieldwork site or by the educational program.

B.10.18. Document a mechanism for evaluating the effectiveness of supervision (e.g., student evaluation of fieldwork) and for providing resources for enhancing supervision (e.g., materials on supervisory skills, continuing education opportunities, articles on theory and practice).

B.10.19. Ensure that supervision provides protection of consumers and opportunities for appropriate role modeling of occupational therapy practice. Initially, supervision should be direct and then decrease to less direct supervision as is appropriate for the setting, the severity of the client's condition, and the ability of the student.

B.10.20. Ensure that supervision provided in a setting where no occupational therapy services exist includes a documented plan for provision of occupational therapy assistant services and supervision by a currently licensed or credentialed occupational therapist or an occupational therapy assistant (under the direction of an occupational therapist) with at least 3 years of professional experience. Supervision must include a minimum of 8 hours per week. Supervision must be initially direct and then may be decreased to less direct supervision as is appropriate for the setting, the client's needs, and the ability of the student. An occupational therapy supervisor must be available, via a variety of contact measures, to the student during all working hours. An on-site supervisor designee of another profession must be assigned while the occupational therapy supervisor is off site.

B.10.21. Document mechanisms for requiring formal evaluation of student performance on Level II fieldwork (e.g., the American Occupational Therapy Association *Fieldwork Performance Evaluation for the Occupational Therapy Assistant Student* or equivalent).

B.10.22. Ensure that students attending Level II fieldwork outside the United States are supervised by an occupational therapist who graduated from a program approved by the World Federation of Occupational Therapists and has 1 year of experience in practice. Such fieldwork must not exceed 8 weeks.

Concept Papers

A Descriptive Review of Occupational Therapy Education

Introduction

In an August 2002 Commission on Education (COE) meeting, COE members decided to design and write a *Guide to Occupational Therapy Education*. With the advent and passing of Resolution J—which became Resolution 670-99 at the 1999 Representative Assembly meeting of the American Occupational Therapy Association (Accreditation Council for Occupational Therapy Education [ACOTE], 1999b)—and new degree structures within the profession (i.e., professional/clinical doctorate), a guide to occupational therapy education is warranted. This guide, retitled *A Descriptive Review of Occupational Therapy Education*, is intended for practitioners, academicians, and potential occupational therapy program applicants to augment their understanding of occupational therapy education.

Organization of Review

The review is organized into eight sections. The first, the introductory section, describes the process of the development of the Descriptive Review. The second section distinguishes between professional and graduate education. This information provides the background and foundational groundwork for the Review. The next section includes the underpinning information that describes the levels of education in the United States as used by most colleges and universities. It is the common language used in all degree majors and programs and should be the guide for occupational therapy education language so that degrees in occupational therapy can be recognized and understood by fields other than occupational therapy.

The fourth section delineates the levels of education in occupational therapy in the United States from the technical level of education to the doctoral level, using the previous foundational information as the basis of the descriptions. The Review then lists suggested factors that should be considered when choosing an occupational therapy program.

The Review was written to describe the present state of occupational therapy education within the American educational system and is limited to this perspective only. It is purposefully written in a factual format and does not intend to promote one occupational therapy degree over any other, nor is it intended to resolve the multiple issues regarding the various degree levels or entry-level competencies. Those issues need to be addressed by a broad-based consensus group or other professional bodies.

Professional and Graduate Education

The terms *professional education* and *graduate education* are often used synonymously. Educational institutions have the prerogative to house degree programs in any appropriate organizational structure. For example, some master's-degree programs award the degree under the auspices of the graduate school, whereas others offer the degree from a professional school. However, a distinction between *graduate* and *professional* education is needed to understand the nature of the organizational context of occupational therapy educational programs within colleges and universities. Although there is a paucity of literature distinguishing the two types of education, Mayhew and Ford's (1974) *Reform in Graduate and Professional Education* was a welcomed resource to higher educational planners. Mayhew and Ford eloquently articulated the purposes and problems of both graduate and professional education.

Professional Education

Professional education is a term used to describe educational programs in which students are enrolled to study service delivery of a particular profession (e.g., dentistry, medicine, nursing, pharmacy, veterinary science). Studying a profession is different from studying a discipline (e.g., physics, theology, mathematics, biology, sociology) (Mayhew & Ford, 1971). A discipline has its own "unique epistemology" that serves as its foundation for autonomy (Knowles, 1977, p. 2209). Professional programs are highly influenced by the professions they serve. The professional standards are at a minimally acceptable level, and governance from the institution often requires higher and different standards (e.g., requirement of thesis, capstone project, electives, additional coursework, interdisciplinary classes).

The purpose of professional education is to admit and educate a sufficient number of students who meet minimum theoretical knowledge and practice skill competencies to practice a profession (Mayhew & Ford, 1974). "Professional education should be directed toward significant objectives, including professional competence, understanding of society, ethical behavior, and scholarly concern" (Mayhew & Ford, 1974, p. 3).

Graduate Education

Graduate education comprises the master's (e.g., MA, MS) degree and doctor of philosophy (PhD) degree (Carmichael, 1961). The graduate school is the organizational authority within colleges and universities that houses graduate educational programs. Traditionally, graduate education focused on advanced study and scholarship within a discipline; however, more recently, some graduate programs in professional fields have emerged (e.g., master's degree in nursing, PhD in rehabilitation).

Historically, graduate education was intended for four purposes (Mayhew & Ford, 1974). The first purpose of graduate education was character formation—to produce broadly learned graduates. The second purpose, preparation of college teachers, was traditionally the primary purpose of PhD programs. The paradox of this intent was that traditional PhD graduate education focused primarily on producing independent researchers and rarely addressed preparation for college teaching. A third purpose of graduate education was "to prepare people for research and scholarship in a specialized field" (Mayhew & Ford, 1974, p. 94). The fourth purpose of graduate education was to have graduates enter the work force and apply their research competencies in professional fields.

Levels of Education in the United States

One of the hallmarks of higher education in the United States is the diversity of institutions, degrees, and programs available. Levels of education are represented by the academic degree conferred to graduates. A degree is a credential or title "conferred by a college or university as official recognition for the completion of a program of studies" (Shafritz, Koeppe, & Soper, 1988, p. 145). Academic degree levels include associate, baccalaureate, master's, and doctoral.

Associate Degree

According to the National Center for Education Statistics, an *associate degree* is "an award that requires the completion of at least 2 but less than 4 full-time equivalent academic years of college-level work in an academic or occupationally specified field of study, and which meets institutional standards for otherwise satisfying the requirements for this degree level" (U.S. Department of Education [USDE], 2002, p. A-63).

Baccalaureate

A *baccalaureate degree* is an award requiring completion of 4 to 5 full-time equivalent academic years of college-level work in an academic or occupationally specific field of study, and which satisfies institutional standards of the requirement of the degree level (USDE, 2002, p. A-63). Two common baccalaureate degrees are the bachelor of arts (BA or AB, for the Latin *atrium baccalareus*) for programs in the humanities and the bachelor of science (BS) for programs in the sciences. Some institutions offer baccalaureate degrees in specialized areas, for example, bachelor of music (BMus) or bachelor of education (BEd) (Unger, 1996).

Master's

A *master's degree* typically requires approximately 36 credits of postbaccalaureate education in a subject field. Three master's degrees are commonly awarded. One type includes both the master of arts (MA) and the master of science (MS). MA and MS degrees are "awarded in liberal arts and sciences for advanced scholarship in a subject field or discipline and demonstrated ability to perform scholarly research" (USDE, 2002, p. 298). A second type of master's degree is conferred for completion of a professional entry-level program; for example, an MEd in education, an MBA in business administration, or an MFA in fine arts. In occupational therapy, the MOT, or master of occupational therapy, degree is awarded by some institutions. The third type of master's degree includes the award in professional fields for study beyond the first-professional (entry-level) degree, such as the master of laws (LLM) and the master of science (MS) in various medical professions. Occupational therapy has typically referred to this level of degree as a post-professional master's degree.

Various classifications of master's degrees exist, including *academic, professional,* and *experiential* (Glazer, 1988). Curricular requirements for master's degrees vary from institution to institution and from state to state. The diversity in master's degree curricula makes comparison of degree programs, fields, and credentials difficult (Glazer, 1988). For example, some master's-degree programs require a thesis, whereas others do not. The master's degree must be approached "as a class of degrees rather than as a generic model, and as a credential sought increasingly for its own merits rather than in relation to the bachelor's or doctoral degree" (Glazer, 1988, p. 1).

Historically, the purpose of a master's degree was to produce graduates with beginning research or inquiry skills. Not all professions offer a degree at the doctoral level, and thus the master's degree may be the *terminal degree* (highest degree conferred) for some professions.

During the 1980s, master's-degree programs were challenged by more convenient educational alternatives that were shorter in duration and less expensive (e.g., certificate programs). Such certificate alternatives typically did not result in the conferral of a graduate degree. To compete with certificate programs, some master's-degree programs were oriented toward practice rather than research. Currently, approximately 85% of all master's-degree programs in the United States are considered to be practice-oriented or professional degrees (LaPidus, 2000). These programs are specialized in their focus, applied in terms of their content, and decentralized in that they are frequently not housed under the auspices of a graduate school (LaPidus, 2000).

Doctorate: Professional and Research

A *doctoral degree* is the highest degree conferred by an institution of higher education. Most doctoral degrees require the equivalent of 3 years of full-time postbaccalaureate study (Kapel, Gifford, & Kapel, 1991). Commonly, universities require a minimum of 72 hours of postbaccalaureate study plus a residence requirement. "Doctorate entitles bearers to be addressed as 'Doctor' and to append their names with the appropriate letters of their degrees—that is, PhD (doctor of philosophy) or MD (doctor of medicine)" (Unger, 1996, p. 305). There are two types of doctoral degrees: the *research doctorate* and the *professional doctorate* (Shafritz et al., 1988; Unger, 1996). The professional doctorate is also referred to as a *clinical doctorate* in many health professions (Pierce & Peyton, 1999).

The *research doctorate* (also called the *academic doctorate*), or PhD, was originally awarded for the study of philosophy in the mid- to late 19th century. However, the degree was extended to include many disciplines of the humanities and sciences, with each PhD simply modified to indicate the field of study; for example, PhD in engineering, PhD in history, or PhD in chemistry. The purpose of the PhD degree is to develop graduates who are independent researchers and are knowledgeable in a specific area of study. Requirements for the PhD degree usually include a course of didactic study, followed by written or oral comprehensive examinations (upon passing, one applies for candidacy), and the completion of a dissertation in some area of new knowledge as deemed appropriate by a committee of senior faculty after an oral defense of the research (Shafritz et al., 1988).

The *doctor of science* (ScD) is an alternative doctoral degree similar to the PhD. Its curriculum is focused on the study of an applied science, such as audiology, occupational therapy, and so forth. ScD degree programs commonly include didactic coursework focused on the study of an applied science, an advanced clinical practicum, and a supervised clinical research project (Kidd, Cox, & Matthies, 2003). Other alternative doctoral degrees include the doctor of education (EdD) and the doctor of public health (DPH).

The professional doctorate reflects academic attainment and seldom requires a master's degree or dissertation (Unger, 1996). Unlike the PhD's focus on developing independent researchers, "sophisticated practice competencies" (Pierce & Peyton, 1999, p. 64) are emphasized in the professional doctorate degree. A person with a professional doctorate, such as an MD or doctor of jurisprudence (JD), must pass state or national qualifying examinations to obtain a license to practice (Unger, 1996). In the health sciences, the term *clinical doctorate* is synonymous with the term *professional doctorate* and the program of study typically requires "mentored advanced clinical experiences for autonomous practice competencies" (Edens & Labadie, 1987; Faut-Callahan, 1992; Hummer, Hunt, & Figuers, 1994; Pierce & Peyton, 1999; Watson, 1988).

Postdoctoral Education

With the growing complexity of knowledge and the need for scholars trained to high, creative levels, postdoctoral education has become increasingly popular to meet work demands in universities, industries, and government (Carmichael, 1961). However, postdoctoral education is widely misunderstood because there is little uniformity.

The adjective *postdoctoral* is frequently used to describe the variety of postdoctoral educational experiences. For example, terms such as *postdoctoral fellow, postdoctoral research associate,* and *postdoctoral trainee* are typically used. Despite the lack of uniformity among terms, postdoctoral is used to denote a *research* appointment after a doctoral degree has been awarded within a discipline or profession (Knowles, 1977).

Residencies

Although residencies are not common practice in occupational therapy, they are a form of postdoctoral education. "The purpose of postprofessional residency education is to advance the resident's preparation as a provider of patient care services in a defined (specialized) area of clinical practice" (DiFabio, 1999, p. 81). Residency training activities are designed to promote the integration of practice, research, and scholarly inquiry (Medeiros, 1998). Professions such as medicine, pharmacy (American Society of Health-System Pharmacists, 2001; Miller & Clarke, 2002), and physical therapy (DiFabio, 1999; Farrell, 1996; Medeiros, 2000) offer postdoctoral specialty residencies to qualified practitioners.

Levels of Education in Occupational Therapy Within the United States

Technical Level

OTA

Occupational therapy assistant (OTA) programs are classified as technical and obtain accreditation from the Accreditation Council for Occupational Therapy Education (ACOTE®). OTA programs are commonly offered at community colleges, private junior colleges, and some 4-year colleges and universities. All OTA programs must adhere to the *Standards for an Accredited Educational Program for the Occupational Therapy Assistant.* As articulated in the Preamble of the Standards, an entry-level OTA must

- Have acquired an educational foundation in the liberal arts and sciences, including a focus on issues related to diversity;

- Be educated as a generalist, with a broad exposure to the delivery models and systems utilized in settings where occupational therapy is currently practiced and where it is emerging as a service;

- Have achieved entry-level competence through a combination of academic andfieldwork education;

- Be prepared to work under the supervision of and in cooperation with the occupational therapist;

- Be prepared to articulate and apply occupational therapy principles, intervention approaches and rationales, and expected outcomes as these relate to occupation;

- Be prepared to be a lifelong learner and keep current with best practice;

- Uphold the ethical standards, values, and attitudes of the occupational therapy profession (ACOTE, 1999b, p. 583).

After completing the OTA didactic and fieldwork requirements, the OTA graduate is eligible to sit for the national certification examination for OTAs. On successful completion, the certified occupational therapy assistant (COTA) may apply for the appropriate state credential and, under specified supervision, render occupational therapy services at the technical level of practice.

Professional Level

Master's: Entry-Level and Postprofessional

As of January 2007, the master's degree is the lowest degree level at which one can enter the profession as an occupational therapist. In occupational therapy education, there are entry-level (or sometimes referred to as the *first professional degree*) and postprofessional master's-degree programs. Distinguishing between entry-level and postprofessional master's-degree programs is not typical in other professions and disciplines (Rogers, 1980a, 1980b). Entry-level master's-degree programs are the entrance into the profession of occupational therapy and are accredited by ACOTE. Some entry-level programs may require students to earn a baccalaureate degree in a related field before entering the master's-degree program in occupational therapy. Other entry-level programs may require extensive prerequisite coursework but not mandate a baccalaureate degree. For example, the course of study may be a 5-year program leading to a master's degree; or, in other programs, the study comprises two semesters beyond an undergraduate degree in a major such as occupational science. Coursework that may be considered remedial or prerequisite is not generally included in the total credits required for the master's degree. On successful completion of the academic and fieldwork requirements, the graduate is eligible to take the national certification examination, then apply for state licensure and provide occupational therapy services at the professional level.

Postprofessional master's-degree programs are available to individuals who have a professional degree in occupational therapy (e.g., baccalaureate, entry-level master's, or an entry-level doctorate degree). Such postprofessional degrees are typical of master's-degree programs in other disciplines with a range of 30 to 36 credits. Postprofessional programs are developed to enhance occupational therapy skills in a specific area (e.g., pediatrics, assistive technology, gerontology). Other master's-degree programs may provide a general program with a curricular emphasis (e.g., leadership or research).

Doctorate: Professional and Research

Currently, doctoral-level occupational therapy offerings include the professional (or clinical) and research doctorates. Some programs offer the PhD degree in occupational therapy. Other doctoral-degree programs related to occupational therapy exist, such as the PhD degree in rehabilitation sciences or occupational science or the ScD. Although many of these programs focus on the application of occupational therapy, it is beyond the scope of this document to describe the variations of doctoral programs closely aligned with occupational therapy.

The professional or clinical doctorate degree in occupational therapy confers the degree of *doctor of occupational therapy* (OTD) or *doctor of occupational therapy* (DrOT) degree to graduates. Two pathways exist for pursuing the clinical doctorate degree. The first is available to postprofessional students, that is, students who have an entry-level degree in occupational therapy. The second pathway leading to the clinical doctorate degree is an entry-level program. Entry-level clinical doctorate degree programs are available for individuals who do not have an entry-level degree in occupational therapy but who have completed specified prerequisite coursework and, as of 2010, a baccalaureate degree.

Although the clinical-doctorate-degree programs vary in philosophy and curriculum, typically the post-professional clinical-doctorate programs are shorter in duration than the entry-level clinical-doctorate programs. The rationale for the difference in program length is that postprofessional clinical-doctorate students have previously completed an entry-level occupational therapy degree.

Several occupational therapy programs offer the PhD degree in occupational therapy. These doctoral programs focus on preparing graduates who are independent researchers and who will develop original knowledge pertinent to occupational therapy.

Accreditation

There are two types of accreditation: institutional (or regional) accreditation and program (or specialized) accreditation (Kaplin & Lee, 1995). Accreditation of occupational therapy programs is completed by ACOTE, which is part of a larger accreditation context (Kramer & Graves, 2005).

Institutional Accreditation

Regional or national accrediting bodies do not accredit programs but rather accredit institutions. "Institutional accreditation applies to the entire institution and all its programs, departments, and schools" (Kaplin & Lee, 1995, p. 873). There are 6 regional agencies that accredit institutions located in distinct geographical areas. Accreditation standards from regional or national accrediting bodies influence ACOTE in that their standards must be aligned with requirements from the USDE and the Council for Higher Education Accreditation (CHEA) (Kramer & Graves, 2005). In postprofessional OT programs, there is no specialized accrediting body. However, institutional accrediting bodies can require a focus visit of a particular program. A focus visit does not result in the accrediting of a specific program.

Program or Specialized Accreditation

Program or specialized accreditation "applies to a particular school, department or program within the institution" and "may also apply to an entire institution if it is a free-standing, specialized institution … whose curriculum is all in the same program area" (Kaplin & Lee, 1995, p. 873). The USDE and the CHEA afford ACOTE "the distinction of being reflected as a national recognized accrediting agency that is seen as a reliable authority about the quality of education offered by the occupational therapy and occupational therapy assistant programs it accredits" (Kramer & Graves, 2005, p. 1). Currently, ACOTE accredits OTA and entry-level or first professional-degree programs in occupational therapy. Such accreditation endeavors are considered specialized, because the accrediting body, ACOTE, reviews OT and OTA programs to ensure quality and that educational standards are met. The educational standards are developed through ACOTE with input from stakeholders.

Suggested Considerations When Choosing an Occupational Therapy Educational Program

When choosing an occupational therapy educational program, important factors must be considered (see Table 1).

A variety of resources can help one to obtain information about specific education programs. Institutional Web sites can be helpful in acquiring information about the program's curriculum and faculty. Brochures, catalogs, and bulletin descriptions often present the program's mission, philosophy, curriculum, or policies. These materials can be requested from the admissions office of each institution. Contacting faculty within the program is frequently useful to answer specific questions. Prospective students may request contact with a current student or alumni to gain a consumer's perspective of the program.

Table 1. Considerations for Occupational Therapy Entry-Level and Postprofessional Education

- Location of program
- Tuition
- Length of program
- Availability of student scholarships
- Full- or part-time programs
- On-campus or distance-formatted programs
- Admission requirements
  - Interview
  - Entrance exams (e.g., Miller's Analogy, Graduate Record Exam)
  - Letters of recommendation, essays
  - Prerequisite classes or degree
  - Observation hours in occupational therapy
- Type of program
  - Degree awarded (e.g., AA, MS, MA, MOT, PhD, ScD, OTD)
  - Thesis requirement
  - Dissertation requirement
  - Curriculum (e.g., courses offered, course descriptions printed in catalog)
  - Program mission and philosophical grounding
  - Specialization (e.g., gerontology, pediatrics, entrepreneurialism)
  - Experiential components
    - Fieldwork, internships, rotations, etc.
    - Length of clinical preparation
    - Opportunities for postdegree experiences (e.g., residencies/fellowships)
- Institutional variables
  - Carnegie classification
  - Library resources
  - Information technology/computer support
  - Stability of program
  - Graduate or professional school
  - Ratings and rankings of programs
- Graduate/alumni accomplishments
  - Graduation rate
  - Employment rates, sites
  - Employer satisfaction with graduates
  - Consumer satisfaction with graduate performance
- Faculty
  - Faculty credentials (e.g., doctorally prepared, specialty certified)
  - Faculty-to-student ratios
  - Faculty accessibility
  - Faculty projects (e.g., grants, publications)
  - Faculty clinical practice

In addition, it is important to answer the following questions:
- What are my future career goals?
- Does the degree offered contribute to accomplishing my short-term and long-term goals?
- If considering an online program, do I have the necessary skills to be successful (e.g., motivation, self-initiative, technical skills)?

References and Resources

Accreditation Council for Occupational Therapy Education. (1999a, August). *ACOTE Motion* and *Resolution J* [Minutes at the meeting of the Accreditation Council for Occupational Therapy Education]. Bethesda, MD: Author.

Accreditation Council for Occupational Therapy Education. (1999b). Standards for an accredited educational program for the occupational therapy assistant. *American Journal of Occupational Therapy, 53,* 583–589.

American Occupational Therapy Association. (2001). *ACOTE sets timeline for post baccalaureate degree programs.* Retrieved June 19, 2001, from http://www.aota.org/nonmembers/area13/links/LINK16.asp

American Society of Health-System Pharmacists. (2001). *The residency learning system (RLS) model* (2nd ed.). Bethesda, MD: Author.

Carmichael, O. C. (1961). *Graduate education: A critique and a program.* New York: Harper & Brothers.

DiFabio, R. P. (1999). Clinical expertise and the DPT: A need for residency training. *Journal of Orthopaedic and Sports Physical Therapy, 29,* 80–82.

Edens, G. E., & Labadie, G. C. (1987). Opinions about the professional doctorate in nursing. *Nursing Outlook, 35,* 136–140.

Farrell, J. P. (1996). In search of clinical excellence. *Journal of Orthopaedic and Sports Physical Therapy, 24,* 115–121.

Faut-Callahan, M. (1992). Graduate education for nurse anesthetists: Master's versus a clinical doctorate. *Journal of the American Association of Nurse Anesthetists, 60,* 98–103.

Glazer, J. S. (1988). *The master's degree* (Report No. EDO-HE-88-3). Washington, DC: Office of Educational Research and Improvement. (ERIC Document Reproduction Service No. ED301140)

Hummer, L. A., Hunt, K. S., & Figuers, C. C. (1994). Predominant thought regarding entry-level doctor of physical therapy programs. *Journal of Physical Therapy Education, 8,* 60–66.

Kapel, D. E., Gifford, C. S., & Kapel, M. B. (1991). *American educators' encyclopedia* (rev. ed.). Westport, CT: Greenwood.

Kaplin, W. A., & Lee, B. A. (1995). *The law of higher education* (3rd ed.). San Francisco: Jossey-Bass.

Kidd, G. D., Cox, C. C., & Matthies, M. L. (2003). Boston University doctor of science degree program: Clinical doctorate in audiology. *American Journal of Audiology, 12,* 3–6.

Knowles, A. S. (1977). Postdoctoral education. In *The international encyclopedia of higher education* (Vol. 5, pp. 1923–1928). San Francisco: Jossey-Bass.

Kramer, P., & Graves, S. (2005, March). Accreditation 101: Understanding the broad world of accreditation. *Education Special Interest Section Quarterly, 15,* 1–2.

LaPidus, J. B. (2000). Postbaccalaureate and graduate education: A dynamic balance. In K. Kohl & J. LaPidus (Eds.), *Postbaccalaureate futures* (pp. 3–9). Phoenix, AZ: Oryx.

Mayhew, L. B., & Ford, P. J. (1971). *Changing the curriculum.* San Francisco: Jossey-Bass.

Mayhew, L. B., & Ford, P. J. (1974). *Reform in graduate and professional education.* San Francisco: Jossey-Bass.

Medeiros, J. M. (1998). Post professional clinical residency programs. *Journal of Manual and Manipulative Therapy, 6,* 10.

Medeiros, J. M. (2000). Educational standards for residency education. *Journal of Manual and Manipulative Therapy, 8,* 50.

Miller, S., & Clarke, A. (2002). Impact of postdoctoral specialty residencies in drug information on graduates' career paths. *American Journal of Health-System Pharmacy, 59,* 961–963.

Pierce, D., & Peyton, C. (1999). A historical cross-disciplinary perspective on the professional doctorate in occupational therapy. *American Journal of Occupational Therapy, 53,* 64–71.

Rogers, J. C. (1980a). Design of the master's degree in occupational therapy, part 1. A logical approach. *American Journal of Occupational Therapy, 34,* 113–118.

Rogers, J. C. (1980b). Design of the master's degree in occupational therapy, part 2. An empirical approach. *American Journal of Occupational Therapy, 34,* 176–184.

Shafritz, J. M., Koeppe, R. P., & Soper, E. W. (1988). *American educators' encyclopedia.* Westport, CT: Greenwood Press.

Unger, H. G. (1996). *Encyclopedia of American education.* New York: Facts on File.

U.S. Department of Education. (2002). *Classification of instructional programs: 2000 edition.* Washington, DC: Office of Educational Research and Improvement.

Watson, J. (1988). *The professional doctorate as an entry level into practice. Perspectives in nursing—1987–1989.* New York: National League for Nursing.

Authors
Brenda M. Coppard, PhD, OTR/L
Creighton University, Omaha, NE
Member, AOTA Commission on Education, 2002–2007
Anne Dickerson, PhD, OTR/L, FAOTA
East Carolina University, Greenville, NC
Member, AOTA Commission on Education, 2000–2006

for

The Commission on Education
Linda Fazio, PhD, OTR/L, FAOTA, *Chairperson*
Brenda M. Coppard, PhD, OTR/L, *Postprofessional Academic Educator*
Donna Costa, MS, OTR/L, *Academic Fieldwork Educator*
Linda Musselman, PhD, OTR, FAOTA, *Professional Program Director*
David Haynes, MBA, OTR/L, *OTA Program Director*
Kelly Fischer, OTR/L, *Fieldwork Educator*
Terrianne Jones, MA, OTR/L, *OTA Academic Educator*
Marc Freedman, *ASD Liaison*
Shirley Marino, COTA, AP, *OTA Educator*
Jaime Muñoz, PhD, OTR/L, FAOTA, *Professional Academic Educator*
René Padilla, PhD, OTR/L, FAOTA, *Chair-Elect*
Jyothi Gupta, PhD, OTR/L, *EDSIS Liaison*

Adopted by the Representative Assembly 2007C11

The Role of Occupational Therapy in Disaster Preparedness, Response, and Recovery

When a societal crisis occurs, individuals, families, communities, institutions, and society as a whole become "disabled"—that is, limited in their ability to perform normal daily activities; restricted by environmental barriers; prohibited from participating in usual social roles; threatened by personal and financial losses, and subject to a variety of psychological reactions, including fear, helplessness, and loss of confidence (Scaffa, 2003). Along with everyone else, occupational therapy practitioners are victims and survivors of these experiences. However, they also have the opportunity to be part of the solution. They can use their understanding of the importance of occupation to increase readiness, to enhance the effectiveness of response, and ultimately to promote health and recovery.

Occupational therapy theorists have proposed seven ways in which occupation can mediate the effects of stressful situations and promote health (McColl, 2002). Occupation can contribute to a person's sense of mastery, and it can reinforce identity. It can restore habits and normalcy, and it can provide diversion. Many occupations (such as rest, exercise, and nutrition) are health-promoting activities, which are essential in responding to and recovering from trauma. Finally, occupation is a means through which people support themselves and others, and through which they are reminded of their connection with a spiritual force.

This paper provides a definition of disaster and a staged model for thinking about occupational therapy's contribution in times of disaster.[1] Further, it identifies 10 premises that inform occupational therapy practitioners'[2] participation in disaster relief. These premises extend occupational therapy practitioners' usual roles as therapists to persons with disabilities and help them to expand their role in relation to families, communities, and organizations that are "disabled" by disaster. The paper makes a cogent case for an occupational therapy role in all three stages of disaster relief, and it leaves occupational therapy practitioners with the challenge of how and where to become involved.

Purpose

Natural and technological disasters are common occurrences throughout the world. Disasters have a significant negative impact, both short- and long-term, on the occupational performance of individuals and communities. The focus of occupational therapy is to facilitate engagement in occupation in order to support participation in valued life roles and activities and to enhance the quality of life. Therefore, occupational therapy practitioners have an important role in responding to disasters.

The purpose of this concept paper is to provide occupational therapy practitioners with a basic understanding of disasters and the support that they can provide to individuals and communities across the spectrum of disaster preparedness, response, and recovery. The paper focuses on the impact of disasters

---

[1]This paper, the product of a collaboration between civilian and military personnel and American and Canadian occupational therapists, arose from the work of the American Occupational Therapy Foundation's Task Force on Occupation in Societal Crises.

[2]*Occupational therapy practitioner:* An individual initially certified to practice as an occupational therapist or occupational therapy assistant or licensed or regulated by a state, district, commonwealth, or territory of the United States to practice as an occupational therapist or occupational therapy assistant and who has not had that certification, license, or regulation revoked due to disciplinary action (American Occupational Therapy Association [AOTA], 1998).

on occupational performance, the benefits of occupational engagement during disasters, and the contribution of occupational therapy in those times.

Definitions and Background

In 1961, Charles E. Fritz, a pioneer in disaster research, defined *disasters* as

> actual or threatened accidental or uncontrollable events that are concentrated in time and space, in which a society or a relatively self-sufficient subdivision of a society undergoes severe danger, and incurs such losses to its members and physical appurtenances that the social structure is disrupted and the fulfillment of all or some of the essential functions of the society, or its subdivision, is prevented (p. 655).

This definition describes not only the physical damage and personal injuries that are typically sustained during a disaster but also the potential widespread social and economic disruption of daily-life routines.

Typically, disasters are classified into two categories: *natural* and *technological* (or *human-made*). Natural disasters include hurricanes, earthquakes, tornadoes, volcanoes, floods, landslides, and winter storms. Technological disasters include mass transportation accidents, nuclear power plant accidents, accidents involving hazardous materials (e.g., oil spills), and massively destructive fires. Newer forms of technological disasters are emerging, among them massive power failures; the spread of computer viruses; assault with biological, nuclear, or chemical weapons; and terrorism (Fischer, 1998; Schneid & Collins, 2001).

Disasters progress through five stages, each requiring different behavioral and organizational responses. In the first stage, the *pre-impact period*, a warning of impending disaster may allow for preparation. For example, the National Weather Service may issue a hurricane warning. In some cases, though, there is no warning, and the pre-impact stage is short or nonexistent.

The second stage, the *impact period*, is the shortest in duration but the most dangerous in the life cycle of a disaster. In this stage the disaster is experienced in full force. Research has shown that widespread panic, looting, price gouging, and deviant behavior during disasters are largely myth. More often, altruism is the norm. People tend to share food, equipment, and supplies and assist one another in recovery efforts (Fischer, 1998).

In the third stage, the *immediate post-impact period*, search-and-rescue efforts are initiated, the media generate increasing coverage of the event, and emergency organizations begin to respond.

During the fourth stage, the *recovery period*, clearance of debris is completed, essential services such as electricity and water are restored, preliminary reconstruction plans are initiated, and daily-life routines begin to normalize.

The fifth and final stage, the *reconstruction period*, may last from several months to several years depending on the scope and the severity of the disaster. Reconstruction involves the rebuilding not only of structures but also of individual lifestyles and a sense of community. The mental health effects of disasters often last longer than the physical manifestations (Fischer, 1998).

Premises

This paper is based on the following 10 premises:

1. Natural and technological disasters are common occurrences throughout the world.

2. Disasters can adversely affect the adaptive occupational performance of individuals and communities across all areas of occupation (Rosenfeld, 1982, 1989).

3. Disaster situations generate significant personal loss and environmental changes that can directly disrupt occupational roles, habit patterns, and routines (Rosenfeld, 1989). Performance patterns may be disrupted through the loss of loved ones, changed living situations, loss of employment, or loss of the ability to engage in other previously valued occupations.

4. Disasters also can generate significant traumatic stress. Traumatic stress affects survivors emotionally, cognitively, physically, and interpersonally (Young, Ford, Ruzek, Friedman, & Gusman, 1998).

5. Disaster victims' usual coping strategies may prove inadequate for the overwhelming stress of disaster situations (Rosenfeld, 1982; Young et al., 1998).

6. Engagement in occupation can have a moderating effect on disaster response and recovery (McColl, 2002).

7. Occupational therapy practitioners can assist individuals and communities in coping with disaster situations and in returning to optimal occupational performance (Rosenfeld, 1982, 1989).

8. In disaster situations, the focus of occupational therapy is to facilitate engagement in occupation in order to support participation in adaptive disaster recovery and resumption of valued life roles and activities (AOTA, 2002).

9. The occupational therapist and the occupational therapy assistant (under the supervision of the therapist) can identify disruptions in clients' previously adaptive occupational performance patterns and help clients develop new effective patterns of performance (Rosenfeld, 1982).

10. The role of the occupational therapy practitioner in disaster response is to enhance the effective occupational performance of disaster survivors by facilitating the process of occupational adaptation (Rosenfeld, 1982).

Discussion: Occupational Therapy Contributions in Times of Disaster

Occupational therapy practitioners can and should be involved in the three aspects of disaster preparedness, response, and recovery. In working with individuals and communities affected by disasters, practitioners bring a set of core practice skills founded on the importance of occupational engagement. Working together with the client, occupational therapists and occupational therapy assistants can plan and implement interventions that enable people to reestablish balance in daily life in activities of daily living, work, leisure, and social participation by

- Analyzing occupations and activities to determine the underlying requisites for effective performance;

- Evaluating occupational performance (functional abilities) in relation to specific activities, tasks, and occupations; and

- Configuring physical and psychological environments to maximize function and social integration.

In addition, occupational therapy practitioners have mental health skills in common with other professionals that are useful in disaster management and response. Possession of these skills facilitates inclusion of occupational therapy practitioners on mental health intervention teams in times of disaster.

The following are examples of potential occupational therapy contributions in disaster preparedness, response, and recovery.

Occupational Therapy Contributions in Disaster Preparedness

Disaster preparedness involves actions taken before a disaster that enable a community to respond effectively. This requires planning at the community, organizational, and household levels. Disaster planning roles, by definition, continue over time and must respond to changing levels of threat. To meet this need for flexibility, some roles may be long-term, while others will be specific to an issue and may be long- or short-term. Planned interventions designed to address system-level concerns, as well as direct service interventions for the individual, are necessary to accomplish safety and normalization. Organizations and businesses must develop emergency response plans, train employees in how to handle emergency situations, acquire needed supplies and equipment, and conduct response drills and exercises (Tierney, Lindell, & Perry, 2001). Individuals must know what these plans entail so that they can proactively remain safe or seek help, when needed, in a timely and efficient way. In essence, disaster planning requires an activity analysis of what will be expected of individuals and agencies when a disaster occurs. Interventions must be designed to be meaningful and purposeful to those engaged in them, and they must support the individual or the agency in performing what the context of the disaster requires.

Knowing the hierarchical structure of agencies and organizations involved in planning, response, and recovery from disasters is important. The National Disaster Medical System is a section within the U.S. Department of Homeland Security, Federal Emergency Management Agency (FEMA). It is responsible for managing and coordinating the federal medical response to major emergencies and federally declared disasters. Its focus is to ensure medical response to a disaster area in the form of teams, supplies, and equipment; move injured people from disaster sites to unaffected areas; and identify the types of medical care available at participating hospitals in unaffected areas. All states are divided into local regions with Disaster Medical Assistance Teams. These teams develop and implement plans to meet physical and mental health needs during disasters in their areas. State, county, and local agencies; businesses; and individuals may assist these teams in planning and in disaster response and recovery. Becoming affiliated with local and national organizations, such as the American Red Cross, mental health crisis services, critical incident stress management (CISM) teams, and employee assistance programs, prior to a disaster increases one's credibility and facilitates involvement when a disaster occurs.

Occupational therapy practitioners can select roles that fit their personal availability and activity preferences at the system level just identified or within their personal context. Because so many occupational therapy practitioners work in health care facilities, they can easily expand a discussion of existing policies, procedures, and occupational therapy roles for the safety of clients during a fire or severe weather conditions to a consideration of what to do when these conditions continue for an extended period. For example, when a predicted hurricane arrives, plans are already in place for securing facilities, moving those with special needs, and providing food and shelter and necessary medications for the short term. But if the storm is fierce, and if there is great destruction, then staff need to be able to design and adapt spaces, modify expectations, create new physical and psychological environments, and provide support services for those under their care for an unknown period of time.

Knowledge of available resources and understanding of local plans for responding to such disasters is critical if the therapist is to facilitate rapid humanitarian responses. Sensitivity to occupational performance needs becomes the marker of the services provided by occupational therapy practitioners, unlike any that are likely to be provided by other members of the response team. It is also essential that practitioners have in place appropriate plans for their family's care during the extended period when they may need to remain on duty at their institution. This will help to prevent conflicting demands on their energies and emotions.

If in the event of a disaster, people with mobility or sensory disabilities are to be moved to a temporary emergency location not specifically designed to accommodate their needs, occupational therapy practitioners can—within their skill level and arena of practice—modify and adapt environments to promote more independent function. Occupational therapy practitioners planning system-level interventions can ensure that planned emergency sites are organized in ways that minimize environmental barriers. For example, they can ensure that people with mobility limitations will be located near restrooms to facilitate independence in self-care. Such planning also decreases the number of environmental modifications or kinds of adaptive equipment that will be required to address self-care needs and privacy concerns. In addition, occupational therapy practitioners can help employers design plans to evacuate workers with disabilities effectively in the event of an emergency, and they can train staff and volunteers to work in shelters for people with special needs.

Occupational Therapy Contributions in Disaster Response

Emergency response involves actions taken just prior to, during, and shortly after disaster impact to address the immediate needs of victims and to reduce damage, destruction, and disruption. Emergency response activities include detection of threats, dissemination of warnings, and evacuation of vulnerable populations. In addition, they include search for and rescue of victims, provision of emergency medical care, and furnishing of food and shelter for displaced persons (Tierney et al., 2001).

During times of disaster or emergency, all professionals are called on to provide their expertise voluntarily in the service of others. Occupational therapy practitioners can provide a variety of services to individuals and families who have evacuated their homes and workplaces and are living in emergency shelters, or who are "sheltering in place" (i.e., remaining in their personal homes or other residences, such as assisted-living facilities, foster and group homes, and long-term-care facilities). In addition, specially trained occupational therapists and occupational therapy assistants under the supervision of an occupational therapist can provide supportive mental health services to first responders and volunteers.

Occupational therapy practitioners are qualified to provide disaster response services to people with special needs. FEMA defines "special needs populations" as people in the community with physical, mental, or medical care needs who may require assistance before, during, or after a disaster or an emergency, after exhausting their usual resources and support network. During a disaster, people with special needs may be moved to regular shelters or shelters for people with special needs, or they may shelter in place. Occupational therapy services may include supervising staff and volunteers at special-needs shelters, making home visits or telephone calls to those sheltering in place, and facilitating support groups designed to reduce anxiety and stress. Occupational therapy practitioners also may provide support for displaced, confused adults and children until their caregivers can be identified and located.

People who are displaced from their homes and workplaces to emergency shelters face a variety of challenges. People of different cultures and races with different beliefs and habits often are forced to live in one large room with no privacy. Children are bored, a general sense of uneasiness pervades, and stress levels increase. Using a client-centered approach, occupational therapy practitioners can evaluate the needs of people in the shelter and provide appropriate services. Interventions might include providing structure in daily routines, identifying and emphasizing people's strengths, encouraging creative expression of feelings, coordinating age-appropriate play for children, and providing opportunities for stress management (Newton, 2000).

Occupational therapy is based on the premise that engagement in occupations facilitates adaptation. Occupation can help disaster survivors reestablish their lost sense of control. Focused, constructive activity, such as helping others, moves people beyond shock and denial. This strategy is especially effective for survivors who are being disruptive. By focusing on occupations that help such people take charge of their life as active participants in their ongoing survival and adjustment to change, occupational therapy practitioners can help them regain their sense of mastery and overcome any sense of guilt from a perceived failure to prepare for the disaster or to protect their family. By engaging in play, vigorous physical activity, or valued leisure occupations, survivors can get a brief respite from recurring thoughts, worries, and concerns about the future.

First responders, including firefighters, police, and emergency medical personnel, also may benefit from occupational therapy. These individuals work long hours under difficult circumstances and often are away from home. Occupational therapists can observe first responders and volunteers for signs of distress, and together with occupational therapy assistants, can provide respite or other appropriate interventions (Newton, 2000). Supportive mental health services may take the form of *critical incident stress debriefings* (CISDs). A CISD is a seven-step, small-group technique for crisis intervention that is part of a larger *critical incident stress management* (CISM) program (Mitchell, 2003). CISDs involve structured discussions of the traumatic events, designed to help people cope with the stressors they have experienced. Such debriefings are thought to lessen the harmful effects of traumatic events. Special training in CISM is required to conduct CISD sessions (Mitchell, 2003). The U.S. military has used these debriefings for many years, and occupational therapists are one of the professional groups trained to conduct them (Newton, 2000).

Occupational Therapy Contributions in Disaster Recovery

Postdisaster recovery involves repair and rebuilding of property, reestablishment of public utilities, and restoration of disrupted social and economic activities and routines. It also includes efforts to enhance the psychosocial well-being and the quality of life of the community members affected (Tierney et al., 2001).

Following disasters, many survivors experience acute stress reactions (see Table 1). Some survivors may suffer lasting psychological effects from the traumatic stress of their experience. These posttraumatic stress symptoms may be severe enough to manifest themselves as depression or an anxiety disorder. One such anxiety disorder is posttraumatic stress disorder (PTSD). Characteristic of PTSD is persistent reexperiencing of the event (e.g., in nightmares and flashbacks), avoidance of reminders of the trauma and numbing of emotions (e.g., difficulty recalling aspects of the trauma and detachment from others), and heightened physiological arousal (e.g., insomnia, irritability, and an exaggerated startle response), all lasting more than 1 month (American Psychiatric Association, 1994). In addition, and of greatest concern to the occupational therapy practitioner, a person with PTSD may experience significant occupational dysfunction.

Table 1. Common Acute Stress Reactions to Disaster

Emotional Effects	Cognitive Effects
Shock	Impaired concentration
Anger	Impaired decision-making ability
Despair	Memory impairment
Emotional numbing	Disbelief
Terror	Confusion
Guilt	Distortion
Grief or sadness	Decreased self-esteem
Irritability	Decreased self-efficacy
Helplessness	Self-blame
Loss of derived pleasure from regular activities	Intrusive thoughts and memories
Dissociation (e.g., perceptual experience seems "dreamlike," "tunnel vision," "spacey," or on "automatic pilot")	Worry

Physical Effects	Interpersonal Effects
Fatigue	Alienation
Insomnia	Social withdrawal
Sleep disturbance	Increased conflict within relationships
Hyperarousal	Vocational impairment
Somatic complaints	School impairment
Impaired immune response	
Headaches	
Gastrointestinal problems	
Decreased appetite	
Decreased libido	
Startle response	

Note. From *Disaster Mental Health Services: A Guidebook for Clinicians and Administrators*, by B. H. Young, J. D. Ford, J. I. Ruzek, M. J. Friedman, & F. D. Gusman, 1998, Menlo Park, CA: National Center for Post-Traumatic Stress Disorder, Department of Veterans Affairs. Available at www.ncptsd.org/publications/disaster/.

Both for short-term, "normal" stress reactions and those that persist over time, occupational therapy practitioners can provide supportive, informative, and educational counseling, as well as crisis intervention to help survivors deal with the consequences of their experience (Roberts, 1995). Clarke (1999) supports this notion that the "use of self" is integral to occupational therapy and that "there appears to be no question that occupational therapists use counseling skills every day in practice" (p. 137). However, occupational therapy is a triadic relationship consisting of the client, the therapist, and the activity. Without the use of activity, occupational therapy does not occur (Clarke, 1999). This differentiates occupational therapy from other mental health approaches.

Occupation and activity can help clients cope with traumatic stress and meet survival needs. Occupational engagement provides diversion from stressful events and helps reestablish a sense of mastery in a situation in which a person feels a loss of control. Participation in occupation facilitates restoration of adaptive habits, supports a person's sense of identity, and helps establish a spiritual connection in the disaster situation (McColl, 2002). The military has long used occupational therapy to help soldiers overcome occupational dysfunction due to the stress of war (Ellsworth, Laedtke, & McPhee, 1993; Laedtke, 1996), to support their role identity, and to restore their confidence in their ability to function (Gerardi, 1996, 1999; Gerardi & Newton, 2004).

For persons diagnosed with PTSD, occupation can be used to recover and enhance skills required by one's daily life roles. Such interventions may focus on activities of daily living to enhance independent living; coping skills (relaxation, biofeedback, etc.) to deal with stress, anxiety, and physiological arousal; and socialization skills to decrease emotional and social withdrawal and to increase socialization (Davis & Kutter, 1998; Froelich, 1992; Rosenfeld, 1982, 1989; Short-Degraff & Engelman, 1992). Expressive media can be used to help clients reexperience their trauma in a safe, supportive environment. This enables them to explore and discover how they have been affected by the event and to practice skills to deal more effectively with their physiological and emotional responses (Davis, 1999; Froelich, 1992; Morgan & Johnson, 1995; Short-Degraff & Engelman, 1992).

As part of the intervention team, occupational therapy practitioners can help clients develop coping skills to deal with the aftereffects of their experience. Additionally, through engagement in occupation, disaster survivors can restructure their habits and routines to cope more effectively with stress and anxiety, to enhance their sense of mastery over their environment, and to participate in their valued life roles.

Conclusion

In summary, occupational therapy practitioners can have a significant role in disaster preparedness, response, and recovery. For example, in preparation for disaster, practitioners can

- Participate in facility-level and community-wide planning efforts,
- Design special-needs shelters and train staff and volunteers, and
- Assist businesses and employers in developing plans for evacuating employees with disabilities.

During the disaster response, practitioners can

- Provide supportive mental health services to victims and their families;
- Provide supportive mental health services to first responders, such as police, firefighters, and military personnel;
- Manage special needs shelters;
- Provide supportive services by telephone or visits to those sheltering in place;

Table 2. Common Acute Stress Reactions to Disaster

Title	Web Address	Description
Disaster Preparedness for Persons With Disabilities	www.redcross.org/services/disaster/beprepared/disability.html	Booklet
Disaster Preparedness for Seniors by Seniors	www.redcross.org/services/disaster/beprepared/seniors.html	Booklet
Disaster Preparedness for Persons With Disabilities	www.accessiblesociety.org/topics/independentliving/disasterprep.htm	Web site prepared by June Isaacson Kailes, vice-president of the Access Board
National Center on Emergency Preparedness for Persons With Disabilities	www.disabilitypreparedness.org/	Web site focused on ensuring that all people are included in development of plans for protection from natural and technological disasters
Disaster Mental Health Services: A Guidebook for Clinicians and Administrators	www.ncptsd.org/publications/disaster/	Publication of National Center for Post-Traumatic Stress Disorder
Training Manual for Mental Health and Human Service Workers in Major Disasters	www.mentalhealth.org/publications/allpubs/ADM90-538/Default.asp	Training manual developed by the U.S. Department of Health and Human Services, Substance Abuse and Mental Health Services Administration, Center for Mental Health Services
Federal Emergency Management Agency (FEMA)	www.fema.gov	Web site of FEMA, a formerly independent agency that became part of the U.S. Department of Homeland Security in March 2003; responsible for responding to, planning for, recovering from, and mitigating against disasters
Emergency Management Institute (EMI)	www.training.fema.gov/EMIWeb/index.asp	Web site of EMI, a nationwide training program of resident and nonresident courses to enhance U.S. emergency management practices
A Citizen Guide to Disaster Preparedness	http://purl.access.gpo.gov/GPO/LPS31779	Booklet prepared by FEMA and published by the Federal Citizen Information Center, General Services Administration (2003)
International Critical Incident Stress Foundation (ICISF)	www.icisf.org/	Web site of ICISF, a nonprofit, open-membership foundation dedicated to prevention and mitigation of disabling stress through provision of education, training, and support services for all emergency medical service professions; continuing education and training in emergency mental health services; and consultation in establishment of Crisis and Disaster Response Programs for varied organizations and communities worldwide
Emergency Planning and Special Needs Populations	http://training.fema.gov/EMIWeb/pub/register.html	Course materials for training program sponsored by EMI
National Disaster Medical System	http://ndms.dhhs.gov	Web site of the National Disaster Medical System, a section within U.S. Department of Homeland Security that has responsibility for managing and coordinating federal medical response to major emergencies and federally declared disasters

- Provide occupational interventions in shelters; and

- Facilitate psychoeducational support groups to decrease anxiety and stress.

Throughout the disaster recovery phase, practitioners can provide occupation-based and psychoeducational mental health services for persons with acute stress reactions and PTSD.

Occupational therapy has much to offer individuals and communities affected by disaster. The profession's holistic approach and its focus on occupational engagement and adaptation constitute its contribution to disaster management. However, to be effective in this arena, occupational therapy practitioners must

- Define and establish their role in disaster preparedness, response, and recovery (McDaniel, 1960);

- Be aware of existing hospital, institutional, work site, and community disaster plans;

- Be knowledgeable about how national, state, and local governments and private agencies involved in disaster management are organized and how to gain entry into these systems;

- Develop skills and train for their role in disaster response and recovery; and

- Be personally and professionally prepared to respond effectively to disaster situations (see Table 2).

Occupational therapy practitioners can use their professional expertise and the power of occupational engagement to restore control, order, and quality of life and to normalize lives in crisis when individuals, families, and communities are disrupted by natural or technological disasters.

A quote from C. S. Lewis written for another time remains relevant today as occupational therapy practitioners think about their response to disaster, both as private individuals and as professionals. It reminds them of the power of occupation to restore and uphold humanity in stressful times:

> The first action to be taken is to pull ourselves together. If we are to be destroyed by an atomic bomb, let that bomb, when it comes, find us doing sensible and human things—praying, working, teaching, reading, listening to music, bathing the children, playing tennis, chatting to our friends over a pint and a game of darts—not huddled together like frightened sheep and thinking about bombs. (Lewis, 1986, pp. 73–74)

References

American Occupational Therapy Association. (1998). Policy 1.44: Categories of occupational therapy personnel. In *American Occupational Therapy Association policy manual*. Bethesda, MD: Author.

American Occupational Therapy Association. (2002). Occupational therapy practice framework: Domain and process. *American Journal of Occupational Therapy, 56,* 609–639.

American Psychiatric Association. (1994). *Diagnostic and statistical manual of mental disorders* (4th ed.). Washington, DC: Author.

Clarke, C. (1999). Treating post-traumatic stress disorder: Occupational therapist or counselor? *British Journal of Occupational Therapy, 62,* 136–138.

Davis, J. (1999). Effects of trauma on children: Occupational therapy to support recovery. *Occupational Therapy International, 6,* 126–142.

Davis, J., & Kutter, C. J. (1998). Independent living skills and posttraumatic stress disorder in women who are homeless: Implications for future practice. *American Journal of Occupational Therapy, 52,* 39–44.

Ellsworth, P. D., Laedtke, M. E., & McPhee, S. D. (1993). Utilization of occupational therapy in combat stress control during the Persian Gulf War. *Military Medicine, 158,* 381–385.

Fischer, H. W. (1998). *Response to disaster: Fact versus fiction and its perpetuation: The sociology of disaster* (2nd ed.). Lanham, MD: University Press of America.

Fritz, C. E. (1961). Disasters. In R. K. Merton & R. A. Nisbet (Eds.), *Contemporary social problems* (pp. 651–694). New York: Harcourt.

Froelich, J. (1992). Occupational therapy interventions with survivors of sexual abuse. *Occupational Therapy in Health Care, 8*(2/3), 1–25.

Gerardi, S. M. (1996). The management of battle-fatigued soldiers: An occupational therapy model. *Military Medicine, 161*, 483–488.

Gerardi, S. M. (1999). Part I. Work hardening for warriors: Occupational therapy for combat stress casualties. *Work, 13*, 185–195.

Gerardi, S. M., & Newton, S. M. (2004, July–September). The role of the occupational therapist in CSC (combat stress control) operations. *U.S. Army Medical Department Journal,* pp. 20–27.

Laedtke, M. E. (1996). Occupational therapy and the treatment of combat stress. In J. A. Martin, L. R. Sparacinco, & G. Belenky (Eds.), *The Gulf War and mental health: A comprehensive guide* (pp. 145–152). Westport, CT: Praeger.

Lewis, C. S. (1986). *Present concerns: A compelling collection of timely journalistic essays.* London: C. S. Lewis PTE, Ltd.

McColl, M. A. (2002). Occupation in stressful times. *American Journal of Occupational Therapy, 56*, 350–353.

McDaniel, M. L. (1960). The role of the occupational therapist in natural disaster situations. *American Journal of Occupational Therapy, 14*, 195–198.

Mitchell, J. T. (2003). Major misconceptions in crisis intervention. *International Journal of Emergency Mental Health, 5*, 185–198.

Morgan, C. A., & Johnson, D. R. (1995). Use of a drawing task in the treatment of nightmares in combat-related post-traumatic stress disorder. *Art Therapy: Journal of the American Art Therapy Association, 12*, 244–247.

Newton, S. (2000, November). *Matching occupational therapy skills to new opportunities: Working on a natural disaster.* Poster session presented at the annual meeting of the Occupational Therapy Association of California.

Roberts, G. W. (1995). Trauma following major disasters: The role of the occupational therapist. *British Journal of Occupational Therapy, 58*, 204–208.

Rosenfeld, M. S. (1982). A model for activity intervention in disaster-stricken communities. *American Journal of Occupational Therapy, 36*, 229–235.

Rosenfeld, M. S. (1989). Occupational disruption and adaptation: A study of house fire victims. *American Journal of Occupational Therapy, 43*, 89–96.

Scaffa, M. (2003, Spring). Competence, mastery, and independence: Our cultural heritage. *American Occupational Therapy Foundation Connection, 10*(1), 6–7.

Schneid, T. D., & Collins, L. (2001). *Disaster management and preparedness.* Boca Raton, FL: Lewis Publishers.

Short-Degraff, M. A., & Engelman, T. (1992). Activities in the treatment of combat-related post-traumatic stress disorder. *Occupational Therapy in Health Care, 8*(2/3), 27–47.

Tierney, K. J., Lindell, M. K., & Perry, R. W. (Eds.). (2001). *Facing the unexpected: Disaster preparedness and response in the United States.* Washington, DC: Joseph Henry Press & National Academy of Sciences.

Young, B. H., Ford J. D., Ruzek, J. I., Friedman, M. J., & Gusman, F. D. (1998). *Disaster mental health services: A guidebook for clinicians and administrators*. Menlo Park, CA: National Center for Post-Traumatic Stress Disorder, Department of Veterans Affairs. Available at www.ncptsd.org/publications/disaster/

Authors

Marjorie E. Scaffa, PhD, OTR/L, FAOTA
Steven Gerardi, MS, OTR/L, CHT
Georgiana Herzberg, PhD, OTR/L
Mary Ann McColl, PhD

for

The Commission on Practice
Sara Jane Brayman, PhD, OTR/L, FAOTA, *Chairperson*

and

The American Occupational Therapy Foundation
Martha M. Kirkland, OTR, *Executive Director*
Jane Davis Rourk, OTR/L, FAOTA, *Chairperson, Task Force on Societal Crises*

Adopted by the Representative Assembly 2005CO304

Scholarship in Occupational Therapy

In this document, we present the position of the American Occupational Therapy Association (AOTA) on the importance of scholarship to the growth, development, and vitality of the profession, and we describe the range of scholarly activities that will advance the profession. In addition, this document serves to inform both internal and external audiences concerning the expectations for—and the role of—scholarship in occupational therapy practices..

It is important to distinguish between scholarly practice and scholarship. *Scholarly practice* involves using the knowledge base of the profession or discipline in one's practice. As occupational therapy practitioners we, call this scholarly practice *evidence-based practice.* When engaged in scholarly teaching, educators draw on the "knowledge base on teaching and learning" (McKinney, 2007, p. 9) and their discipline or professional knowledge bases. Occupational therapy practitioners engaged in scholarly practice or scholarly teaching are reflective practitioners who assess and discuss their actions in light of the current knowledge base (McKinney, 2007; Schön, 1983). In contrast, *scholarship* or *research* is "a systematic investigation… designed to develop or to contribute to generalizable knowledge" (U.S. Department of Health and Human Services, 2005). Scholarship is made public, subject to review, and part of the discipline or professional knowledge base (Glassick, Huber, & Maeroff, 1997). It allows others to build on it and further advance the field.

Occupational therapy practitioners view scholarship as a vitally important contribution to the profession, the academy, and ultimately to society. Hence, practitioners see that engaging in scholarship is a professional responsibility. Every occupational therapy practitioner should contribute independently or collaboratively to building the evidence base for occupational therapy practice and occupational therapy education (Accreditation Council for Occupational Therapy Education, 2008; AOTA, 2007).

Occupational therapy practitioners are committed to engagement in scholarship that honors societal ethical standards and adheres to the standards of rigor accepted by the scientific community. Occupational therapy scholars value empiricism as the means by which knowledge must emerge, recognizing that through a variety of experimental and naturalistic means one may achieve knowledge and understanding (DePoy & Gitlin, 2005; Kielhofner, 2006). Moreover, they recognize that knowledge is not established in isolation but through interdisciplinary collaboration and intellectual discourse (Yerxa, 1987). As providers of therapeutic and educational services, occupational therapy practitioners are committed to continually developing foundational and theoretical knowledge that underlies practice; understanding the process and outcomes of service; and finally, establishing evidence of efficacious therapy and educational outcomes (Kielhofner, 2006).

The profession recognizes the necessity of a broad range of scholarly endeavors that will serve to describe and interpret the scope of the profession, establish new knowledge, interpret and appropriately apply this knowledge to practice, and engage learners in their development and understanding of the profession. Therefore, we acknowledge the relevance and legitimacy of the variety of scholarly approaches as described by Boyer (1990): the Scholarship of Discovery, the Scholarship of Integration, the Scholarship of Application, and the Scholarship of Teaching. This range of scholarship is particularly relevant considering the diversity in the field of occupational therapy represented by stakeholders with varying educational backgrounds. The four types of scholarship are discussed in the order Boyer (1990) presented them in *Scholarship Reconsidered: Priorities for the Professoriate.* He did not identify a hierarchy among the four types of scholarship and none is intended in this document.

Scholarship of Discovery

According to Boyer (1990), the *Scholarship of Discovery* is the engagement in activity that leads to the development of "knowledge for its own sake" (p. 17). The Scholarship of Discovery encompasses original research that contributes to expanding the knowledge base of a discipline. It is the type of research that the academic community most easily recognizes and accepts, and as such, is often the expected vehicle for intellectual discourse within the academy. Traditionally, faculty members who are trained to be independent researchers in research universities conduct discovery scholarship. Such scholars are, according to Golde (2006), stewards of the discipline responsible for "*generating* new knowledge and defending knowledge claims against challenges and criticism; of *conserving* the most important ideas and findings that are a legacy of past and current work; and of *transforming* knowledge that has been generated and conserved by teaching well to a variety of audiences, including those outside formal classrooms."

Clearly, there is a need for scholarship in occupational therapy that expands overall understanding of the engagement in and meaning of human occupation and its role in attaining and maintaining health. Clark (2006) noted that the profession needed a critical mass of the scholarship of discovery to continue to build the theoretical and knowledge base for occupational therapy, to foster intellectual vitality, and to maintain and strengthen the central tenets of the discipline.

Scholarship of Integration

The *Scholarship of Integration* is concerned with making creative connections both within and across disciplines to integrate, synthesize, interpret, and create new perspectives and theories. This form of scholarship is the most similar to the Scholarship of Discovery, but the difference lies in the nature of the research questions. In this form of inquiry, the scholars' aim is to find the meaning of research findings and interpret the findings in ways that synthesize isolated facts from within and outside of the discipline and integrate them to provide a richer and more thorough understanding of the issues. In light of the complex nature of contemporary issues confronting the individual and society, the profession needs the scholarship of integration, which lies in the intersections of disciplinary boundaries, to generate new knowledge for occupational therapy to better understand and meet societal needs.

Scholarship of Application

Through the Scholarship of Application, practitioners apply the knowledge generated by Scholarship of Discovery or Integration to address real problems at all levels of society. In occupational therapy, an example would be the application of theoretical knowledge to practice interventions or to teaching in the classroom. Another example may be using knowledge about the value of occupations as a health determinant to address health disparities of populations. Some authors, in focusing their efforts on application, have coined the term *Scholarship of Practice* (Braveman, Helfrich, & Fisher, 2001; Kielhofner, 2005), which focuses on program development and occupational therapy intervention. Another dimension of the Scholarship of Application is the *Scholarship of Engagement* (1990), which focuses on an interactive, participatory scholarship with persons and organizations (Barker, 2004; Boyer, 1996). In this form of scholarship, multiple stakeholders, including community members, produce knowledge. Regardless of differing terms, these activities fit best under Boyer's (1990) scholarship of application.

Scholarship of Teaching and Learning

Boyer (1990) identified a fourth area of scholarship, the *Scholarship of Teaching*. Over time it has been expanded to the *Scholarship of Teaching and Learning*, recognizing the interrelatedness of teaching and learning. The Scholarship of Teaching and Learning implies a "research agenda," and "involves the systematic study of teaching and/or learning and the public sharing and review of such work through presentations, publications, and performances" (McKinney, 2007, p. 10). Contributions must meet the rigorous standards of all forms of scholarship, be public, and be open to critical review.

Scholarship and Practice Roles

Scholarship must be generated, evaluated, and used to inform the many practice roles of occupational therapy. All occupational therapists and occupational therapy assistants, regardless of their individual practice roles, have the professional responsibility to not only use that evidence to inform their professional decision making but also to generate new evidence through independent or collaborative research, or both. For example, research through the Scholarships of Discovery and of Integration will contribute to the improved understanding of the constructs, processes, and theories (e.g., occupation and its therapeutic use) that provide the foundation for meeting society's complex occupational needs. At other times, through the Scholarship of Application, practitioners will establish evidence concerning the effectiveness of a specific intervention or the reliability, validity, and utility of an assessment tool and appropriately use the intervention or assessment on the basis of the strength of that evidence. Finally, they may develop and use evidence derived from the Scholarship of Teaching and Learning in client education to support participation in meaningful occupations. Practitioners challenge occupational therapy educators—including academic educators, academic fieldwork educators, and fieldwork educators—to find better ways to prepare diverse students to be competent professionals who advance the profession. Through the Scholarship of Teaching and Learning and the Scholarship of Application, they can empirically determine and apply better instructional methodologies to prepare students to meet the demands of a rapidly changing and increasingly complex health care environment, where consumers expect evidence-based practice and continuous professional development of all practitioners. Finally, administrators can contribute to, and benefit from, evidence produced through the Scholarship of Application when determining how best to meet the needs of clients in a cost-effective manner or how to better mentor or supervise others. Additional examples and benchmarks of scholarship are provided in Appendix A.

References

Accreditation Council for Occupational Therapy Education. (2008). *Accreditation Council for Occupational Therapy Education standards and interpretive guidelines.* Retrieved November 14, 2008, from http://www.aota.org/Educate/Accredit/StandardsReview/guide/42369.aspx

American Occupational Therapy Association. (2007). *AOTA's Centennial Vision.* Retrieved November 14, 2008, from http://www.aota.org/News/Centennial.aspx

Barker, D. (2004). The scholarship of engagement: A taxonomy of five emerging practices. *Journal of Higher Education Outreach and Engagement, 9,* 123–137.

Boyer, E. L. (1990). *Scholarship reconsidered: Priorities of the professoriate.* San Francisco: Jossey-Bass.

Boyer, E. L. (1996). The scholarship of engagement. *Journal of Public Service and Outreach, 1,* 11–20.

Braveman, B. H., Helfrich, C. A., & Fisher, G. S. (2001). Developing and maintaining community partnerships within "A Scholarship of Practice." *Occupational Therapy in Health Care, 15,* 109–125.

Clark, F. (2006). One person's thoughts on the future of occupational science. *Journal of Occupational Science, 13*(3), 167–179.

DePoy, E., & Gitlin, L. N. (2005). *Introduction to research: Understanding and applying multiple strategies* (3rd ed.). St. Louis, MO: Elsevier/Mosby.

Glassick, C. E., Huber, M. T., & Maeroff, G. I. (1997). *Scholarship assessed: Evaluation of the professoriate.* San Francisco: Jossey-Bass.

Golde, C. (2006). *Preparing stewards of the discipline.* The Carnegie Foundation for the advancement of teaching. Retrieved September, 2008 from http://www.carnegiefoundation.org/perspectives/sub.asp?key=245&subkey=1811

Kielhofner, G. (2005). A scholarship of practice: Creating discourse between theory, research, and practice. *Occupational Therapy in Health Care, 19,* 7–16.

Kielhofner, G. (2006). *Research in occupational therapy: Methods of inquiry for enhancing practice.* Philadelphia: F. A. Davis.

McKinney, K. (2007). *Enhancing learning through the scholarship of teaching and learning.* San Francisco: Jossey-Bass.

Schön, D. A. (1983). *The reflective practitioner.* New York: Basic Books.

U.S. Department of Health Human Services. (2005). Part 46—Protection of human subjects. Code of Federal Regulations Title 45—Public Welfare. Available online at http://www.hhs.gov/ohrp/documents/OHRPRegulation.pdf

Yerxa, E. (1987). Research: The key to the development of occupational therapy as an academic discipline. *American Journal of Occupational Therapy, 41,* 415–419.

The Commission on Education:
René Padilla, PhD, OTR/L, FAOTA, *Chairperson*
Andrea Bilics, PhD, OTR/L
Judith C. Blum, MS, OTR/L
Paula C. Bohr, PhD, OTR/L, FAOTA
Jennifer C. Coyne, COTA/L
Jyothi Gupta, PhD, OTR/L
Linda Musselman, PhD, OTR, FAOTA
Linda Orr, MPA, OTR/L
Abbey Sipp (ASD)
Patricia Stutz-Tanenbaum, MS, OTR
Neil Harvison, PhD, OTR/L, *Staff Liaison*

Adopted by the Representative Assembly 2009FebCS114

This document replaces the document *Scholarship and Occupational Therapy* 2003M42T.

Appendix A.
Characteristics of Scholarship in Occupational Therapy

Type of Scholarship	Examples	Demonstration of Scholarship	Documentation
Scholarship of Discovery Contributes to the development or creation of new knowledge	• Primary empirical research • Historical research • Theory development • Methodological studies • Philosophical inquiry	• Peer-reviewed publications of research, theory, or philosophical essays • Peer-reviewed/invited professional presentations of research, theory, or philosophical essays • Grant awards in support of research or scholarship • Positive peer evaluations of the body of work	• Bibliographic citation of the accomplishments • Positive external evaluation of the body of work
Scholarship of Integration Contributes to the critical analysis and review of knowledge within disciplines or the creative synthesis of insights contained in different disciplines or fields of study	• Inquiry that advances knowledge across a range of theories, practice areas, techniques, or methodologies • Includes works that interface among occupational therapy and a variety of disciplines, including but not limited to occupational science	• Peer-reviewed publications of research, policy analysis, case studies, integrative reviews of the literature, and others • Copyrights, licenses, patents, or products • Published books • Positive peer evaluations of contributions to integrative scholarship • Reports of interdisciplinary programs or services • Interdisciplinary grant awards • Peer-reviewed/invited professional presentations • Policy papers designed to influence organizations or governments • Service on editorial board or as peer reviewer	• Bibliographic citation of the accomplishments • Positive external evaluation of the body of work • Documentation of role in editorial/review processes

(continued)

Appendix A.
Characteristics of Scholarship in Occupational Therapy *(cont.)*

Type of Scholarship	Examples	Demonstration of Scholarship	Documentation
Scholarship of Application, Practice, or Engagement Applies findings generated through the Scholarship of Integration or discovery to solve real problems in the professions, industry, government, and community	• Development of clinical knowledge • Application of technical or research skills to address problems • Participatory action research involving collaboration with community groups • Efficacy of treatment approach • Developing valid outcome measures	• Peer-reviewed publications of research, policy analysis, case studies, integrative reviews of the literature, and others • Activities related to the faculty member's area of expertise (e.g., consultation, technical assistance, policy analysis, program evaluation, development of practice patterns) • Peer-reviewed/invited professional presentations related to practice • Consultation reports • Reports compiling and analyzing patient or health services outcomes • Products, patents, license copyrights • Peer reviews of practice • Grant awards in support of practice • Reports of meta-analyses related to practice problems • Reports of clinical demonstration projects • Policy papers related to practice	• Formal documentation of a record of the activity and positive formal evaluation by users of the work • Bibliographic citation of the accomplishments • Positive external evaluation of the body of work • Documentation of role in multi-authored products

Appendix A.
Characteristics of Scholarship in Occupational Therapy *(cont.)*

Type of Scholarship	Examples	Demonstration of Scholarship	Documentation
Scholarship of Teaching and Learning Contributes to the development of critically reflective knowledge about teaching and learning	• Application of knowledge of the discipline or specialty applied in teaching–learning in the academic and/or fieldwork setting • Development of innovative teaching and evaluation methods • Program development and learning outcome evaluation of academic and/or fieldwork education • Professional role modeling	• Peer-reviewed publications of research related to teaching methodology or learning outcomes, case studies related to teaching–learning, learning theory development, and development or testing of educational models or theories • Educational effectiveness studies such as those found in comprehensive programs reports • Successful applications of technology to teaching and learning • Positive peer evaluations of innovations in teaching • Published textbooks or other learning aids • Grant awards in support of teaching and learning • Peer-reviewed/invited professional presentations related to teaching and learning	• Bibliographic citation of the accomplishments • Positive external evaluation of the body of work

Note. Adapted from http://www.clt.uts.edu.au/Scholarship/A.Model.html, http://aacn.nche.edu/Publications/positions/scholar.htm, http://www.apta.org/AM/Template.cfm?Section=CAPTE3&Template=/CM/ContentDisplay.cfm&ContentID=23140

Ethics

Core Values and Attitudes of Occupational Therapy Practice

Introduction

In 1985, the American Occupational Therapy Association (AOTA) funded the Professional and Technical Role Analysis Study (PATRA). This study had two purposes: to delineate the entry-level practice of OTRs and COTAs through a role analysis and to conduct a task inventory of what practitioners actually do. Knowledge, skills, and attitude statements were to be developed to provide a basis for the role analysis. The PATRA study completed the knowledge and skills statements. The Executive Board subsequently charged the Standards and Ethics Commission (SEC) to develop a statement that would describe the attitudes and values that undergird the profession of occupational therapy. The SEC wrote this document for use by AOTA members.

The list of terms used in this statement was originally constructed by the American Association of Colleges of Nursing (AACN) (1986). The PATRA committee analyzed the knowledge statements that the committee had written and selected those terms from the AACN list that best identified the values and attitudes of our profession. This list of terms was then forwarded to SEC by the PATRA Committee to use as the basis for the Core Values and Attitudes paper.

The development of this document is predicated on the assumption that the values of occupational therapy are evident in the official documents of the American Occupational Therapy Association. The official documents that were examined are: (a) *Dictionary Definition of Occupational Therapy* (AOTA, 1986), (b) *The Philosophical Base of Occupational Therapy* (AOTA, 1979), (c) *Essentials and Guidelines for an Accredited Educational Program for the Occupational Therapist* (AOTA, 1991a), (d) *Essentials and Guidelines for an Accredited Educational Program for the Occupational Therapy Assistant* (AOTA, 1991b), and (e) *Occupational Therapy Code of Ethics* (AOTA, 1988). It is further assumed that these documents are representative of the values and beliefs reflected in other occupational therapy literature.

A *value* is defined as a belief or an ideal to which an individual is committed. Values are an important part of the base or foundation of a profession. Ideally, these values are embraced by all members of the profession and are reflected in the members' interactions with those persons receiving services, colleagues, and the society at large. Values have a central role in a profession and are developed and reinforced throughout an individual's life as a student and as a professional.

Actions and attitudes reflect the values of the individual. An attitude is the disposition to respond positively or negatively toward an object, person, concept, or situation. Thus, there is an assumption that all professional actions and interactions are rooted in certain core values and beliefs.

Seven Core Concepts

In this document, the *core values and attitudes* of occupational therapy are organized around seven basic concepts—altruism, equality, freedom, justice, dignity, truth, and prudence. How these core values and attitudes are expressed and implemented by occupational therapy practitioners may vary depending upon the environments and situations in which professional activity occurs.

Altruism is the unselfish concern for the welfare of others. This concept is reflected in actions and attitudes of commitment, caring, dedication, responsiveness, and understanding.

Equality requires that all individuals be perceived as having the same fundamental human rights and opportunities. This value is demonstrated by an attitude of fairness and impartiality. We believe that we should respect all individuals, keeping in mind that they may have values, beliefs, or lifestyles that are different from our own. Equality is practiced in the broad professional arena but is particularly important in day-to-day interactions with those individuals receiving occupational therapy services.

Freedom allows the individual to exercise choice and to demonstrate independence, initiative, and self-direction. There is a need for all individuals to find a balance between autonomy and societal membership that is reflected in the choice of various patterns of interdependence with the human and nonhuman environment. We believe that individuals are internally and externally motivated toward action in a continuous process of adaptation throughout the life span. Purposeful activity plays a major role in developing and exercising self-direction, initiative, interdependence, and relatedness to the world. Activities verify the individual's ability to adapt, and they establish a satisfying balance between autonomy and societal membership. As professionals, we affirm the freedom of choice for each individual to pursue goals that have personal and social meaning.

Justice places value on the upholding of such moral and legal principles as fairness, equity, truthfulness, and objectivity. This means we aspire to provide occupational therapy services for all individuals who are in need of these services and that we will maintain a goal-directed and objective relationship with all those served. Practitioners must be knowledgeable about and have respect for the legal rights of individuals receiving occupational therapy services. In addition, the occupational therapy practitioner must understand and abide by the local, state, and federal laws governing professional practice.

Dignity emphasizes the importance of valuing the inherent worth and uniqueness of each person. This value is demonstrated by an attitude of empathy and respect for self and others. We believe that each individual is a unique combination of biologic endowment, sociocultural heritage, and life experiences. We view human beings holistically, respecting the unique interaction of the mind, body, and physical and social environment. We believe that dignity is nurtured and grows from the sense of competence and self-worth that is integrally linked to the person's ability to perform valued and relevant activities. In occupational therapy we emphasize the importance of dignity by helping the individual build on his or her unique attributes and resources.

Truth requires that we be faithful to facts and reality. Truthfulness or veracity is demonstrated by being accountable, honest, forthright, accurate, and authentic in our attitudes and actions. There is an obligation to be truthful with ourselves, those who receive services, colleagues, and society. One way that this is exhibited is through maintaining and upgrading professional competence. This happens, in part, through an unfaltering commitment to inquiry and learning, to self-understanding, and to the development of an interpersonal competence.

Prudence is the ability to govern and discipline oneself through the use of reason. To be prudent is to value judiciousness, discretion, vigilance, moderation, care, and circumspection in the management of one's affairs, to temper extremes, make judgments, and respond on the basis of intelligent reflection and rational thought.

Summary

Beliefs and values are those intrinsic concepts that underlie the core of the profession and the professional interactions of each practitioner. These values describe the profession's philosophy and provide the basis for defining purpose. The emphasis or priority that is given to each value may change as one's professional career evolves and as the unique characteristics of a situation unfold. This evolution of values is developmental in nature. Although we have basic values that cannot be violated, the degree to which certain values will take priority at a given time is influenced by the specifics of a situation and the environment in which it occurs. In one instance dignity may be a higher priority than truth; in another, prudence may be chosen over freedom. As we process information and make decisions, the weight of the values that we hold may change. The practitioner faces dilemmas because of conflicting values and is required to engage in thoughtful deliberation to determine where the priority lies in a given situation.

The challenge for us all is to know our values, be able to make reasoned choices in situations of conflict, and be able to clearly articulate and defend our choices. At the same time, it is important that all members of the profession be committed to a set of common values. This mutual commitment to a set of beliefs and principles that govern our practice can provide a basis for clarifying expectations between the recipient and the provider of services. Shared values empower the profession and, in addition, build trust among ourselves and with others.

References

American Association of Colleges of Nursing. (1986). *Essentials of college and university education for professional nursing* (Final report). Washington, DC: Author.

American Occupational Therapy Association. (1979). Resolution C, 531–79. The philosophical base of occupational therapy. *American Journal of Occupational Therapy, 33,* 785.

American Occupational Therapy Association. (1986, April). *Dictionary definition of occupational therapy.* Adopted and approved by the Representative Assembly to fulfill Resolution 596-83. (Available from AOTA, 4720 Montgomery Lane, Bethesda, MD 20814.)

American Occupational Therapy Association. (1988). Occupational therapy code of ethics. *American Journal of Occupational Therapy, 42,* 795–796.

American Occupational Therapy Association. (1991a). Essentials and guidelines for an accredited educational program for the occupational therapist. *American Journal of Occupational Therapy, 45,* 1077–1084.

American Occupational Therapy Association. (1991b). Essentials and guidelines for an accredited educational program for the occupational therapy assistant. *American Journal of Occupational Therapy, 45,* 1085–1092.

Prepared by

Elizabeth Kanny, MA, OTR, *Education Representative (1990–1996) for the Standards and Ethics Commission*

Ruth A. Hansen, PhD, OTR, FAOTA, *Chairperson (1988–1994)*

Approved by the Representative Assembly June 1993

Note. This AOTA *Core Values and Attitudes of Occupational Therapy Practice* is one of three documents that constitute the "Ethics Standards." The other two are the *Occupational Therapy Code of Ethics (2005)* and the *Guidelines to the Occupational Therapy Code of Ethics (2006).*

Enforcement Procedures for the *Occupational Therapy Code of Ethics*

1. Introduction

The American Occupational Therapy Association (AOTA) and its members are committed to furthering each individual's ability to function fully within his or her total environment. To this end, the occupational therapist and occupational therapy assistant render services to clients in all phases of health and illness, to institutions, to organizations, to other professionals and colleagues, to students, and to the public.

The AOTA's *Occupational Therapy Code of Ethics*, its *Guidelines*, and its *Core Values* (hereinafter jointly referred to as "Ethics Standards") are public statements of values and principles to use as a guide in promoting and maintaining high standards of behavior in occupational therapy.

The Ethics Standards apply to occupational therapy personnel at all levels. They apply to professional roles such as those of practitioner, educator, fieldwork educator or coordinator, clinical supervisor, manager, administrator, consultant, faculty, program director, researcher/scholar, private practice owner, entrepreneur, student, and other professional roles, including elective and appointed volunteer roles within the AOTA. More broadly, these Ethics Standards apply not only to conduct within occupational therapy roles but also to conduct that may affect the performance of occupational therapy or the reputation of the profession. The principal purposes of the Ethics Standards are to help protect the public and to reinforce its confidence in the occupational therapy profession rather than to resolve private business, legal, or other disputes for which there are other more appropriate forums.

To ensure compliance with the Ethics Standards, these *Enforcement Procedures* are established and maintained by the Ethics Commission and (hereinafter referred to as the "EC"). Acceptance of membership in the AOTA commits members to adherence to the Ethics Standards and cooperation with its Enforcement Procedures. The EC urges particular attention to the following issues.

1.1. **Professional Responsibility, Other Processes**—All occupational therapy personnel have an obligation to maintain the standards of ethics of their profession and to promote and support these standards among their colleagues. Each member must be alert to practices that undermine these standards and is obligated to take action that is appropriate in the circumstances. At the same time, members must carefully weigh their judgments as to potentially unethical practice to ensure that they are based on objective evaluation and not on personal bias or prejudice, inadequate information, or simply differences of professional viewpoint. It is recognized that individual occupational therapy personnel may not have the authority or ability to address or correct all situations of concern. Whenever feasible and appropriate, members should first pursue other corrective steps within the relevant institution or setting before resorting to the AOTA ethics complaint process.

1.2. **Jurisdiction**—The Code of Ethics (hereinafter referred to as the "Code") applies to persons who are or were members of the AOTA at the time of the conduct in question. Later nonrenewal or relinquishment of membership does not affect AOTA jurisdiction. The Code that is applicable to any complaint shall be the Code in force at the time the alleged act or omission occurred, unless the date of the alleged act or omission cannot be precisely determined. In that case, the conduct shall be judged by the Code in force on the date of the complaint.

1.3. Disciplinary Actions/Sanctions (Pursuing a Complaint)—If the EC determines that unethical conduct has occurred, it may impose sanctions, including reprimand, censure, probation, suspension, or permanent revocation of membership in the AOTA. In all cases, except those involving only reprimand, the AOTA will report the conclusions and sanctions in its official publications and will also communicate to any appropriate persons or entities. The potential sanctions are defined as follows:

1.3.1. Reprimand—A formal expression of disapproval of conduct communicated privately by letter from the Chairperson of the EC that is nondisclosable and noncommunicative to other bodies (e.g., state regulatory boards [SRBs]; National Board for Certification in Occupational Therapy, hereinafter known as "NBCOT®").

1.3.2. Censure—A formal expression of disapproval that is public.

1.3.3. Probation of membership subject to terms—Failure to meet terms will subject a member to any of the disciplinary actions or sanctions.

1.3.4. Suspension—Removal of membership for a specified period of time.

1.3.5. Revocation—Permanent denial of membership.

1.3.5.1. If an individual is on either the Roster of Fellows (ROF) or the Roster of Honor (ROH), the chairperson of the EC (via the EC staff liaison) shall notify the Chairperson of the Recognitions Committee (and Executive Director) of their membership revocation. That individual shall have their name removed from either the ROF or the ROH and no longer has the right to use the designated credential of FAOTA or ROH.

1.4. Educative Letters—If the EC determines that the alleged conduct, even if proven, does not appear to be unethical but may not be completely in keeping with the aspirational nature of the Code or within the prevailing standards of practice or good professionalism, the EC may send a letter to educate the Respondent only regarding standards of practice and/or good professionalism. In addition, a different educative letter, if appropriate, may be sent to the Complainant.

1.5. Advisory Opinions—The EC may issue general advisory opinions on ethical issues to inform and educate the membership. These opinions shall be publicized to the membership.

1.6. Rules of Evidence—The EC proceedings shall be conducted in accordance with fundamental fairness. However, formal rules of evidence that are employed in legal proceedings do not apply to these *Enforcement Procedures*. The Disciplinary Council (see Section 5) and the Appeal Panel (see Section 6) can consider any evidence that they deem appropriate and pertinent.

1.7. Confidentiality and Disclosure—The EC develops and adheres to strict rules of confidentiality in every aspect of its work. Maintaining confidentiality throughout the investigation and enforcement process of a formal ethics complaint is essential in order to ensure fairness to all parties involved. These rules of confidentiality pertain not only to the EC but also apply to others involved in the complaint process. Beginning with the EC staff liaison and support staff, strict rules of confidentiality are followed. These same rules of confidentiality apply to complainants, respondents and their attorneys, and witnesses involved with the EC's investigatory process. Due diligence must be exercised by everyone involved in the investigation to avoid compromising the confidential nature of the process. Any AOTA member who breaches these rules of confidentiality may become subject to an ethics complaint/investigatory process himself or herself. Non–AOTA members may lodge an ethics complaint against an AOTA member, and these individuals are still expected to adhere to AOTA's confidentiality rules. The AOTA reserves the right to take appropriate action against non–AOTA members who violate confidentiality rules, including notification of their appropriate licensure boards, etc.

1.7.1. Disclosure—When the EC investigates a complaint, it may request information from a variety of sources. The process of obtaining additional information is carefully executed in order to maintain confidentiality. The EC may request information from a variety of sources, including state licensing agencies, academic councils, courts, employers, and other persons and entities. It is within the EC's purview to determine what disclosures are appropriate for particular parties in order to effectively implement its investigatory obligations. Public sanctions by the EC, Disciplinary Council, or Appeal Panel will be publicized as provided in these Procedures. Normally, the EC does not disclose information or documentation reviewed in the course of an investigation unless the EC determines that disclosure is necessary to obtain additional, relevant evidence or to administer the ethics process or is legally required.

Individuals who file a complaint (i.e., complainant) and those who are the subject of one (i.e., respondent) must not disclose to anyone their role in an ethics complaint. Disclosing this information in and of itself may jeopardize the ethics process and violate the rules of fundamental fairness by which all parties are protected. Disclosure of information related to any case under investigation by the EC is prohibited and, if done, will lead to repercussions as outlined in these Procedures (see Section 2.2.3.).

2. Complaints

2.1. Interested Party Complaints

2.1.1. Complaints stating an alleged violation of the Code may originate from any individual, group, or entity within or outside the Association. All complaints must be in writing, signed by the complainant(s), and submitted to the Chairperson of the EC at the address of the AOTA's headquarters. Complainants must complete the Formal Statement of Complaint Form at the end of this document. All complaints shall identify the person against whom the complaint is directed (the respondent), the ethical principles that the complainant believes have been violated, and the key facts of the alleged violations. If lawfully available, supporting documentation should be attached.

2.1.2. Within 90 days of receipt of a complaint, the EC shall make a preliminary assessment of the complaint and decide whether it presents sufficient questions as to a potential ethics violation that an investigation is warranted. Commencing an investigation does not imply a conclusion that an ethical violation has in fact occurred or any judgment as to the ultimate sanction, if any, which may be appropriate. In the event the EC determines that the complaint does not rise to the level of an ethical violation, the EC may direct the parties to utilize *Roberts Rules* and/or other conflict resolution resources via an educative letter. This applies to all complaints including those involving elected/volunteer leadership of the Association related to their official roles.

2.2. Complaints Initiated by the EC

2.2.1. The EC itself may initiate a complaint (a "sua sponte" complaint) when it receives information from a governmental body, certification or similar body, public media, or other source indicating that a person subject to its jurisdiction may have committed acts that violate the Code. AOTA will ordinarily act promptly after learning of the basis of a sua sponte complaint, but there is no specified time limit.

If the EC passes a motion to initiate a sua sponte complaint, the members of the EC will complete the Formal Statement of Complaint Form (at the end of this document) and will describe the nature of the factual allegations that led to the complaint and the manner in which the EC learned of the matter. The Complaint Form will be signed by the Chairperson of the EC on behalf of the EC. The form will be given to the EC staff liaison.

2.2.2. *De Jure* Complaints—*De jure* sua sponte complaints will proceed as follows:

a. The EC staff liaison will present to the EC any findings from external sources (as described above) pertaining to members of AOTA that come to his or her attention and that may warrant sua sponte complaints.

b. Since *de jure* complaints are based upon the findings of fact or conclusions of another official body, the EC will decide whether or not to act based on such findings or conclusions and will not ordinarily initiate another investigation, absent clear and convincing evidence that such findings and conclusions were erroneous or not supported by substantial evidence. Based upon the information presented by the EC staff liaison, the EC will determine whether the findings of the public body also are sufficient to demonstrate an egregious violation of the Code and therefore warrant an ethics charge.

c. If the EC decides that a formal charge is warranted, the Chairperson of the EC will notify the respondent in writing of the formal charge and the proposed education and/or disciplinary action. In response to the *de jure* sua sponte charge by the EC, the respondent may either

1. Accept the decision of the EC (as to both the ethics violation and the sanction) based solely upon the findings of fact and conclusions of the EC or the public body, or

2. Accept the charge that the respondent committed unethical conduct but within 30 days submit to the EC a statement setting forth the reasons why any sanction should not be imposed or reasons why the sanction should be mitigated or reduced, or

3. Within 30 days, present information showing the findings of fact of the official body relied upon by the EC to initiate the charge is clearly erroneous and request reconsideration by the EC. The EC may have the option of opening an investigation or modifying the sanction in the event they find clear and convincing evidence that the findings and the conclusions of the other body are erroneous.

d. In cases of *de jure* complaints, a Disciplinary Council hearing can later be requested (pursuant to Section 5 below) only if the respondent has first exercised Option 2 or 3.

2.2.3. The EC shall have the jurisdiction to investigate, charge, or sanction any matter or person for violations based on information learned in the course of investigating a complaint under Section 2.2.2.

2.3. **Continuation of Complaint Process**—If a member relinquishes membership, fails to renew membership, or fails to cooperate with the ethics investigation, the EC shall nevertheless continue to process the complaint, noting in its report the circumstances of the respondent's action. Such actions shall not deprive the EC of jurisdiction.

3. EC Review and Investigations

3.1. **Initial Action**—The purpose of the preliminary review is to decide whether or not the information submitted with the complaint warrants opening the case. If in its preliminary review of the complaint the EC determines that an investigation is not warranted, the complainant will be so notified.

3.2. **Dismissal of Complaints**—The EC may at any time dismiss a complaint for any of the following reasons:

3.2.1. **Lack of Jurisdiction**—The EC determines that it has no jurisdiction over the respondent (e.g., a complaint against a person who is or was not a member at the time of the alleged incident or who has never been a member).

3.2.2. Absolute Time Limit/Not Timely Filed—The EC determines that the violation of the Code is alleged to have occurred more than 7 years prior to the filing of the complaint.

3.2.3. Subject to Jurisdiction of Another Authority—The EC determines that the complaint is based on matters that are within the authority of and are more properly dealt with by another governmental or nongovernmental body, such as an SRB, NBCOT, an AOTA component other than the EC, an employer, or a court (e.g., accusing a superior of sexual harassment at work, accusing someone of anticompetitive practices subject to the antitrust laws).

3.2.4. No Ethics Violation—The EC finds that the complaint, even if proven, does not state a basis for action under the Code (e.g., simply accusing someone of being unpleasant or rude on an occasion).

3.2.5. Insufficient Evidence—The EC determines that there clearly would not be sufficient factual evidence to support a finding of an ethics violation.

3.2.6. Corrected Violation—The EC determines that any violation it might find already has been or is being corrected, and that this is an adequate result in the given case.

3.2.7. Other good cause.

3.3. Investigator (Avoidance of Conflict of Interest)—The investigator chosen shall not have a conflict of interest (i.e., shall never have had a substantial professional, personal, financial, business, or volunteer relationship with either the complainant or the respondent). In the event that the EC staff liaison has such a conflict, the EC Chairperson shall appoint an alternate investigator who has no conflict of interest.

3.4. Investigation—If an investigation is deemed warranted, the EC Chairperson shall do the following within 15 days: Appoint the EC staff liaison at the AOTA headquarters to investigate the complaint and notify the respondent (by certified, return-receipt mail) that a complaint has been received and an investigation is being conducted. A copy of the complaint and supporting documentation shall be enclosed with this notification. The complainant will also receive notification by certified, return-receipt mail that the complaint is being investigated.

3.4.1. Ordinarily, the investigator will send questions formulated by the EC to be answered by the complainant and/or the respondent.

3.4.2. The complainant shall be given 30 days from receipt of the questions to respond in writing to the investigator.

3.4.3. The respondent shall be given 30 days from receipt of the questions to respond in writing to the investigator.

3.4.4. The EC ordinarily will notify the complainant of any substantive new evidence adverse to the complainant's initial complaint that is discovered in the course of the ethics investigation and allow the complainant to respond to such adverse evidence. In such cases, the complainant will be given a copy of such evidence and will have 14 days in which to submit a written response. If the new evidence clearly shows that there has been no ethics violation, the EC may terminate the proceeding. In addition, if the investigation includes questions for both the respondent and the complainant, the evidence submitted by each party in response to the investigatory questions shall be available to the other party upon their request. The EC may request reasonable payment for copying expenses depending on the volume of material to be sent.

3.4.5. The investigator, in consultation with the EC, may obtain evidence directly from third parties.

3.5. Investigation Timeline—The investigation will be completed within 90 days after receipt of notification by the respondent or his/her designee that an investigation is being conducted, unless the EC determines that special circumstances warrant additional time for the investigation. All timelines noted here can be extended for good cause at the discretion of the EC, including the EC's schedule and additional requests of the respondent. The respondent and the complainant shall be notified in writing if a delay occurs or if the investigational process requires more time.

3.6. Report—The investigator's report shall include the complaint and any documentation on which the EC relied in initiating the investigation and shall state findings without recommendations.

3.7. Cooperation by Member—Every AOTA member has a duty to cooperate reasonably with enforcement processes under the Code. Failure of the respondent to participate and/or cooperate with the investigative process of the EC shall not prevent continuation of the ethics process, and this behavior itself may constitute a violation of the Code.

3.8. Referral of Complaint—The EC may at any time refer a matter to NBCOT, SRB, or other recognized authorities for appropriate action. Despite such referral to an appropriate authority, the EC shall retain jurisdiction. EC action may be stayed for a reasonable period pending notification of a decision by that authority, at the discretion of the EC (and such delays will extend the time periods under these Procedures). A stay in conducting an investigation shall not constitute a waiver by the EC of jurisdiction over the matters. The EC shall provide written notice by mail (requiring signature and proof of date of receipt) to the respondent and the complainant of any such stay of action.

4. EC Review and Decision

4.1. Charges—The EC shall review the investigator's report and shall render a decision on whether a charge by the EC is warranted within 90 days of receipt of the report. The EC may, in the conduct of its review, take whatever further investigatory actions it deems necessary. If the EC determines that an ethics complaint warrants a charge, the EC shall proceed with a disciplinary proceeding by promptly sending a notice of the charge(s) to the respondent and complainant by mail with signature and proof of date received. The notice of the charge(s) shall describe the alleged conduct that, if proven in accordance with these *Procedures,* would constitute a violation of the Code. The notice of charge(s) shall describe the conduct in sufficient detail to inform the respondent of the nature of the unethical behavior that is alleged. The EC may indicate in the notice its preliminary view (absent contrary facts or mitigating circumstances) as to what sanction would be warranted if the violation is proven in accordance with these *Procedures.*

4.2. Respondent's Response—Within 30 days of notification of the EC's decision to charge, and proposed sanction, if any, the respondent shall either

4.2.1. Advise the EC Chairperson in writing that he or she accepts the EC's charge of an ethics violation and the proposed sanction and waives any right to a Disciplinary Council hearing, or

4.2.2. Advise the EC Chairperson in writing that he or she accepts the EC's charge of an ethics violation but believes the sanction is not justified and requests a hearing before the Council on that matter alone, or

4.2.3. Advise the EC Chairperson in writing that he or she contests the EC's charge and the proposed sanction and requests a hearing before the Disciplinary Council.

Failure of the respondent to take one of these actions within the time specified will be deemed to constitute acceptance of the charge and proposed sanction. If the respondent requests a Disciplinary Council hearing, it will be scheduled. If the respondent does not request a Disciplinary Council hearing but accepts the decision, the EC will notify all relevant parties and implement the sanction.

5. The Disciplinary Council

5.1. Purpose—The purpose of the Disciplinary Council (hereinafter to be known as "the Council") hearing is to provide the respondent an opportunity to present evidence and witnesses to answer and refute the charge and/or the proposed sanction and to permit the EC Chairperson or designee (the "EC Chair") to present evidence and witnesses in support of his or her charge. The Council shall consider the matters alleged in the complaint; the matters raised in defense; and other relevant facts, ethical principles, and federal or state law, if applicable. The Council may question the parties concerning and determine ethical issues arising from the factual matters in the case even if those specific ethical issues were not raised by the complainant. The Council also may choose to apply Principles (from the AOTA *Occupational Therapy Code of Ethics*) and Guidelines not originally identified by the EC. The Council may affirm the decision of the EC or reverse or modify it if it finds that the decision was clearly erroneous or a material departure from its written procedure.

5.2. Parties—The parties to a Council Hearing are the respondent and the EC Chairperson.

5.3. Criteria and Process for Selection of Council Chairperson

5.3.1. Criteria

5.3.1.1. Must currently be a member of a Disciplinary Council or a former EC member who has been off the EC for at least 3 years.

5.3.1.2. Must have experience in analyzing/reviewing cases.

5.3.1.3. May be selected from the pool of candidates for the Council.

5.3.1.4. The EC Chairperson shall not serve as the Council chairperson.

5.3.2. Process

5.3.2.1. The Assembly Speaker (in consultation with EC staff liaison) will select the Council chairperson.

5.3.2.2. If the Assembly Speaker needs to be recused from this duty the Vice Speaker will select the chairperson.

5.4. Criteria and Process for Selection of Council Members:

5.4.1. Criteria

5.4.1.1. Association Administrative SOP guidelines in Policy 2.6 shall be considered in the selection of qualified potential candidates for the Council and it shall be composed of qualified individuals and AOTA members drawn from a pool of candidates who meet the criteria outlined below.

5.4.1.2. Members ideally will have some knowledge or experience in the areas of activity that are at issue in the case. They will also have experience in disciplinary hearings and/or general knowledge about ethics as demonstrated by education, presentations, and/or publications.

5.4.1.3. No conflict of interest may exist with either the complainant or the respondent (refer to AOTA Policy 1.22–Conflict of Interest for guidance).

5.4.1.4. No individual may serve on the Disciplinary Council who is currently a member of the EC or the Board of Directors.

5.4.1.5. No individual may serve on the Disciplinary Council who has previously been the subject of an ethics complaint that resulted in a specific EC disciplinary action.

5.4.1.6. The public member on the Disciplinary Council shall have knowledge of the profession and ethical issues.

5.4.1.7. The public member shall not be an occupational therapy practitioner.

5.4.2. Process

5.4.2.1. Potential candidates for the Disciplinary Council pool will be recruited through public postings in Association publications and via the listservs, etc. AOTA leadership will be encouraged to recruit qualified candidates. Potential members of the Council shall be interviewed to ascertain:

(a) Willingness to serve on the Council and availability for a period of 3 years

(b) Qualifications per criteria outlined in section 5.3.1.

5.4.2.2. The President and EC staff liaison will maintain a pool of no less than six (6) and no more than twelve (12) qualified individuals.

5.4.2.3. The President and EC staff liaison will select from the pool the members of each Council within 30 days of notification by a respondent that a Council is being requested.

5.4.2.4. Each council shall be composed of three (3) AOTA members in good standing and a public member.

5.4.2.5. The EC staff liaison will remove anyone with a potential conflict of interest in a particular case from the potential Disciplinary Council pool.

5.5. Notification of Parties (EC Chairperson, Complainant, Respondent, Council Members)

5.5.1. The Council Chairperson shall schedule a hearing date in coordination with the EC staff liaison.

5.5.2. The Council (via the EC staff liaison) shall notify all parties at least forty-five (45) days prior to the hearing of the date, time, and place of hearing.

5.5.3. Case material will be sent to all parties and the Council members by national delivery service or mail with signature required and proof of date received with return receipt.

5.6. Hearing Witnesses, Materials, and Evidence

5.6.1. Within 30 days of notification of the hearing, the respondent shall submit to the Council a written response to the charges, including a detailed statement as to the reasons that he or she is appealing the decision and a list of potential witnesses (if any) with a statement indicating the subject matter they will be addressing.

5.6.2. The complainant before the Council also will submit a list of potential witnesses (if any) to the Council with a statement indicating the subject matter they will be addressing. Only under limited circumstances may the Council consider additional material evidence from the Respondent or the Complainant not presented or available prior to the issuance of their proposed sanction. Such new or additional evidence may be considered by the Council if the Council is satisfied that the Respondent or the Complainant has demonstrated the new evidence was previously unavailable and provided it is submitted to all parties in writing no later than 15 days prior to the hearing.

5.6.3. The Council Chairperson may permit testimony by conference call (at no expense to the participant), limit participation of witnesses in order to curtail repetitive testimony, or prescribe other reasonable arrangements or limitations. The Respondent may elect to appear (at Respondent's own expense) and present testimony.

5.7. Counsel—The Respondent may be represented by legal counsel at his or her own expense. The AOTA legal counsel shall advise and represent the Association at the hearing. The AOTA legal counsel also may advise the Council regarding procedural matters to ensure fairness to all parties. All parties and legal counsel (at the request of the EC or the Council) shall have the opportunity to question witnesses.

5.8. Hearing

5.8.1. The Disciplinary Council hearing shall be recorded by a professional transcription service and shall be limited to two (2) hours.

5.8.2. The Council Chairperson will conduct the hearing and does not vote except in the case of a tie.

5.8.3. Each person present shall be identified for the record and the Chairperson will describe the procedures for the Council hearing. An oral affirmation of truthfulness will be requested from each participant who gives factual testimony in the Council hearing.

5.8.4. The Council Chairperson shall allow for questions.

5.8.5. The EC Chairperson shall present the ethics charge, a summary of the evidence resulting from the investigation and the EC recommendation(s) for disciplinary action against the respondent.

5.8.6. The respondent may present a defense to the charges(s) after the EC presents its case.

5.8.7. Each party and/or their legal representative shall have the opportunity to call witnesses to present testimony and to question any witnesses, including the EC Chairperson or their designee. The Council chairperson shall be entitled to provide reasonable limits on the extent of any witnesses' testimony or any questioning.

5.8.8. The Chairperson may recess the hearing at any time.

5.8.9. The Council Chairperson shall call for final statements from each party before concluding the hearing.

5.8.10. Decisions of the Council will be by majority vote.

5.9. Disciplinary Council Decision

5.9.1. An official copy of the transcript shall be sent to each Council member, the EC Chairperson, AOTA legal counsel, the EC staff liaison, and the respondent and his/her counsel as soon as it is available from the transcription company.

5.9.2. The Chairperson of the Disciplinary Council shall work with the EC staff liaison and the AOTA legal counsel in preparing the text of the final decision.

5.9.3. The Council shall issue a decision in writing to the AOTA Executive Director within thirty (30) days of receiving the written transcription of the hearing (unless special circumstances warrant additional time). The Council decision shall be based on the record and evidence presented and may affirm, modify, or reverse the decision of the EC, including increasing or decreasing the level of sanction or determining that no disciplinary action is warranted.

5.10. Action, Notification, and Timeline Adjustments

5.10.1. A copy of the Disciplinary Council's official decision and appeal process (Section 6) is sent to the respondent, the EC Chairperson, and other appropriate parties within fifteen (15) working days via mail (with signature and proof of date received) after notification of the AOTA Executive Director.

5.10.2. The time limits specified in the *Enforcement Procedures for the Occupational Therapy Code of Ethics* may be extended by mutual consent of the respondent, complainant, and Disciplinary Council Chairperson for good cause by the Chairperson.

5.10.3. Other features of the preceding *Procedures* may be adjusted in particular cases in light of extraordinary circumstances, consistent with fundamental fairness.

5.11. Appeal—Within 30 days after notification of the Council's decision, a respondent upon whom a sanction was imposed may appeal the decision as provided in Section 6. Within 30 days after notification of the Council's decision, the EC may also appeal the decision as provided in Section 6. If no appeal is filed within that time, the Executive Director shall notify appropriate bodies within the Association and make any other notifications deemed necessary.

6. Appeal Process

6.1. Appeals—Either the EC or the respondent may appeal. Appeals shall be written, signed by the appealing party, and sent by certified mail to the Executive Director c/o the Ethics Office of AOTA. The grounds for the appeal shall be fully explained in this document. When an appeal is requested, the other party will be notified.

6.2. Grounds for Appeal—Appeals shall generally address only the issues, procedures, or sanctions that are part of the record before the Disciplinary Council. However, in the interest of fairness, the Appeal Panel may consider newly available evidence relating to the original charge only under extraordinary circumstances.

6.3. Composition and Leadership of Appeal Panel—The Vice-President, Secretary, and Treasurer of the Association shall constitute the Appeal Panel. In the event of vacancies in these positions or the existence of a conflict of interest, the Vice President shall appoint replacements drawn from among the other Board members. If the entire Board of Directors has a conflict of interest (e.g., the Complainant or Respondent is or was recently a member of the Board of Directors), the Board Appeal process shall be followed. The President shall not serve on the Appeal Panel. No individual may serve on the Council who has previously been the subject of an ethics complaint that resulted in a specific EC disciplinary action.

The chair of the Appeal Panel will be selected by its members from among themselves.

6.4. Appeal Process—The Executive Director shall forward any letter of appeal to the Appeal Panel within 15 days of receipt. Within 45 days after the Appeal Panel receives the appeal, the Panel shall determine whether a hearing is warranted according to the Board of Directors policy on appeals (unless it is an EC appeal). If the Panel decides that a hearing is warranted, timely notice for such hearing shall be given to the parties. Participants at the hearing shall be limited to the Respondent and legal counsel (if so desired), the EC Chairperson, Disciplinary Council Chairperson, AOTA legal counsel, or others approved in advance by the Appeal Panel as necessary to the proceedings.

6.5. Decision

6.5.1. The Appeal Panel shall have the power to (a) affirm the decision, or (b) modify the decision, or (c) reverse or remand to the EC, but only if there were procedural errors materially prejudicial to the outcome of the proceeding or if the Disciplinary Council decision was against the clear weight of the evidence.

6.5.2. Within 45 days after receipt of the appeal if no hearing was granted, or within 30 days after receipt of the transcript if a hearing was held, the Appeal Panel shall notify the AOTA Executive Director of its decision. The Executive Director shall promptly notify the respondent, the original complainant, appropriate bodies of the Association, and any other parties deemed appropriate. For Association purposes, the decision of the Appeal Panel shall be final.

7. Notifications

All notifications referred to in these *Procedures* shall be in writing and shall be delivered by national delivery service or mail with signature and proof of date of receipt required.

8. Records and Reports

At the completion of the Ethics process, the written records and reports that state the initial basis for the complaint, material evidence, and the disposition of the complaint shall be retained in the Ethics Office for a period of 5 years. Electronic files will be kept indefinitely.

9. Publication

Final decisions will be publicized only after any Appeal Panel process has been completed.

10. Modification

AOTA reserves the right to (a) modify the time periods, procedures, or application of these Procedures for good cause consistent with fundamental fairness in a given case and (b) modify its Code of Ethics and/or these *Procedures*, with such modifications to be applied only prospectively.

Adopted by the Representative Assembly 2006CO458 as Attachment A of the Standard Operating Procedures (SOPs) of the Commission on Standards and Ethics (SEC).

Reviewed by BPPC 1/04, 1/05, 9/06, 1/07

Adopted by RA 4/96, 5/04, 5/05, 11/06, 4/07

Revised by SEC 4/98, 4/00, 1/02, 1/04, 12/04, 9/06

Revised by EC 12/06, 2/07

Note: The Commission on Standards and Ethics (SEC) changed to Ethics Commission (EC) in September 2005 as per AOTA Bylaws.

AMERICAN OCCUPATIONAL THERAPY ASSOCIATION
ETHICS COMMISSION

Formal Complaint of Alleged Violation of the
Occupational Therapy Code of Ethics

If an investigation is deemed necessary, a copy of this form will be provided to the individual against whom the complaint is filed.

DATE _____

COMPLAINANT: (Information regarding individual filing the complaint)

NAME _____ SIGNATURE _____

ADDRESS _____ TELEPHONE _____

_____ E-MAIL ADDRESS _____

RESPONDENT: (Information regarding individual against whom the complaint is directed)

NAME _____ TELEPHONE _____

ADDRESS _____ E-MAIL ADDRESS _____

_____

1. Indicate the Ethical Principle(s) you believe have been violated:

2. Summarize in an attachment the **facts and circumstances, including dates and events, warranting the complaint.** Attach documentation that you think would help the Ethics Commission in its assessment of this complaint. **Please sign and date all documents you have written and are submitting.** *Do not include confidential documents such as patient or employment records.* (Statements from witnesses are not necessary at this time.)

3. If you have filed a complaint about this same matter to any other agency (e.g., NBCOT; SRB; academic institution; any federal, state, or local official), indicate to whom it was submitted and the approximate date(s).

4. What steps have been taken to resolve this complaint?

I CERTIFY THAT THE STATEMENTS/INFORMATION WITHIN THIS COMPLAINT ARE CORRECT AND TRUTHFUL TO THE BEST OF MY KNOWLEDGE.

SIGNATURE _____

Send completed form, with accompanying documentation, IN AN ENVELOPE MARKED *CONFIDENTIAL* to:

Ethics Commission
American Occupational Therapy Association, Inc.
Attn: Staff Liaison to the EC/Ethics Office
4720 Montgomery Lane, PO Box 31220
Bethesda, MD 20824-1220

Office Use Only:
Membership Verified? ❏ Yes ❏ No
By: _____

EC/forms/complaint form, Revised: 1/04

Guidelines to the
Occupational Therapy Code of Ethics

Professional Behaviors	Principles From Code
1. **HONESTY:** *Professionals must be honest with themselves, must be honest with all whom they come in contact with, and must know their strengths and limitations.*	
1.1. In education, research, practice, and leadership roles, individuals must be honest in receiving and disseminating information by providing opportunities for informed consent and for discussion of available options.	Veracity
1.2. Occupational therapy practitioners must be certain that informed consent has been obtained prior to the initiation of services, including evaluation. If the service recipient cannot give informed consent, the practitioner must be sure that consent has been obtained from the person who is legally responsible for the service recipient.	Autonomy, Veracity
1.3. Occupational therapy practitioners must be truthful about their individual competencies as well as the competence of those under their supervision. In some cases the therapist may need to refer the client to another professional to assure that the most appropriate services are provided.	Duty, Veracity
1.4. Referrals to other health care specialists shall be based exclusively on the other provider's competence and ability to provide the needed service.	Beneficence
1.5. All documentation must accurately reflect the nature and quantity of services provided.	Veracity
1.6. Occupational therapy practitioners terminate services when they do not meet the needs and goals of the recipient or when services no longer produce a measurable outcome.	Procedural Justice, Beneficence
1.7. All marketing and advertising must be truthful and carefully presented to avoid misleading the client or the public.	Veracity

Professional Behaviors	Principles From Code
1.8. All occupational therapy personnel shall accurately represent their credentials and roles.	Veracity
1.9. Occupational therapy personnel shall not use funds for unintended purposes or misappropriate funds.	Duty, Veracity
2. COMMUNICATION: *Communication is important in all aspects of occupational therapy. Individuals must be conscientious and truthful in all facets of written, verbal, and electronic communication.*	
2.1. Occupational therapy personnel do not make deceptive, fraudulent, or misleading statements about the nature of the services they provide or the outcomes that can be expected.	Veracity
2.2. Professional contracts for occupational therapy services shall explicitly describe the type and duration of services as well as the duties and responsibilities of all involved parties.	Veracity, Procedural Justice
2.3. Documentation for reimbursement purposes shall be done in accordance with applicable laws, guidelines, and regulations.	Veracity, Procedural Justice
2.4. Documentation shall accurately reflect the services delivered and the outcomes. It shall be of the kind and quality that satisfies the scrutiny of peer reviews, legal proceedings, payers, regulatory bodies, and accrediting agencies.	Veracity, Procedural Justice, Duty
2.5. Occupational therapy personnel must be honest in gathering and giving fact-based information regarding job performance and fieldwork performance. Information given shall be timely and truthful, accurate, and respectful of all parties involved.	Veracity, Fidelity
2.6. Documentation for supervisory purposes shall accurately reflect the factual components of the interactions and the expected outcomes.	Veracity
2.7. Occupational therapy personnel must give credit and recognition when using the work of others.	Veracity, Procedural Justice
2.8. Occupational therapy personnel do not fabricate data, falsify information, or plagiarize.	Veracity, Procedural Justice
2.9. Occupational therapy personnel refrain from using biased or derogatory language in written, verbal, and electronic communication about clients, students, research participants, and colleagues.	Nonmaleficence, Fidelity

Professional Behaviors	Principles From Code
2.10. Occupational therapy personnel who provide information through oral and written means shall emphasize that ethical and appropriate service delivery for clients cannot be done without proper individualized evaluations and plans of care.	Beneficence
3. ENSURING THE COMMON GOOD: *Occupational therapy personnel are expected to increase awareness of the profession's social responsibilities to help ensure the common good.*	
3.1. Occupational therapy personnel take steps to make sure that employers are aware of the ethical principles of the profession and occupational therapy personnel's obligation to adhere to those ethical principles.	Duty
3.2. Occupational therapy personnel shall be diligent stewards of human, financial, and material resources of their employers. They shall refrain from exploiting these resources for personal gain.	Fidelity
3.3. Occupational therapy personnel should actively work with their employer to prevent discrimination and unfair labor practices. They should also advocate for employees with disabilities to ensure the provision of reasonable accommodations.	Procedural Justice
3.4. Occupational therapy personnel should actively participate with their employer in the formulation of policies and procedures. They should do this to ensure that these policies and procedures are legal, in accordance with regulations governing aspects of practice, and consistent with the AOTA Occupational Therapy Code of Ethics.	Procedural Justice
3.5. Occupational therapy personnel in educational settings are responsible for promoting ethical conduct by students, faculty, and fieldwork colleagues.	Duty, Fidelity
3.6. Occupational therapy personnel involved in or preparing to be involved in research, including education and policy research, need to obtain all necessary approvals prior to initiating research.	Procedural Justice

Professional Behaviors	Principles From Code
4. COMPETENCE: *Occupational therapy personnel are expected to work within their areas of competence and to pursue opportunities to update, increase, and expand their competence.*	
4.1. Occupational therapy personnel developing new areas of competence (skills, techniques, approaches) must engage in appropriate study and training, under appropriate supervision, before incorporating new areas into their practice.	Duty
4.2. When generally recognized standards do not exist in emerging areas of practice, occupational therapy personnel must take responsible steps to ensure their own competence.	Duty
4.3. Occupational therapy personnel shall develop an understanding and appreciation for different cultures in order to be able to provide culturally competent service. Culturally competent practitioners are aware of how service delivery can be affected by economic, age, ethnic, racial, geographic, gender, gender identity, religious, and political factors, as well as marital status, sexual orientation, and disability.	Beneficence, Duty
4.4. In areas where the ability to communicate with the client is limited (e.g., aphasia, different language, literacy), occupational therapy personnel shall take appropriate steps to facilitate meaningful communication and comprehension.	Autonomy
4.5. Occupational therapy personnel must ensure that skilled occupational therapy interventions or techniques are performed only by qualified persons.	Duty, Beneficence, Nonmaleficence
4.6. Occupational therapy administrators (academic, research, and clinical) are responsible for ensuring the competence and qualifications of personnel in their employment.	Beneficence, Nonmaleficence
5. CONFIDENTIAL AND PROTECTED INFORMATION: *Information that is confidential must remain confidential. This information cannot be shared verbally, electronically, or in writing without appropriate consent. Information must be shared on a need-to-know basis only with those having primary responsibilities for decision making.*	
5.1. All occupational therapy personnel shall respect the confidential nature of information gained in any occupational therapy interaction. The only exceptions are when a practitioner or staff member believes that an individual is in serious, foreseeable, or imminent harm. In this instance, laws and regulations require disclosure to appropriate authorities without consent.	Confidentiality

Professional Behaviors	Principles From Code
5.2. Occupational therapy personnel shall respect the clients' and colleagues' right to privacy.	Confidentiality
5.3. Occupational therapy personnel shall maintain the confidentiality of all verbal, written, electronic, augmentative, and non-verbal communications (as required by HIPAA).	Confidentiality

6. CONFLICT OF INTEREST: *Avoidance of real or perceived conflict of interest is imperative to maintaining the integrity of interactions.*

6.1. Occupational therapy personnel shall be alert to and avoid any action that would interfere with the exercise of impartial professional judgment during the delivery of occupational therapy services.	Nonmaleficence
6.2. Occupational therapy personnel shall not take advantage of or exploit anyone to further their own personal interests.	Nonmaleficence
6.3. Gifts and remuneration from individuals, agencies, or companies must be reported in accordance with employer policies as well as state and federal guidelines.	Veracity, Procedural Justice
6.4. Occupational therapy personnel shall not accept obligations or duties that may compete with or be in conflict with their duties to their employers.	Veracity, Fidelity
6.5. Occupational therapy personnel shall not use their position or the knowledge gained from their position in such a way that knowingly gives rise to real or perceived conflict of interest between themselves and their employers, other association members or bodies, and/or other organizations.	Veracity, Fidelity

7. IMPAIRED PRACTITIONER: *Occupational therapy personnel who cannot competently perform their duties after reasonable accommodation are considered to be impaired. The occupational therapy practitioner's basic duty to students, patients, colleagues, and research subjects is to ensure that no harm is done. It is difficult to report a professional colleague who is impaired. The motive for this action must be to provide for the protection and safety of all, including the person who is impaired.*

7.1. Occupational therapy personnel shall be aware of their own personal problems and limitations that may interfere with their ability to perform their job competently. They should know when these problems have the potential to cause harm to clients, colleagues, students, research participants, or others.	Nonmaleficence

Professional Behaviors	Principles From Code
7.2. The individual should seek the appropriate professional help and take steps to remedy personal problems and limitations that interfere with job performance.	Nonmaleficence
7.3. Occupational therapy personnel who believe that a colleague's impairment interferes with safe and effective practice should, when possible, discuss their questions and concerns with the individual and assist their colleague in seeking appropriate help or treatment.	Nonmaleficence
7.4. When efforts to assist an impaired colleague fail, the occupational therapy practitioner is responsible for reporting the individual to the appropriate authority (e.g., employer, agency, licensing or regulatory board, certification body, professional organization).	Nonmaleficence
8. SEXUAL RELATIONSHIPS: *Sexual relationships that occur during any professional interaction are forms of misconduct.*	
8.1. Because of potential coercion or harm to former clients, students, or research participants, occupational therapy practitioners are responsible for ensuring that the individual with whom they enter into a romantic/sexual relationship has not been coerced or exploited in any way.	Nonmaleficence
8.2. Sexual relationships with current clients, employees, students, or research participants are not permissible, even if the relationship is consensual.	Nonmaleficence
8.3. Occupational therapy personnel must not sexually harass any persons.	Nonmaleficence
8.4. Occupational therapy personnel have full responsibility to set clear and appropriate boundaries in their professional interactions.	Nonmaleficence
9. PAYMENT FOR SERVICES AND OTHER FINANCIAL ARRANGEMENTS: *Occupational therapy personnel shall not guarantee or promise specific outcomes for occupational therapy services. Payment for occupational therapy services shall not be contingent on successful outcomes.*	
9.1. Occupational therapy personnel shall only collect fees legally. Fees shall be fair and reasonable and commensurate with services delivered.	Procedural Justice

Professional Behaviors	Principles From Code
9.2. Occupational therapy personnel do not ordinarily participate in bartering for services because of potential exploitation and conflict of interest. However, such an arrangement may be appropriate if it is not clinically contraindicated, if the relationship is not exploitative, and if bartering is a culturally appropriate custom.	Beneficence
9.3. Occupational therapy practitioners can render pro bono ("for the good," free of charge) or reduced-fee occupational therapy services for selected individuals only when consistent with guidelines of the business/facility, third-party payer, or government agency.	Beneficence, Procedural Justice
9.4. Occupational therapy personnel may engage in volunteer activities to improve access to occupational therapy or by providing individual service and expertise to charitable organizations.	Beneficence
9.5. Occupational therapy personnel who participate in a business arrangement as owner, stockholder, partner, or employee have an obligation to maintain the ethical principles and standards of the profession. They also shall refrain from working for or doing business with organizations that engage in illegal or unethical business practices (e.g., fraudulent billing).	Procedural Justice
10. RESOLVING ETHICAL ISSUES: *Occupational therapy personnel should utilize any and all resources available to them to identify and resolve conflicts and/or ethical dilemmas.*	
10.1. Occupational therapy personnel are obligated to be familiar with the Code and its application to their respective work environments. Occupational therapy practitioners are expected to share the Code with their employer and other employees and colleagues. Lack of familiarity with and knowledge of the Code is not an excuse or a defense against a charge of ethical misconduct.	Duty
10.2. Occupational therapy personnel who are uncertain of whether a specific action would violate the Code have a responsibility to consult with knowledgeable individuals, ethics committees, or other appropriate authorities.	Duty
10.3. When conflicts occur in professional organizations, members must clarify the nature of the conflict and, where possible, seek to resolve the conflict in a way that permits the fullest adherence to the Code.	Fidelity

Professional Behaviors	Principles From Code
10.4. Occupational therapy personnel shall attempt to resolve perceived violations of the Code within institutions by utilizing internal resources.	Fidelity
10.5. If the informal resolution is not appropriate or is not effective, the next step is to take action by consultation with or referral to institutional, local, district, territorial, state, or national groups who have jurisdiction over occupational therapy practice.	Fidelity
10.6. Occupational therapy personnel shall cooperate with ethics committee proceedings and comply with resulting requirements. Failure to cooperate is, in itself, an ethical violation.	Procedural Justice
10.7. Occupational therapy personnel shall file only formal ethics complaints aimed at protecting the public or promoting professional conduct rather than harming or discrediting a colleague.	Fidelity

Authors
Ethics Commission (EC)

S. Maggie Reitz, PhD, OTR/L, FAOTA, *Chairperson*
Darryl John Austin, MS, OT/L
Lea C. Brandt, OTD, OTR/L
Betsy DeBrakeleer, COTA/L, AP, ROH
Linda Gabriel Franck, PHD, OTR/L
Donna F. Homenko, RDH, PhD
Lorie J. McQuade, MEd, CRC
Deborah Yarett Slater, MS, OT/L, FAOTA, *Staff Liaison*

Note: Commission on Standards and Ethics (SEC) changed to Ethics Commission (EC) in September 2005 per AOTA Bylaws. This document was developed by the EC in 2005 and replaces the 1998 document of the same name.

A previous edition was published and copyrighted in 1998 in the *American Journal of Occupational Therapy, 52,* 881–884.

Copyright © 2006, by the American Occupational Therapy Association. Previously published in the *American Journal of Occupational Therapy, 60,* 652–658.

Note. This AOTA *Guidelines to the Occupational Therapy Code of Ethics* is one of the three documents that constitute the "Ethics Standards." The other two are the *Occupational Therapy Code of Ethics (2005)* and the *Core Values and Attitudes of Occupational Therapy Practice* (1993).

Occupational Therapy Code of Ethics (2005)

Preamble

The American Occupational Therapy Association (AOTA) *Occupational Therapy Code of Ethics (2005)* is a public statement of principles used to promote and maintain high standards of conduct within the profession and is supported by the *Core Values and Attitudes of Occupational Therapy Practice* (AOTA, 1993). Members of AOTA are committed to promoting inclusion, diversity, independence, and safety for all recipients in various stages of life, health, and illness and to empower all beneficiaries of occupational therapy. This commitment extends beyond service recipients to include professional colleagues, students, educators, businesses, and the community.

Fundamental to the mission of the occupational therapy profession is the therapeutic use of everyday life activities (occupations) with individuals or groups for the purpose of participation in roles and situations in home, school, workplace, community, and other settings. "Occupational therapy addresses the physical, cognitive, psychosocial, sensory, and other aspects of performance in a variety of contexts to support engagement in everyday life activities that affect health, well-being and quality of life" (*Definition of Occupational Therapy Practice for the AOTA Model Practice Act,* 2004). Occupational therapy personnel have an ethical responsibility first and foremost to recipients of service as well as to society.

The historical foundation of this Code is based on ethical reasoning surrounding practice and professional issues, as well as empathic reflection regarding these interactions with others. This reflection resulted in the establishment of principles that guide ethical action. Ethical action goes beyond rote following of rules or application of principles; rather, it is a manifestation of moral character and mindful reflection. It is a commitment to beneficence for the sake of others, to virtuous practice of artistry and science, to genuinely good behaviors, and to noble acts of courage. It is an empathic way of being among others, which is made every day by all occupational therapy personnel.

The AOTA *Occupational Therapy Code of Ethics (2005)* is an aspirational guide to professional conduct when ethical issues surface. Ethical decision making is a process that includes awareness regarding how the outcome will impact occupational therapy clients in all spheres. Applications of Code principles are considered situation-specific, and where a conflict exists, occupational therapy personnel will pursue responsible efforts for resolution.

The specific purpose of the AOTA *Occupational Therapy Code of Ethics (2005)* is to:

1. Identify and describe the principles supported by the occupational therapy profession

2. Educate the general public and members regarding established principles to which occupational therapy personnel are accountable

3. Socialize occupational therapy personnel new to the practice to expected standards of conduct

4. Assist occupational therapy personnel in recognition and resolution of ethical dilemmas.

The AOTA *Occupational Therapy Code of Ethics* (2005) defines the set principles that apply to occupational therapy personnel at all levels:

Principle 1. Occupational therapy personnel shall demonstrate a concern for the safety and well-being of the recipients of their services. (BENEFICENCE)

Occupational therapy personnel shall

A. Provide services in a fair and equitable manner. They shall recognize and appreciate the cultural components of economics, geography, race, ethnicity, religious and political factors, marital status, age, sexual orientation, gender identity, and disability of all recipients of their services.

B. Strive to ensure that fees are fair and reasonable and commensurate with services performed. When occupational therapy practitioners set fees, they shall set fees considering institutional, local, state, and federal requirements, and with due regard for the service recipient's ability to pay.

C. Make every effort to advocate for recipients to obtain needed services through available means.

D. Recognize the responsibility to promote public health and the safety and well-being of individuals, groups, and/or communities.

Principle 2. Occupational therapy personnel shall take measures to ensure a recipient's safety and avoid imposing or inflicting harm. (NONMALEFICENCE)

Occupational therapy personnel shall

A. Maintain therapeutic relationships that shall not exploit the recipient of services sexually, physically, emotionally, psychologically, financially, socially, or in any other manner.

B. Avoid relationships or activities that conflict or interfere with therapeutic professional judgment and objectivity.

C. Refrain from any undue influences that may compromise provision of service.

D. Exercise professional judgment and critically analyze directives that could result in potential harm before implementation.

E. Identify and address personal problems that may adversely impact professional judgment and duties.

F. Bring concerns regarding impairment of professional skills of a colleague to the attention of the appropriate authority when or if attempts to address concerns are unsuccessful.

Principle 3. Occupational therapy personnel shall respect recipients to assure their rights. (AUTONOMY, CONFIDENTIALITY)

Occupational therapy personnel shall

A. Collaborate with recipients, and if they desire, families, significant others, and/or caregivers in setting goals and priorities throughout the intervention process, including full disclosure of the nature, risk, and potential outcomes of any interventions.

B. Obtain informed consent from participants involved in research activities and ensure that they understand potential risks and outcomes.

C. Respect the individual's right to refuse professional services or involvement in research or educational activities.

D. Protect all privileged confidential forms of written, verbal, and electronic communication gained from educational, practice, research, and investigational activities unless otherwise mandated by local, state, or federal regulations.

Principle 4. Occupational therapy personnel shall achieve and continually maintain high standards of competence. (DUTY)

Occupational therapy personnel shall

A. Hold the appropriate national, state, or any other requisite credentials for the services they provide.

B. Conform to AOTA standards of practice and official documents.

C. Take responsibility for maintaining and documenting competence in practice, education, and research by participating in professional development and educational activities.

D. Be competent in all topic areas in which they provide instruction to consumers, peers, and/or students.

E. Critically examine available evidence so they may perform their duties on the basis of current information.

F. Protect service recipients by ensuring that duties assumed by or assigned to other occupational therapy personnel match credentials, qualifications, experience, and scope of practice.

G. Provide appropriate supervision to individuals for whom they have supervisory responsibility in accordance with Association official documents; local, state, and federal or national laws and regulations; and institutional policies and procedures.

H. Refer to or consult with other service providers whenever such a referral or consultation would be helpful to the care of the recipient of service. The referral or consultation process shall be done in collaboration with the recipient of service.

Principle 5. Occupational therapy personnel shall comply with laws and Association policies guiding the profession of occupational therapy. (PROCEDURAL JUSTICE)

Occupational therapy personnel shall

A. Familiarize themselves with and seek to understand and abide by institutional rules; applicable Association policies; and local, state, and federal/national/international laws.

B. Be familiar with revisions in those laws and Association policies that apply to the profession of occupational therapy and shall inform employers, employees, and colleagues of those changes.

C. Encourage those they supervise in occupational therapy–related activities to adhere to the Code.

D. Take reasonable steps to ensure employers are aware of occupational therapy's ethical obligations, as set forth in this Code, and of the implications of those obligations for occupational therapy practice, education, and research.

E. Record and report in an accurate and timely manner all information related to professional activities.

Principle 6. Occupational therapy personnel shall provide accurate information when representing the profession. (VERACITY)

Occupational therapy personnel shall

A. Represent their credentials, qualifications, education, experience, training, and competence accurately. This is of particular importance for those to whom occupational therapy personnel provide their services or with whom occupational therapy personnel have a professional relationship.

B. Disclose any professional, personal, financial, business, or volunteer affiliations that may pose a conflict of interest to those with whom they may establish a professional, contractual, or other working relationship.

C. Refrain from using or participating in the use of any form of communication that contains false, fraudulent, deceptive, or unfair statements or claims.

D. Identify and fully disclose to all appropriate persons errors that compromise recipients' safety.

E. Accept responsibility for their professional actions that reduce the public's trust in occupational therapy services and those that perform those services.

Principle 7. Occupational therapy personnel shall treat colleagues and other professionals with respect, fairness, discretion, and integrity. (FIDELITY)

Occupational therapy personnel shall

A. Preserve, respect, and safeguard confidential information about colleagues and staff, unless otherwise mandated by national, state, or local laws.

B. Accurately represent the qualifications, views, contributions, and findings of colleagues.

C. Take adequate measures to discourage, prevent, expose, and correct any breaches of the Code and report any breaches of the Code to the appropriate authority.

D. Avoid conflicts of interest and conflicts of commitment in employment and volunteer roles.

E. Use conflict resolution and/or alternative dispute resolution resources to resolve organizational and interpersonal conflicts.

F. Familiarize themselves with established policies and procedures for handling concerns about this Code, including familiarity with national, state, local, district, and territorial procedures for handling ethics complaints. These include policies and procedures created by AOTA, licensing and regulatory bodies, employers, agencies, certification boards, and other organizations having jurisdiction over occupational therapy practice.

Glossary

Autonomy
The right of an individual to self-determination. The ability to independently act on one's decisions for one's own well-being (Beauchamp & Childress, 2001).

Beneficence
Doing good for others or bringing about good for them. The duty to confer benefits to others.

Confidentiality
Not disclosing data or information that should be kept private to prevent harm and to abide by policies, regulations, and laws.

Dilemma
A situation in which one moral conviction or right action conflicts with another. It exists because there is no one, clear-cut, right answer.

Duty
Actions required of professionals by society or actions that are self-imposed.

Ethics
A systematic study of morality (i.e., rules of conduct that are grounded in philosophical principles and theory).

Fidelity

Faithfully fulfilling vows and promises, agreements, and discharging fiduciary responsibilities (Beauchamp & Childress, 2001).

Justice

Three types of justice are

> **Compensatory justice**—Making reparation for wrongs that have been done.
>
> **Distributive justice**—The act of distributing goods and burdens among members of society.
>
> **Procedural justice**—Assuring that processes are organized in a fair manner and policies or laws are followed.

Morality

Personal beliefs regarding values, rules, and principles of what is right or wrong. Morality may be culture-based or culture-driven.

Nonmaleficence

Not harming or causing harm to be done to oneself or others; the duty to ensure that no harm is done.

Veracity

A duty to tell the truth; avoid deception.

References

American Occupational Therapy Association. (1993). Core values and attitudes of occupational therapy practice. *American Journal of Occupational Therapy, 47,* 1085–1086.

American Occupational Therapy Association. (1998). Guidelines to the occupational therapy code of ethics. *American Journal of Occupational Therapy, 52,* 881–884.

American Occupational Therapy Association. (2004). Association policies. *American Journal of Occupational Therapy, 58,* 694–695.

Beauchamp, T. L., & Childress, J. F. (2001). *Principles of biomedical ethics* (5th ed.). New York: Oxford University Press.

Definition of Occupational Therapy Practice forthe AOTA Model Practice Act. (2004). Retrieved April 9, 2005, from www.aota.org/members/area4/docs/defotpractice.pdf

Authors

Commission on Standards and Ethics (SEC):

S. Maggie Reitz, PhD, OTR/L, FAOTA, *Chairperson*
Melba Arnold, MS, OTR/L
Linda Gabriel Franck, PhD, OTR/L
Darryl J. Austin, MS, OT/L
Diane Hill, COTA/L, AP, ROH
Lorie J. McQuade, MEd, CRC
Daryl K. Knox, MD
Deborah Yarett Slater, MS, OT/L, FAOTA, *Staff Liaison*

With contributions to the Preamble by

Suzanne Peloquin, PhD, OTR, FAOTA

Adopted by the RepresentativeAssembly 2005C202

Note. This document replaces the 2000 document, *Occupational Therapy Code of Ethics (2000) (American Journal of Occupational Therapy, 54,* 614–616).

Prepared 4/7/2000, revised draft 1/2005, second revision 4/2005 by SEC.

Note: Commission on Standards and Ethics (SEC) changed to Ethics Commission (EC) in September 2005 per AOTA Bylaws.

Note. This AOTA *Occupational Therapy Code of Ethics* is one of three documents that constitute the "Ethics Standards." The other two are the *Core Values and Attitudes of Occupational Therapy Practice* (1993) and the *Guidelines to the Occupational Therapy Code of Ethics* (2006).

Guidelines

Guidelines for Documentation of Occupational Therapy

Documentation is necessary whenever professional services are provided to a client. Occupational therapists and occupational therapy assistants[1] determine the appropriate type of documentation and document the services provided within their scope of practice. This document, based on the *Occupational Therapy Practice Framework: Domain and Process* (American Occupational Therapy Association [AOTA], 2002, 2008), describes the components and the purpose of professional documentation used in occupational therapy. AOTA's *Standards of Practice for Occupational Therapy* (2005) state that an occupational therapy practitioner[2] documents the occupational therapy services and "abides by the time frames, format, and standards established by the practice settings, government agencies, external accreditation programs, payers, and AOTA documents" (p. 664). In this document, *client* may refer to an individual, organization, or population.

The purpose of documentation is to

- Articulate the rationale for provision of occupational therapy services and the relationship of this service to the client's outcomes

- Reflect the occupational therapy practitioners' clinical reasoning and professional judgment

- Communicate information about the client from the occupational therapy perspective

- Create a chronological record of client status, occupational therapy services provided to the client, and client outcomes.

Types of Documentation

Box 1 outlines common types of reports. Depending on the service delivery and setting, reports may be named differently or combined and reorganized to meet the specific needs of the setting. Occupational therapy documentation should always record the professional's activity in the areas of evaluation, intervention, and outcomes (AOTA, 2002, 2008).

Box 1. Common Types of Occupational Therapy Reports

Process Areas	Type of Report
I. Evaluation	A. Evaluation or Screening Report
	B. Reevaluation Report
II. Intervention	1. Intervention Plan
	2. Occupational Therapy Service Contacts
	3. Progress Report
	4. Transition Plan
III. Outcomes	5. Discharge/Discontinuation Report

[1]*Occupational therapists* are responsible for all aspects of occupational therapy service delivery and are accountable for the safety and effectiveness of the occupational therapy service delivery process. *Occupational therapy assistants* deliver occupational therapy services under the supervision of and in partnership with an occupational therapist (AOTA, 2004).

[2]When the term occupational therapy practitioner is used in this document, it refers to both occupational therapists and occupational therapy assistants (AOTA, 2006).

Content of Reports

I. Evaluation

A. Evaluation or Screening Report

    1. Documents the referral source and data gathered through the evaluation process, including

        a. Description of the client's occupational profile

        b. Analysis of occupational performance and identification of factors that hinder and support performance in areas of occupation

        c. Delineation of specific areas of occupation and occupational performance that will be targeted for intervention and outcomes expected.

    2. An abbreviated evaluation process (e.g., screening) documents only limited areas of occupation and occupational performance applicable to the client and to the situation.

    3. Suggested content with examples includes

        a. *Client information*—name/agency, date of birth, gender, health status, applicable medical/educational/developmental diagnoses, precautions, and contraindications

        b. *Referral information*—date and source of referral, services requested, reason for referral, funding source, and anticipated length of service

        c. *Occupational profile*—client's reason for seeking occupational therapy services, current areas of occupation that are successful and problematic, contexts and environments that support and hinder occupations, medical/educational/work history, occupational history (e.g., patterns of living, interest, values), client's priorities, and targeted outcomes

        d. *Assessments used and results*—types of assessments used and results (e.g., interviews, record reviews, observations, standardized or nonstandardized assessments), and confidence in test results

        e. *Analysis of occupational performance*—description of and judgment about performance skills, performance patterns, contexts and environments, features of the activities, and client factors that facilitate and inhibit performance

        f. *Summary and analysis*—interpretation and summary of data as it is related to occupational profile and referring concern

        g. *Recommendation*—judgment regarding appropriateness of occupational therapy services or other services.

    Note: Intervention goals addressing anticipated outcomes, objectives, and frequency of therapy are listed on the Intervention Plan (see below).

B. Reevaluation Report

    1. Documents the results of the reevaluation process. Frequency of reevaluation depends on the needs of the setting and the progress of the client.

    2. Suggested content with examples include

        a. *Client information*—name/agency, date of birth, gender, applicable medical/educational/developmental diagnoses, precautions, and contraindications

b. *Occupational profile*—updates on current areas of occupation that are successful and problematic, contexts and environments that support or hinder occupations, summary of any new medical/educational/work information, and updates or changes to client's priorities and targeted outcomes

c. *Reevaluation results*—focus of reevaluation, specific types of assessments used, and client's performance and subjective responses

d. *Summary and analysis*—interpretation and summary of data as related to referring concern and comparison of results with previous evaluation results

e. *Recommendations*—changes to occupational therapy services, revision or continuation of goals and objectives, frequency of occupational therapy services, and recommendation for referral to other professionals or agencies where applicable.

II. Intervention

A. Intervention Plan

1. Documents the goals, intervention approaches, and types of interventions to be used to achieve the client's identified targeted outcomes based on results of evaluation or reevaluation processes. Includes recommendations or referrals to other professionals and agencies.

2. Suggested content with examples include

   a. *Client information*—name/agency, date of birth, gender, precautions, and contraindications

   b. *Intervention goals*—measurable goals and short-term objectives directly related to the client's ability and need to engage in desired occupations

   c. *Intervention approaches and types of interventions to be used*—intervention approaches that include create/promote, establish/restore, maintain, modify, and prevent; types of interventions that include consultation process, education process, advocacy, therapeutic use of occupations or activities, and therapeutic use of self

   d. *Service delivery mechanisms*—service provider, service location, and frequency and duration of services

   e. *Plan for discharge*—discontinuation criteria, location of discharge, and follow-up care

   f. *Outcome measures*—outcomes that include improved occupational performance, adaptation, role competence, improved health and wellness, prevention of further difficulties, improved quality of life, self-advocacy, and occupational justice

   g. *Professionals responsible and date of plan*—names and positions of persons overseeing plan, date plan was developed, and date when plan was modified or reviewed.

B. Occupational Therapy Service Contacts

1. Documents contacts between the client and the occupational therapy practitioner. Records the types of interventions used and client's response. Includes telephone contacts, interventions, and meetings with others.

2. Suggested content with examples include

   a. *Client information*—name/agency, date of birth, gender, diagnosis, precautions, and contraindications

   b. *Therapy log*—date, type of contact, names/positions of persons involved, summary or significant information communicated during contacts, client attendance and participation in intervention, reason service is missed, types of interventions used, client's response, environmental or task modification, assistive or adaptive devices used or fabricated, statement of any training education or consultation provided, and the persons present.

C. Progress Report

1. Summarizes intervention process and documents client's progress toward goals achievement. Includes new data collected; modifications of treatment plan; and statement of need for continuation, discontinuation, or referral.

2. Suggested content with examples include

a. *Client information*—name/agency, date of birth, gender, diagnosis, precautions, and contraindications

b. *Summary of services provided*—brief statement of frequency of services and length of time services have been provided; techniques and strategies used; environmental or task modifications provided; adaptive equipment or orthotics provided; medical, educational, or other pertinent client updates; client's response to occupational therapy services; and programs or training provided to the client or caregivers

c. *Current client performance*—client's progress toward the goals and client's performance in areas of occupations

d. *Plan or recommendations*—recommendations and rationale as well as client's input to changes or continuation of plan.

D. Transition Plan

1. Documents the formal transition plan and is written when client is transitioning from one service setting to another within a service delivery system.

2. Suggested content with examples include

a. *Client information*—name/agency, date of birth, gender, diagnosis, precautions, and contraindications

b. *Client's current status*—client's current performance in occupations

c. *Transition plan*—name of current service setting and name of setting to which client will transition, reason for transition, time frame in which transition will occur, and outline of activities to be carried out during the transition plan

d. *Recommendations*—recommendations and rationale for occupational therapy services, modifications or accommodations needed, and assistive technology and environmental modifications needed.

III. Outcomes

A. Discharge Report—Summary of Occupational Therapy Services and Outcomes

1. Summarize the changes in client's ability to engage in occupations between the initial evaluation and discontinuation of services and make recommendations as applicable.

2. Suggested content with examples include

a. *Client information*—name/agency, date of birth, gender, diagnosis, precautions, and contraindications

b. *Summary of intervention process*—date of initial and final service; frequency, number of sessions, summary of interventions used; summary of progress toward goals; and occupational therapy outcomes—initial client status and ending status regarding engagement in occupations, client's assessment of efficacy of occupational therapy services

   c. *Recommendations*—recommendations pertaining to the client's future needs; specific follow-up plans, if applicable; and referrals to other professionals and agencies, if applicable.

Each occupational therapy client has a client record maintained as a permanent file. The record is maintained in a professional and legal fashion (i.e., organized, legible, concise, clear, accurate, complete, current, grammatically correct, and objective).

Box 2. Fundamental Elements of Documentation

Elements Present in All Documentation
1   Client's full name and case number (if applicable) on each page of documentation.
2   Date and type of occupational therapy contact.
3   Identification of type of documentation, agency, and department name.
4   Occupational therapy practitioners' signature with a minimum of first name or initial, last name, and professional designation.
5   When applicable on notes or reports, signature of the recorder directly at the end of the note without space left between the body of the note and the signature.
6   Countersignature by an occupational therapist on documentation written by students and occupational therapy assistants when required by law or the facility.
7   Acceptable terminology defined within the boundaries of setting.
8   Abbreviations usage as acceptable within the boundaries of setting.
9   When no facility requirements are listed, errors corrected by drawing a single line through an error and by initialing the correction (liquid correction fluid and erasures are not acceptable).
10   Adherence to professional standards of technology, when used to document occupational therapy services.
11   Disposal of records within law or agency requirements.
12   Compliance with confidentiality standards.
13   Compliance with agency or legal requirements of storage of records.

References

American Occupational Therapy Association. (2002). Occupational therapy practice framework: Domain and process. *American Journal of Occupational Therapy, 56,* 609–639.

American Occupational Therapy Association. (2004). Guidelines for supervision, roles, and responsibilities during the delivery of occupational therapy services. *American Journal of Occupational Therapy, 58,* 663–667.

American Occupational Therapy Association. (2005). Standards of practice for occupational therapy. *American Journal of Occupational Therapy, 59,* 663–665.

American Occupational Therapy Association. (2006). *Policy 1.41. Categories of occupational therapy personnel.* In policy manual (2005 ed.). Bethesda, MD: Author

American Occupational Therapy Association. (2008). Occupational therapy practice framework: Domain and process (2nd ed.) *American Journal of Occupational Therapy, 62.*

Authors

Gloria Frolek Clark, MS, OTR/L, FAOTA
Mary Jane Youngstrom, MS, OTR/L, FAOTA

for

The Commission on Practice
Sara Jane Brayman, PhD, OTR/L, FAOTA, *Chairperson*

Adopted by the Representative Assembly 2003M16

Edited by the Commission on Practice 2007

Received by the Representative Assembly 2007

Guidelines for Supervision, Roles, and Responsibilities During the Delivery of Occupational Therapy Services

This document contains four sections that direct the delivery of occupational therapy services. These sections are General Supervision, Supervision of Occupational Therapists and Occupational Therapy Assistants, Roles and Responsibilities of Occupational Therapists and Occupational Therapy Assistants During the Delivery of Occupational Therapy Services, and Supervision of Occupational Therapy Aides.

General Supervision

These guidelines provide a definition of supervision and outline parameters regarding effective supervision as it relates to the delivery of occupational therapy services. These supervision guidelines are to assist in the appropriate and effective provision of occupational therapy services. The guidelines themselves cannot be interpreted to constitute a standard of supervision in any particular locality. Occupational therapists, occupational therapy assistants, and occupational therapy aides are expected to meet applicable state and federal regulations, adhere to relevant workplace policies and the *Occupational Therapy Code of Ethics* (AOTA, 2005) and participate in ongoing professional development activities to maintain continuing competency.

In these guidelines, *supervision* is viewed as a cooperative process in which two or more people participate in a joint effort to establish, maintain, and or elevate a level of competence and performance. Supervision is based on mutual understanding between the supervisor and the supervisee about each other's competence, experience, education, and credentials. It fosters growth and development, promotes effective utilization of resources, encourages creativity and innovation, and provides education and support to achieve a goal (AOTA, 2004). Within the scope of occupational therapy practice, supervision is a process aimed at ensuring the safe and effective delivery of occupational therapy services and fostering professional competence and development.

Supervision of Occupational Therapists and Occupational Therapy Assistants

Occupational Therapists

Based on their education and training, occupational therapists, after initial certification, are autonomous practitioners who are able to deliver occupational therapy services independently. Occupational therapists are responsible for all aspects of occupational therapy service delivery and are accountable for the safety and effectiveness of the occupational therapy service delivery process. Occupational therapists are encouraged to seek supervision and mentoring to develop best practice approaches and promote professional growth.

Occupational Therapy Assistants

Based on their education and training, occupational therapy assistants must receive supervision from an occupational therapist to deliver occupational therapy services. Occupational therapy assistants deliver occupational therapy services under the supervision of and in partnership with occupational therapists. Occupational therapists and occupational therapy assistants are responsible for collaboratively developing a plan for supervision.

General Principles

1. Supervision involves guidance and oversight related to the delivery of occupational therapy services and the facilitation of professional growth and competence. It is the responsibility of occupational therapists and occupational therapy assistants to seek the appropriate quality and frequency of supervision to ensure safe and effective occupational therapy service delivery.

2. To ensure safe and effective occupational therapy services, it is the responsibility of occupational therapists and occupational therapy assistants to recognize when supervision is needed and to seek supervision that supports current and advancing levels of competence.

3. The specific frequency, methods, and content of supervision may vary by practice setting and are dependent on the

   a. Complexity of client needs,

   b. Number and diversity of clients,

   c. Skills of the occupational therapist and the occupational therapy assistant,

   d. Type of practice setting,

   e. Requirements of the practice setting, and

   f. Other regulatory requirements.

4. Supervision that is more frequent than the minimum level required by the practice setting or regulatory agencies may be necessary when

   a. The needs of the client and the occupational therapy process are complex and changing,

   b. The practice setting provides occupational therapy services to a large number of clients with diverse needs, or

   c. The occupational therapist and occupational therapy assistant determine that additional supervision is necessary to ensure safe and effective delivery of occupational therapy services.

5. A variety of types and methods of supervision should be used. Methods may include direct, face-to-face contact and indirect contact. Examples of methods or types of supervision that involve direct face-to-face contact include observation, modeling, co-treatment, discussions, teaching, and instruction. Examples of methods or types of supervision that involve indirect contact include phone conversations, written correspondence, and electronic exchanges.

6. Occupational therapists and occupational therapy assistants must abide by agency and state requirements regarding the documentation of a supervision plan and supervision contacts. Documentation may include the

   a. Frequency of supervisory contact,

   b. Method(s) or type(s) of supervision,

   c. Content areas addressed,

   d. Evidence to support areas and levels of competency, and

   e. Names and credentials of the persons participating in the supervisory process.

7. Supervision related to professional growth, such as leadership and advocacy development, may differ from that needed to provide occupational therapy services. The person providing this supervision, as

well as the frequency, method, and content of supervision, should be responsive to the supervisee's advancing levels of professional growth.

Supervision Outside the Delivery of Occupational Therapy Services

The education and expertise of occupational therapists and occupational therapy assistants prepare them for employment in arenas other than those related to the delivery of occupational therapy. In these other arenas, supervision may be provided by non–occupational therapy professionals.

1. The guidelines of the setting, regulatory agencies, and funding agencies direct the supervision requirements.

2. The occupational therapist and occupational therapy assistant should obtain and use credentials or job titles commensurate with their roles in these other employment arenas.

3. The following are used to determine whether the services provided are related to the delivery of occupational therapy:

   a. State practice acts;

   b. Regulatory agency standards and rules;

   c. Domain of occupational therapy practice; and

   d. Written and verbal agreement among the occupational therapist, the occupational therapy assistant, the client, and the agency or payer about the services provided.

Roles and Responsibilities of Occupational Therapists and Occupational Therapy Assistants During the Delivery of Occupational Therapy Services

General Statement

The focus of occupational therapy is to support the client's "health and participation in life through engagement in occupation" (AOTA, 2008, p. 626). Occupational therapy addresses the needs and goals of the client related to engaging in areas of occupation and considers the performance skills, performance patterns, context and environment, activity demands, and client factors that may influence performance in various areas of occupation.

1. The occupational therapist is responsible for all aspects of occupational therapy service delivery and is accountable for the safety and effectiveness of the occupational therapy service delivery process. The occupational therapy service delivery process involves evaluation, intervention planning, intervention implementation, intervention review, and outcome evaluation.

2. The occupational therapist must be directly involved in the delivery of services during the initial evaluation and regularly throughout the course of intervention and outcome evaluation.

3. The occupational therapy assistant delivers occupational therapy services under the supervision of and in partnership with the occupational therapist.

4. It is the responsibility of the occupational therapist to determine when to delegate responsibilities to an occupational therapy assistant. It is the responsibility of the occupational therapy assistant who performs the delegated responsibilities to demonstrate service competency.

5. The occupational therapist and the occupational therapy assistant demonstrate and document service competency for clinical reasoning and judgment during the service delivery process as well as for the performance of specific techniques, assessments, and intervention methods used.

6. When delegating aspects of occupational therapy services, the occupational therapist considers the following factors:

    a. Complexity of the client's condition and needs;

    b. Knowledge, skill, and competence of the occupational therapy practitioner;

    c. Nature and complexity of the intervention; and

    d. Needs and requirements of the practice setting.

Roles and Responsibilities

Regardless of the setting in which occupational therapy services are delivered, occupational therapists and occupational therapy assistants assume the following generic responsibilities during evaluation, intervention, and outcomes evaluation.

Evaluation

1. The occupational therapist directs the evaluation process.

2. The occupational therapist is responsible for directing all aspects of the initial contact during the occupational therapy evaluation, including

    a. Determining the need for service,

    b. Defining the problems within the domain of occupational therapy that need to be addressed,

    c. Determining the client's goals and priorities,

    d. Establishing intervention priorities,

    e. Determining specific further assessment needs, and

    f. Determining specific assessment tasks that can be delegated to the occupational therapy assistant.

3. The occupational therapist initiates and directs the evaluation, interprets the data, and develops the intervention plan.

4. The occupational therapy assistant contributes to the evaluation process by implementing delegated assessments and by providing verbal and written reports of observations and client capacities to the occupational therapist.

5. The occupational therapist interprets the information provided by the occupational therapy assistant and integrates that information into the evaluation and decision-making process.

Intervention Planning

1. The occupational therapist has overall responsibility for the development of the occupational therapy intervention plan.

2. The occupational therapist and the occupational therapy assistant collaborate with the client to develop the plan.

3. The occupational therapy assistant is responsible for being knowledgeable about evaluation results and for providing input into the intervention plan, based on client needs and priorities.

Intervention Implementation

1. The occupational therapist has overall responsibility for implementing the intervention.

2. When delegating aspects of the occupational therapy intervention to the occupational therapy assistant, the occupational therapist is responsible for providing appropriate supervision.

3. The occupational therapy assistant is responsible for being knowledgeable about the client's occupational therapy goals.

4. The occupational therapy assistant selects, implements, and makes modifications to therapeutic activities and interventions that are consistent with demonstrated competency levels, client goals, and the requirements of the practice setting.

Intervention Review

1. The occupational therapist is responsible for determining the need for continuing, modifying, or discontinuing occupational therapy services.

2. The occupational therapy assistant contributes to this process by exchanging information with and providing documentation to the occupational therapist about the client's responses to and communications during intervention.

Outcome Evaluation

1. The occupational therapist is responsible for selecting, measuring, and interpreting outcomes that are related to the client's ability to engage in occupations.

2. The occupational therapy assistant is responsible for being knowledgeable about the client's targeted occupational therapy outcomes and for providing information and documentation related to outcome achievement.

3. The occupational therapy assistant may implement outcome measurements and provide needed client discharge resources.

Supervision of Occupational Therapy Aides[1]

An *aide,* as used in occupational therapy practice, is an individual who provides supportive services to the occupational therapist and the occupational therapy assistant. Aides do not provide skilled occupational therapy services. An aide is trained by an occupational therapist or an occupational therapy assistant to perform specifically delegated tasks. The occupational therapist is responsible for the overall use and actions of the aide. An aide first must demonstrate competency to be able to perform the assigned, delegated client and non-client tasks.

1. The occupational therapist must oversee the development, documentation, and implementation of a plan to supervise and routinely assess the ability of the occupational therapy aide to carry out non-client- and client-related tasks. The occupational therapy assistant may contribute to the development and documentation of this plan.

2. The occupational therapy assistant can supervise the aide.

3. Non-client-related tasks include clerical and maintenance activities and preparation of the work area or equipment.

4. Client-related tasks are routine tasks during which the aide may interact with the client. The following factors must be present when an occupational therapist or occupational therapy assistant delegates a selected client-related task to the aide:

---

[1]Depending on the setting in which service is provided; aides may be referred to by various names. Examples include, but are not limited to, *rehabilitation aides, restorative aides, extenders, paraprofessionals,* and *rehab techs* (AOTA, 2004).

    a. The outcome anticipated for the delegated task is predictable.

    b. The situation of the client and the environment is stable and will not require that judgment, interpretations, or adaptations be made by the aide.

    c. The client has demonstrated some previous performance ability in executing the task.

    d. The task routine and process have been clearly established.

5. When performing delegated client-related tasks, the supervisor must ensure that the aide

    a. Is trained and able to demonstrate competency in carrying out the selected task and using equipment, if appropriate;

    b. Has been instructed on how to specifically carry out the delegated task with the specific client; and

    c. Knows the precautions, signs, and symptoms for the particular client that would indicate the need to seek assistance from the occupational therapist or occupational therapy assistant.

6. The supervision of the aide needs to be documented. Documentation includes information about frequency and methods of supervision used the content of supervision and the names and credentials of all persons participating in the supervisory process.

Summary

These guidelines about supervision, roles, and responsibilities are to assist in the appropriate utilization of occupational therapists, occupational therapy assistants, and occupational therapy aides and in the appropriate and effective provision of occupational therapy services. It is expected that occupational therapy services are delivered in accordance with applicable state and federal regulations, relevant workplace policies, the *Occupational Therapy Code of Ethics* (AOTA, 2005), and continuing competency and professional development guidelines.

References

American Occupational Therapy Association. (2004). Guidelines for supervision, roles, and responsibilities during the delivery of occupational therapy services. *American Journal of Occupational Therapy, 58,* 663–667.

American Occupational Therapy Association. (2005). Occupational therapy code of ethics (2005). *American Journal of Occupational Therapy, 59,* 639–642.

American Occupational Therapy Association. (2008). Occupational therapy practice framework: Domain and process (2nd ed.). *American Journal of Occupational Therapy, 62,* 625–683.

Additional Reading

American Occupational Therapy Association. (2005). Standards of practice for occupational therapy. *American Journal of Occupational Therapy, 59,* 663–665.

Authors

Sara Jane Brayman, PhD, OTR/L, FAOTA, *Chairperson, 2002–2005*

Gloria Frolek Clark, MS, OTR/L, FAOTA

Janet V. DeLany, DEd, OTR/L

Eileen R. Garza, PhD, OTR, ATP

Mary V. Radomski, MA, OTR/L, FAOTA

Ruth Ramsey, MS, OTR/L

Carol Siebert, MS, OTR/L

Kristi Voelkerding, BS, COTA/L
Patricia D. LaVesser, PhD, OTR/L, *SIS Liaison*
Lenna Aird, *ASD Liaison*
Deborah Lieberman, MHSA, OTR/L, FAOTA, *AOTA Headquarters Liaison*

for

The Commission on Practice
Sara Jane Brayman, PhD, OTR/L, FAOTA, *Chairperson*

Adopted by the Representative Assembly 2004C24

Edited by the Commission on Practice 2009

This replaces the 2004 document *Guidelines for Supervision, Roles, and Responsibilities During the Delivery of Occupational Therapy Services* (previously published and copyrighted in 2004 in the *American Journal of Occupational Therapy, 58,* 663–667).

OCCUPATIONAL THERAPY PRACTICE
FRAMEWORK:
Domain & Process
2nd Edition

Contents

INTRODUCTION

The *Occupational Therapy Practice Framework: Domain and Process, 2nd Edition* (*Framework–II*) is an official document of the American Occupational Therapy Association (AOTA). Intended for internal and external audiences, it presents a summary of interrelated constructs that define and guide **occupational therapy**[1] practice. The *Framework* was developed to articulate occupational therapy's contribution to promoting the **health** and **participation** of people, organizations, and populations through **engagement** in **occupation.** It is not a taxonomy, theory, or model of occupational therapy and therefore must be used in conjunction with the knowledge and evidence relevant to occupation and occupational therapy. The revisions included in this second edition are intended to refine the document and include language and concepts relevant to current and emerging occupational therapy practice.

Implicit within this summary are the profession's core beliefs in the positive relationship between occupation and health and its view of people as occupational beings. "All people need to be able or enabled to engage in the occupations of their need and choice, to grow through what they do, and to experience **independence** or **interdependence,** equality, participation, security, health, and well-being" (Wilcock & Townsend, 2008, p. 198). With this aim, occupational therapy is provided to **clients,** the entity that receives occupational therapy services. Clients may be categorized as

- **Persons,** including families, caregivers, teachers, employers, and relevant others;
- **Organizations,** such as businesses, industries, or agencies; and
- **Populations** within a community, such as refugees, veterans who are homeless, and people with chronic health disabling conditions (Moyers & Dale, 2007).

The *Framework* is divided into two major sections: (1) the ***domain,*** which outlines the profession's purview and the areas in which its mem-

---

[1]Many of the terms that appear in **bold** are defined in the glossary.

"The *Framework* was developed to articulate occupational therapy's contribution to promoting the health and participation of people, organizations, and populations through engagement in occupation."

bers have an established body of knowledge and expertise (see Figure 1), and (2) the dynamic occupation and client-centered *process* used in the delivery of occupational therapy services (see Figure 2). The domain and process of occupational therapy direct occupational therapy practitioners[2] to focus on performance of occupations that results from the dynamic intersection of the client, the context and environment, and the client's occupations (Christiansen & Baum, 1997; Christiansen, Baum, & Bass-Hagen, 2005; Law, Baum, & Dunn, 2005). Although the domain and process are described separately, in actuality, they are inextricably linked in a transactional relationship (see Figure 3).

Numerous resource materials, including an appendix, a glossary, references, and a bibliography, are supplied at the end of the document. Although the *Framework* includes a glossary of defined terms, it does not contain an exhaustive or uniform list of terms used in the profession nor all

of the definitions of these terms discussed in the literature.

Domain of Occupational Therapy
Overview

This edition of the *Framework* begins with a description of the occupational therapy profession's domain. The overarching statement—**supporting health and participation in life through engagement in occupation**—describes the domain in its fullest sense. Within this diverse profession, the defining contribution of occupational therapy is the application of core values, knowledge, and skills to assist clients (people, organizations, and populations) to engage in everyday activities or occupations that they want and need to do in a manner that supports health and participation. Figure 4 identifies the aspects of the domain and illustrates the dynamic interrelatedness among them. All aspects of the domain are of equal value, and together they interact to influence the client's engagement in occupations, participation, and health.

Occupational therapists are educated to evaluate aspects of the occupational therapy domain and their **transactional** relationships. Occupational therapists and occupational therapy assistants are educated about the aspects of the occupational therapy domain and apply this knowledge to the intervention process as they work to support the health and participation of their clients. Occupational therapists are responsible for all aspects of occupational therapy service delivery and are accountable for the safety and effectiveness of that service delivery process. Occupational therapy assistants deliver occupational therapy service under the supervision of and in collaboration with an occupational therapist (AOTA, 2004b).

---

[2]When the term *occupational therapy practitioner* is used in this document, it refers to occupational therapists and occupational therapy assistants (AOTA, 2006).

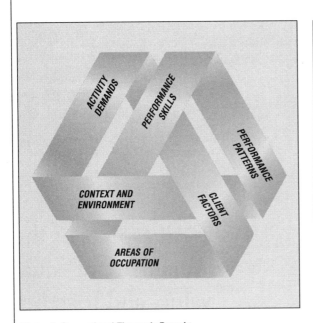

Figure 1. Occupational Therapy's Domain.
Supporting health and participation in life through engagement in occupation.

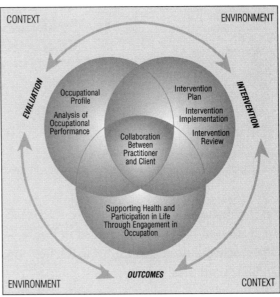

Figure 2. Occupational Therapy's Process.
Collaboration between the practitioner and the client is central to the interactive nature of service delivery.

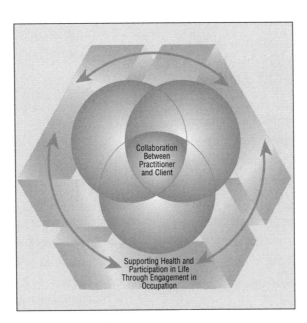

Figure 3. Occupational Therapy.
The domain and process are inextricably linked.

Note: Mobius in figures 1 and 3 originally designed by Mark Dow. Used with permission.

AREAS OF OCCUPATION	CLIENT FACTORS	PERFORMANCE SKILLS	PERFORMANCE PATTERNS	CONTEXT AND ENVIRONMENT	ACTIVITY DEMANDS
Activities of Daily Living (ADL)* Instrumental Activities of Daily Living (IADL) Rest and Sleep Education Work Play Leisure Social Participation	Values, Beliefs, and Spirituality Body Functions Body Structures	Sensory Perceptual Skills Motor and Praxis Skills Emotional Regulation Skills Cognitive Skills Communication and Social Skills	Habits Routines Roles Rituals	Cultural Personal Physical Social Temporal Virtual	Objects Used and Their Properties Space Demands Social Demands Sequencing and Timing Required Actions Required Body Functions Required Body Structures

*Also referred to as *basic activities of daily living (BADL)* or *personal activities of daily living (PADL)*.

Figure 4. Aspects of Occupational Therapy's Domain.
All aspects of the domain transact to support engagement, participation, and health. This figure does not imply a hierarchy.

The discussion that follows provides a brief explanation of each aspect identified in Figure 4. Tables included throughout provide full lists and definitions of terms.

Supporting Health and Participation in Life Through Engagement in Occupation

The profession of occupational therapy uses the term *occupation* to capture the breadth and meaning of "everyday **activity.**" Occupational therapy is founded on an understanding that engaging in occupations structures everyday life and contributes to health and well-being. Occupational therapy practitioners believe that occupations are multidimensional and complex. Engagement in occupation as the focus of occupational therapy intervention involves addressing both subjective (emotional and psychological) and objective (physically observable) aspects of performance. Occupational therapy practitioners understand engagement from this dual and holistic perspective and address all aspects of performance when providing interventions.

Occupational science, a discipline devoted to the study of occupation, informs occupational therapy practice by expanding the understanding of occupation (Zemke & Clark, 1996). Occupations are central to a client's (person, organization, or pop-

"All aspects of the domain are of equal value, and together they interact to influence the client's engagement in occupations, participation, and health."

ulation) identity and sense of competence and have particular meaning and value to the client. They influence how clients spend time making decisions. Several definitions of occupation can be found in the literature that adds to an understanding of this core concept. *Occupation* has been defined as

- "Goal-directed pursuits that typically extend over time, have meaning to the performance, and involve multiple tasks" (Christiansen et al., 2005, p. 548).
- "Daily activities that reflect cultural values, provide structure to living, and meaning to

individuals; these activities meet human needs for self-care, enjoyment, and participation in society" (Crepeau, Cohn, & Schell, 2003, p. 1031).

- "Activities that people engage in throughout their daily lives to fulfill their time and give life meaning. Occupations involve mental abilities and skills and may or may not have an observable physical dimension" (Hinojosa & Kramer, 1997, p. 865).
- "[A]ctivities…of everyday life, named, organized, and given value and meaning by individuals and a culture. Occupation is everything people do to occupy themselves, including looking after themselves…enjoying life…and contributing to the social and economic fabric of their communities" (Law, Polatajko, Baptiste, & Townsend, 1997, p. 32).
- "A dynamic relationship among an occupational form, a person with a unique developmental structure, subjective meanings and purpose, and the resulting occupational performance" (Nelson & Jepson-Thomas, 2003, p. 90).
- "[C]hunks of daily activity that can be named in the lexicon of the culture" (Zemke & Clark, 1996, p. vii).

Sometimes occupational therapy practitioners use the terms *occupation* and *activity* interchangeably to describe participation in daily life pursuits. Some scholars have proposed that the two terms are different (Christiansen & Townsend, 2004; Hinojosa & Kramer, 1997; Pierce, 2001; Reed, 2005). In the *Framework,* the term occupation encompasses activity.

Occupational engagement occurs individually or with others. A client may be considered independent when the client performs or directs the actions necessary to participate regardless of the amount or kind of assistance desired or required. In contrast with narrower definitions of independence, occupational therapy practitioners consider a client as independent whether the client solely performs the activities, performs the activities in an adapted or modified environment, makes use of various devices or alternative strategies, or oversees activity completion by others (AOTA, 2002a). For example, people with a spinal cord injury can direct a personal care assistant to assist them with their activities of daily living (ADLs), demonstrating independence in this essential aspect of their lives.

Occupations often are shared. Those that implicitly involve two or more individuals may be termed *co-occupations* (Zemke & Clark, 1996). Care giving is a co-occupation that involves active participation on the part of the caregiver and the recipient of care. For example, the co-occupations required during mothering, such as the socially interactive routines of eating, feeding, and comforting, may involve the parent, a partner, the child, and significant others (Olsen, 2004). The activities intrinsic to this social interaction are reciprocal, interactive, and nested "co-occupations" (Dunlea, 1996; Esdaile & Olson, 2004). Clients also may perform several occupations simultaneously, enfolding them into one another such as when a caregiver concurrently helps with homework, pays the bills, and makes dinner. Consideration of co-occupation supports an integrated view of the client's engagement in relationship to significant others within context.

Occupational therapy practitioners recognize that health is supported and maintained when clients are able to engage in occupations and activities that allow desired or needed participation in home, school, workplace, and community life. Thus, occupational therapy practitioners are concerned not only with occupations but also the complexity of factors that empower and make possible clients' engagement and participation in positive health-promoting occupations (Wilcock &

Townsend, 2008). In 2003, Townsend applied the concept of **social justice** to occupational therapy's focus and coined the term *occupational justice* to describe the profession's concern with ethical, moral, and civic factors that can support or hinder health-promoting engagement in occupations and participation in home and community life. *Occupational justice* ensures that clients are afforded the opportunity for full participation in those occupations in which they choose to engage (Christiansen & Townsend, 2004, p. 278). Occupational therapy practitioners interested in occupational justice recognize and work to support social policies, actions, and laws that allow people to engage in occupations that provide purpose and meaning in their lives.

Occupational therapy's focus on engaging in occupations and occupational justice complements the World Health Organization's (WHO) perspective of health. WHO, in its effort to broaden the understanding of the effects of disease and disability on health, has recognized that health can be affected by the inability to carry out activities and participate in life situations caused by environmental barriers, as well as by problems that exist with body structures and body functions (WHO, 2001). As members of a global community, occupational therapy practitioners advocate for the well-being of all persons, groups, and populations with a commitment to inclusion and nondiscrimination (AOTA, 2004c).

Areas of Occupation

When occupational therapy practitioners work with clients, they consider the many types of occupations in which clients might engage. The broad range of activities or occupations are sorted into categories called **"areas of occupation"**—*activities of daily living, instrumental activities of daily living, rest and sleep, education, work, play, leisure, and social participation* (see Table 1).

Individual differences in the way in which clients view their occupations reflect the complexity and multidimensionality of each occupation. The client's perspective of how an occupation is categorized varies depending on that client's needs and interests. For example, one person may perceive doing laundry as work, while another may consider it an instrumental activity of daily living (IADL). One population may engage in a quiz game and view their participation as play, while another population may engage in the same quiz game and view it as an educational occupation.

The way in which clients prioritize engagement in areas of occupation may vary at different times. For example, a community psychiatric rehabilitation organization may prioritize member voter registration during a presidential campaign and celebration preparations during holiday periods. The extent and nature of the engagement is as important as the engagement itself; for example, excessive work without sufficient regard to other aspects of life such as sleep or relationships places clients at risk for health problems (Hakansson, Dahlin-Ivanoff, & Sonn, 2006).

Client Factors

Client factors are specific abilities, characteristics, or beliefs that reside within the client and may affect performance in areas of occupation. Because occupational therapy practitioners view clients holistically, they consider client factors that involve the values, beliefs, and spirituality; body functions; and body structures. These underlying client factors are affected by the presence or absence of illness, disease, deprivation, and disability. They affect and are affected by performance skills, performance patterns, activity demands, and contextual and environmental factors.

Despite their importance, the presence or absence of specific body functions and body

TABLE 1. AREAS OF OCCUPATION

Various kinds of life activities in which people, populations, or organizations engage, including ADL, IADL, rest and sleep, education, work, play, leisure, and social participation.

ACTIVITIES OF DAILY LIVING (ADLs)

Activities that are oriented toward taking care of one's own body (adapted from Rogers & Holm, 1994, pp. 181–202). ADL also is referred to as *basic activities of daily living (BADLs)* and *personal activities of daily living (PADLs)*. These activities are "fundamental to living in a social world; they enable basic survival and well-being" (Christiansen & Hammecker, 2001, p. 156).

- **Bathing, showering**—Obtaining and using supplies; soaping, rinsing, and drying body parts; maintaining bathing position; and transferring to and from bathing positions.

- **Bowel and bladder management**—Includes completing intentional control of bowel movements and urinary bladder and, if necessary, using equipment or agents for bladder control (Uniform Data System for Medical Rehabilitation, 1996, pp. III–20, III–24).

- **Dressing**—Selecting clothing and accessories appropriate to time of day, weather, and occasion; obtaining clothing from storage area; dressing and undressing in a sequential fashion; fastening and adjusting clothing and shoes; and applying and removing personal devices, prostheses, or orthoses.

- **Eating**—"The ability to keep and manipulate food or fluid in the mouth and swallow it; *eating* and *swallowing* are often used interchangeably" (AOTA, 2007b).

- **Feeding**—"The process of setting up, arranging, and bringing food [or fluid] from the plate or cup to the mouth; sometimes called *self-feeding*" (AOTA, 2007b).

- **Functional mobility**—Moving from one position or place to another (during performance of everyday activities), such as in-bed mobility, wheelchair mobility, and transfers (e.g., wheelchair, bed, car, tub, toilet, tub/shower, chair, floor). Includes functional ambulation and transporting objects.

- **Personal device care**—Using, cleaning, and maintaining personal care items, such as hearing aids, contact lenses, glasses, orthotics, prosthetics, adaptive equipment, and contraceptive and sexual devices.

- **Personal hygiene and grooming**—Obtaining and using supplies; removing body hair (e.g., use of razors, tweezers, lotions); applying and removing cosmetics; washing, drying, combing, styling, brushing, and trimming hair; caring for nails (hands and feet); caring for skin, ears, eyes, and nose; applying deodorant; cleaning mouth; brushing and flossing teeth; or removing, cleaning, and reinserting dental orthotics and prosthetics.

- **Sexual activity**—Engaging in activities that result in sexual satisfaction.

- **Toilet hygiene**—Obtaining and using supplies; clothing management; maintaining toileting position; transferring to and from toileting position; cleaning body; and caring for menstrual and continence needs (including catheters, colostomies, and suppository management).

INSTRUMENTAL ACTIVITIES OF DAILY LIVING (IADLs)

Activities to support daily life within the home and community that often require more complex interactions than self-care used in ADL.

- **Care of others (including selecting and supervising caregivers)**—Arranging, supervising, or providing the care for others.

- **Care of pets**—Arranging, supervising, or providing the care for pets and service animals.

- **Child rearing**—Providing the care and supervision to support the developmental needs of a child.

- **Communication management**—Sending, receiving, and interpreting information using a variety of systems and equipment, including writing tools, telephones, typewriters, audiovisual recorders, computers, communication boards, call lights, emergency systems, Braille writers, telecommunication devices for the deaf, augmentative communication systems, and personal digital assistants.

- **Community mobility**—Moving around in the community and using public or private transportation, such as driving, walking, bicycling, or accessing and riding in buses, taxi cabs, or other transportation systems.

- **Financial management**—Using fiscal resources, including alternate methods of financial transaction and planning and using finances with long-term and short-term goals.

- **Health management and maintenance**—Developing, managing, and maintaining routines for health and wellness promotion, such as physical fitness, nutrition, decreasing health risk behaviors, and medication routines.

- **Home establishment and management**—Obtaining and maintaining personal and household possessions and environment (e.g., home, yard, garden, appliances, vehicles), including maintaining and repairing personal possessions (clothing and household items) and knowing how to seek help or whom to contact.

- **Meal preparation and cleanup**—Planning, preparing, and serving well-balanced, nutritional meals and cleaning up food and utensils after meals.

- **Religious observance**—Participating in *religion,* "an organized system of beliefs, practices, rituals, and symbols designed to facilitate closeness to the sacred or transcendent" (Moreira-Almeida & Koenig, 2006, p. 844).

- **Safety and emergency maintenance**—Knowing and performing preventive procedures to maintain a safe environment as well as recognizing sudden, unexpected hazardous situations and initiating emergency action to reduce the threat to health and safety.

- **Shopping**—Preparing shopping lists (grocery and other); selecting, purchasing, and transporting items; selecting method of payment; and completing money transactions.

(Continued)

TABLE 1. AREAS OF OCCUPATION
(Continued)

▇ REST AND SLEEP

Includes activities related to obtaining restorative rest and sleep that supports healthy active engagement in other areas of occupation.

- **Rest**—Quiet and effortless actions that interrupt physical and mental activity resulting in a relaxed state (Nurit & Michel, 2003, p. 227). Includes identifying the need to relax; reducing involvement in taxing physical, mental, or social activities; and engaging in relaxation or other endeavors that restore energy, calm, and renewed interest in engagement.

- **Sleep**—A series of activities resulting in going to sleep, staying asleep, and ensuring health and safety through participation in sleep involving engagement with the physical and social environments.

- **Sleep preparation**—(1) Engaging in routines that prepare the self for a comfortable rest, such as grooming and undressing, reading or listening to music to fall asleep, saying goodnight to others, and meditation or prayers; determining the time of day and length of time desired for sleeping or the time needed to wake; and establishing sleep patterns that support growth and health (patterns are often personally and culturally determined).

  (2) Preparing the physical environment for periods of unconsciousness, such as making the bed or space on which to sleep; ensuring warmth/coolness and protection; setting an alarm clock; securing the home, such as locking doors or closing windows or curtains; and turning off electronics or lights.

- **Sleep participation**—Taking care of personal need for sleep such as cessation of activities to ensure onset of sleep, napping, dreaming, sustaining a sleep state without disruption, and nighttime care of toileting needs or hydration. Negotiating the needs and requirements of others within the social environment. Interacting with those sharing the sleeping space such as children or partners, providing nighttime care giving such as breastfeeding, and monitoring the com-

fort and safety of others such as the family while sleeping.

▇ EDUCATION

Includes activities needed for learning and participating in the environment.

- **Formal educational participation**—Including the categories of academic (e.g., math, reading, working on a degree), nonacademic (e.g., recess, lunchroom, hallway), extracurricular (e.g., sports, band, cheerleading, dances), and vocational (prevocational and vocational) participation.

- **Informal personal educational needs or interests exploration (beyond formal education)**—Identifying topics and methods for obtaining topic-related information or skills.

- **Informal personal education participation**—Participating in classes, programs, and activities that provide instruction/training in identified areas of interest.

▇ WORK

Includes activities needed for engaging in remunerative employment or volunteer activities (Mosey, 1996, p. 341).

- **Employment interests and pursuits**—Identifying and selecting work opportunities based on assets, limitations, likes, and dislikes relative to work (adapted from Mosey, 1996, p. 342).

- **Employment seeking and acquisition**—Identifying and recruiting for job opportunities; completing, submitting, and reviewing appropriate application materials; preparing for interviews; participating in interviews and following up afterward; discussing job benefits; and finalizing negotiations.

- **Job performance**—Job performance including work skills and patterns; time management; relationships with co-workers, managers, and customers; creation, production, and distribution of products and services; initiation, sustainment, and completion of work; and compliance with work norms and procedures.

- **Retirement preparation and adjustment**—Determining aptitudes, developing interests and skills, and selecting appropriate avocational pursuits.

- **Volunteer exploration**—Determining community causes, organizations, or opportunities for unpaid "work" in relationship to personal skills, interests, location, and time available.

- **Volunteer participation**—Performing unpaid "work" activities for the benefit of identified selected causes, organizations, or facilities.

▇ PLAY

"Any spontaneous or organized activity that provides enjoyment, entertainment, amusement, or diversion" (Parham & Fazio, 1997, p. 252).

- **Play exploration**—Identifying appropriate play activities, which can include exploration play, practice play, pretend play, games with rules, constructive play, and symbolic play (adapted from Bergen, 1988, pp. 64–65).

- **Play participation**—Participating in play; maintaining a balance of play with other areas of occupation; and obtaining, using, and maintaining toys, equipment, and supplies appropriately.

▇ LEISURE

"A nonobligatory activity that is intrinsically motivated and engaged in during discretionary time, that is, time not committed to obligatory occupations such as work, self-care, or sleep" (Parham & Fazio, 1997, p. 250).

- **Leisure exploration**—Identifying interests, skills, opportunities, and appropriate leisure activities.

- **Leisure participation**—Planning and participating in appropriate leisure activities; maintaining a balance of leisure activities with other areas of occupation; and obtaining, using, and maintaining equipment and supplies as appropriate.

TABLE 1. AREAS OF OCCUPATION
(Continued)

■ **SOCIAL PARTICIPATION**

"Organized patterns of behavior that are characteristic and expected of an individual or a given position within a social system" (Mosey, 1996, p. 340).

• **Community**—Engaging in activities that result in successful interaction at the community level (i.e., neighborhood, organizations, work, school).

• **Family**—Engaging in "[activities that result in] successful interaction in specific

required and/or desired familial roles" (Mosey, 1996, p. 340).

• **Peer, friend**—Engaging in activities at different levels of intimacy, including engaging in desired sexual activity.

Note. Some of the terms used in this table are from, or adapted from, the rescinded *Uniform Terminology for Occupational Therapy—Third Edition* (AOTA, 1994, pp. 1047–1054).

structures do not necessarily ensure a client's success or difficulty with daily life occupations. Factors that influence performance such as supports in the physical or social environment may allow a client to manifest skills in a given area even when body functions or structure are absent or deficient. It is in the process of observing a client engaging in occupations and activities that the occupational therapy practitioner is able to determine the transaction between client factors and performance.

Client factors are substantively different at the person, organization, and population levels. Following are descriptions of client factors for each level.

Person

• **Values, beliefs, and spirituality** influence a client's motivation to engage in occupations and give his or her life meaning. *Values* are principles, standards, or qualities considered worthwhile by the client who holds them. *Beliefs* are cognitive content held as true (Moyers & Dale, 2007, p. 28). *Spirituality* is "the personal quest for understanding answers to ultimate questions about life, about meaning and about relationship with the sacred or transcendent, which may (or may not) lead to or arise from the development of religious rituals and the formation of community" (Moreira-Almeida & Koenig, 2006, p. 844).

• *Body functions* refer to the "physiological function of body systems (including psychological functions)" (WHO, 2001, p. 10). Examples include sensory, mental (affective, cognitive, perceptual), cardiovascular, respiratory, and endocrine functions (see Table 2 for complete list).

• *Body structures* are the "anatomical parts of the body such as organs, limbs, and their components" (WHO, 2001, p. 10). Body structures and body functions are interrelated (e.g., the heart and blood vessels are body structures that support cardiovascular function; see Table 2).

The categorization of body function and body structure client factors outlined in Table 2 is based on the *International Classification of Functioning, Disability, and Health* proposed by the WHO (2001). The classification was selected because it has received wide exposure and presents a language that is understood by external audiences.

Organization

• *Values and beliefs* include the vision statement, code of ethics, value statements, and esprit de corps.

• *Functions* include planning, organizing, coordinating, and operationalizing the mission, products or services, and productivity.

• *Structures* include departments and departmental relationships, leadership and management, performance measures, and job titles.

Population

- *Values and beliefs* can be viewed as including emotional, purposive, and traditional perspectives (Foucault, 1973).
- *Functions* include economic, political, social, and cultural capital (Weber, 1978).
- *Structure* may include constituents such as those with similar genetics, sexual orientation, and health-related conditions (Baum, Bass-Haugen, & Christiansen, 2005, p. 381).

Activity Demands

Activity demands refer to the specific features of an activity that influence the type and amount of effort required to perform the activity. Occupational therapy practitioners analyze activities to understand what is required of the client and determine the relationship of the activity's requirements to engagement in occupation. Activity demands include the specific objects and their properties used in the activity, the physical space requirements of the activity,

---

TABLE 2. CLIENT FACTORS

Client factors include (1) values, beliefs, and spirituality; (2) body functions; and (3) body structures that reside within the client and may affect performance in areas of occupation.

■ VALUES, BELIEFS, AND SPIRITUALITY

Category and Definition	Examples
Values: Principles, standards, or qualities considered worthwhile or desirable by the client who holds them.	**Person** 1. Honesty with self and with others 2. Personal religious convictions 3. Commitment to family. **Organization** 1. Obligation to serve the community 2. Fairness. **Population** 1. Freedom of speech 2. Equal opportunities for all 3. Tolerance toward others.
Beliefs: Cognitive content held as true.	**Person** 1. He or she is powerless to influence others 2. Hard work pays off. **Organization** 1. Profits are more important than people 2. Achieving the mission of providing service can effect positive change in the world. **Population** 1. People can influence government by voting 2. Accessibility is a right, not a privilege.
Spirituality: The "personal quest for understanding answers to ultimate questions about life, about meaning, and the sacred" (Moyers & Dale, 2007, p. 28).	**Person** 1. Daily search for purpose and meaning in one's life 2. Guiding actions from a sense of value beyond the personal acquisition of wealth or fame. **Organization and Population** (see "Person" examples related to individuals within an organization and population).

TABLE 2. CLIENT FACTORS

(Continued)

■ **BODY FUNCTIONS:** "[T]he physiological functions of body systems (including psychological functions)" (WHO, 2001, p. 10). The "Body Functions" section of the table below is organized according to the classifications of the *International Classification of Functioning, Disability, and Health (ICF)* classifications. For fuller descriptions and definitions, refer to WHO (2001).

Categories	Body Functions Commonly Considered by Occupational Therapy Practitioners *(Not intended to be all-inclusive list)*
Mental functions (affective, cognitive, perceptual)	
• **Specific mental functions**	**Specific mental functions**
○ Higher-level cognitive	Judgment, concept formation, metacognition, cognitive flexibility, insight, attention, awareness
○ Attention	Sustained, selective, and divided attention
○ Memory	Short-term, long-term, and working memory
○ Perception	Discrimination of sensations (e.g., auditory, tactile, visual, olfactory, gustatory, vestibular–proprioception), including multi-sensory processing, sensory memory, spatial, and temporal relationships (Calvert, Spence, & Stein, 2004)
○ Thought	Recognition, categorization, generalization, awareness of reality, logical/coherent thought, and appropriate thought content
○ Mental functions of sequencing complex movement	Execution of learned movement patterns
○ Emotional	Coping and behavioral regulation (Schell, Cohn, & Crepeau, 2008)
○ Experience of self and time	Body image, self-concept, self-esteem
• **Global mental functions**	**Global mental functions**
○ Consciousness	Level of arousal, level of consciousness
○ Orientation	Orientation to person, place, time, self, and others
○ Temperament and personality	Emotional stability
○ Energy and drive	Motivation, impulse control, and appetite
○ Sleep (physiological process)	
Sensory functions and pain	**Sensory functions and pain**
• Seeing and related functions, including visual acuity, visual stability, visual field functions	Detection/registration, modulation, and integration of sensations from the body and environment
	Visual awareness of environment at various distances
• Hearing functions	Tolerance of ambient sounds; awareness of location and distance of sounds such as an approaching car
• Vestibular functions	Sensation of securely moving against gravity
• Taste functions	Association of taste
• Smell functions	Association of smell
• Proprioceptive functions	Awareness of body position and space
• Touch functions	Comfort with the feeling of being touched by others or touching various textures such as food
• Pain (e.g., diffuse, dull, sharp, phantom)	Localizing pain
• Temperature and pressure	Thermal awareness

(continued)

TABLE 2. CLIENT FACTORS

(Continued)

▨ BODY FUNCTIONS: *(Continued)*

Categories	Body Functions Commonly Considered by Occupational Therapy Practitioners *(Not intended to be all-inclusive list)*

Neuromusculoskeletal and movement-related functions
• Functions of joints and bones
  ○ Joint mobility
  ○ Joint stability
 	
  ○ Muscle power
  ○ Muscle tone
  ○ Muscle endurance
  ○ Motor reflexes
  ○ Involuntary movement reactions
  ○ Control of voluntary movement
 	
  ○ Gait patterns
	Neuromusculoskeletal and movement-related functions
	
	Joint range of motion
	Postural alignment (this refers to the physiological stability of the joint related to its structural integrity as compared to the motor skill of aligning the body while moving in relation to task objects)
	Strength
	Degree of muscle tone (e.g., flaccidity, spasticity, fluctuating)
	Endurance
	Stretch, asymmetrical tonic neck, symmetrical tonic neck
	Righting and supporting
	Eye–hand/foot coordination, bilateral integration, crossing the midline, fine- and gross-motor control, and oculomotor (e.g., saccades, pursuits, accommodation, binocularity)
	Walking patterns and impairments such as asymmetric gait, stiff gait. (*Note:* Gait patterns are considered in relation to how they affect ability to engage in occupations in daily life activities.)

Cardiovascular, hematological, immunological, and respiratory system function • Cardiovascular system function • Hematological and immunological system function • Respiratory system function • Additional functions and sensations of the cardiovascular and respiratory systems	**Cardiovascular, hematological, immunological, and respiratory system function** Blood pressure functions (hypertension, hypotension, postural hypotension), and heart rate (*Note:* Occupational therapy practitioners have knowledge of these body functions and understand broadly the interaction that occurs between these functions to support health and participation in life through engagement in occupation. Some therapists may specialize in evaluating and intervening with a specific function as it is related to supporting performance and engagement in occupations and activities targeted for intervention.) Rate, rhythm, and depth of respiration Physical endurance, aerobic capacity, stamina, and fatigability
Voice and speech functions • Voice functions • Fluency and rhythm • Alternative vocalization functions **Digestive, metabolic, and endocrine system function** • Digestive system function • Metabolic system and endocrine system function **Genitourinary and reproductive functions** • Urinary functions • Genital and reproductive functions	(*Note:* Occupational therapy practitioners have knowledge of these body functions and understand broadly the interaction that occurs between these functions to support health and participation in life through engagement in occupation. Some therapists may specialize in evaluating and intervening with a specific function, such as incontinence and pelvic floor disorders, as it is related to supporting performance and engagement in occupations and activities targeted for intervention.)

TABLE 2. CLIENT FACTORS

(Continued)

▓ BODY FUNCTIONS: *(Continued)*

Categories	Body Functions Commonly Considered by Occupational Therapy Practitioners *(Not intended to be all-inclusive list)*
Skin and related-structure functions • Skin functions • Hair and nail functions	**Skin and related-structure functions** Protective functions of the skin—presence or absence of wounds, cuts, or abrasions Repair function of the skin—wound healing (*Note:* Occupational therapy practitioners have knowledge of these body functions and understand broadly the interaction that occurs between these functions to support health and participation in life through engagement in occupation. Some therapists may specialize in evaluating and intervening with a specific function as it is related to supporting performance and engagement in occupations and activities targeted for intervention.)

▓ BODY STRUCTURES: *Body structures* are "anatomical parts of the body, such as organs, limbs, and their components [that support body function]" (WHO, 2001, p. 10). The "Body Structures" section of the table below is organized according to the *ICF* classifications. For fuller descriptions and definitions, refer to WHO (2001).

Categories	Examples are not delineated in the "Body Structure" section of this table.
Structure of the nervous system **Eyes, ear, and related structures** **Structures involved in voice and speech** **Structures of the cardiovascular, immunological, and respiratory systems** **Structures related to the digestive, metabolic, and endocrine systems** **Structure related to the genitourinary and reproductive systems** **Structures related to movement** **Skin and related structures**	(*Note:* Occupational therapy practitioners have knowledge of body structures and understand broadly the interaction that occurs between these structures to support health and participation in life through engagement in occupation. Some therapists may specialize in evaluating and intervening with a specific structure as it is related to supporting performance and engagement in occupations and activities targeted for intervention.)

Note. Some data adapted from the *ICF* (WHO, 2001).

TABLE 3. ACTIVITY DEMANDS

The aspects of an activity, which include the objects and their properties, space, social demands, sequencing or timing, required actions and skills, and required underlying body functions and body structure needed to carry out the activity.

Activity Demand Aspects	Definition	Examples
Objects and their properties	Tools, materials, and equipment used in the process of carrying out the activity	• Tools (e.g., scissors, dishes, shoes, volleyball) • Materials (e.g., paints, milk, lipstick) • Equipment (e.g., workbench, stove, basketball hoop) • Inherent properties (e.g., heavy, rough, sharp, colorful, loud, bitter tasting)
Space demands (relates to physical context)	Physical environmental requirements of the activity (e.g., size, arrangement, surface, lighting, temperature, noise, humidity, ventilation)	• Large, open space outdoors required for a baseball game • Bathroom door and stall width to accommodate wheelchair • Noise, lighting, and temperature controls for a library
Social demands (relates to social environment and cultural contexts)	Social environment and cultural contexts that may be required by the activity	• Rules of game • Expectations of other participants in activity (e.g., sharing supplies, using language appropriate for the meeting)

Sequence and timing	Process used to carry out the activity (e.g., specific steps, sequence, timing requirements)	• *Steps to make tea:* Gather cup and tea bag, heat water, pour water into cup, and so forth.
		  ○ *Sequence:* Heat water before placing tea bag in water.
		  ○ *Timing:* Leave tea bag to steep for 2 minutes.
		• *Steps to conduct a meeting:* Establish goals for meeting, arrange time and location for meeting, prepare meeting agenda, call meeting to order.
		  ○ *Sequence:* Have people introduce themselves before beginning discussion of topic.
		  ○ *Timing:* Allot sufficient time for discussion of topic and determination of action items.

Required actions and performance skills	The usual skills that would be required by any performer to carry out the activity. Sensory, perceptual, motor, praxis, emotional, cognitive, communication, and social performance skills should each be considered. The performance skills demanded by an activity will be correlated with the demands of the other activity aspects (e.g., objects, space)	• Feeling the heat of the stove • Gripping handlebar • Choosing the ceremonial clothes • Determining how to move limbs to control the car • Adjusting the tone of voice • Answering a question
Required body functions	"[P]hysiological functions of body systems (including psychological functions)" (WHO, 2001, p. 10) that are required to support the actions used to perform the activity	• Mobility of joints • Level of consciousness
Required body structures	"Anatomical parts of the body such as organs, limbs, and their components [that support body function]" (WHO, 2001, p. 10) that are required to perform the activity	• Number of hands • Number of eyes

the social demands, sequence and timing, the required actions or skills needed to perform the activity, and the required body functions and structures used during the performance of the activity (see Table 3 for definitions and examples.)

Activity demands are specific to each activity. A change in one feature of an activity may change the extent of the demand in another feature. For example, an increase in the number of the steps or sequence of steps in an activity increases the demand on attention skills.

Performance Skills

Various approaches have been used to describe and categorize *performance skills*. The occupational therapy literature from research and practice offers multiple perspectives on the complexity and types of skills used during performance.

According to Fisher (2006), *performance skills* are observable, concrete, goal-directed actions clients use to engage in daily life occupations. Fisher further defines these skills as small, measurable units in a chain of actions that are observed as a person performs meaningful tasks. They are learned and developed over time and are situated in specific contexts and environments. Fisher categorized performance skills as follows: Motor Skills, Process Skills, and Communication/Interaction Skills. Rogers and Holm (2008) have proposed that during task-specific performance skills, various body functions and structures coalesce into unique combinations and emerge to affect performance in real life.

Given that **performance skills** are described and categorized in multiple ways, within the *Occupational Therapy Practice Framework* they are defined as the abilities clients demonstrate in the actions they perform. The categories of a person's performance skills are interrelated and include

- **Motor and praxis skills**
- **Sensory–perceptual skills**
- **Emotional regulation skills**
- **Cognitive skills**
- **Communication and social skills.**

Numerous body functions and structures underlie and enable performance (Rogers & Holm, 2008). Whereas body functions such as mental (affective, cognitive, perceptual), sensory, neuromuscular, and movement-related body functions (WHO, 2001) reflect the capacities that reside within the body, performance skills are the clients' demonstrated abilities. For example, praxis skills can be observed through client actions such as imitating, sequencing, and constructing; cognitive skills can be observed as the client demonstrates organization, time management, and safety; and emotional regulation skills can be observed through the behaviors the client displays to express emotion appropriately. Numerous body functions underlie each performance skill.

Multiple factors, such as the context in which the occupation is performed, the specific demands of the activity being attempted, and the client's body functions and structures, affect the client's ability to acquire or demonstrate performance skills. Performance skills are closely linked and are used in combination with one another to allow the client to perform an occupation. A change in one performance skill can affect other performance skills. In practice and in some literature, performance skills often are labeled in various combinations such as perceptual–motor skills and social–emotional skills. Table 4 provides definitions and selected examples under each category.

Occupational therapy practitioners observe and analyze performance skills in order to understand the transactions among underlying factors that support or hinder engagement in occupations and occupational performance. For example, when observing a person writing a check, the occupational therapy practitioner observes the

TABLE 4. PERFORMANCE SKILLS

Performance skills are the abilities clients demonstrate in the actions they perform.

Skill	Definition	Examples
Motor and praxis skills	*Motor:* Actions or behaviors a client uses to move and physically interact with tasks, objects, contexts, and environments (adapted from Fisher, 2006). Includes planning, sequencing, and executing new and novel movements. *Praxis:* Skilled purposeful movements (Heilman & Rothi, 1993). Ability to carry out sequential motor acts as part of an overall plan rather than individual acts (Liepmann, 1920). Ability to carry out learned motor activity, including following through on a verbal command, visual–spatial construction, ocular and oral–motor skills, imitation of a person or an object, and sequencing actions (Ayres, 1985; Filley, 2001). Organization of temporal sequences of actions within the spatial context, which form meaningful occupations (Blanche & Parham, 2002).	• *Bending* and *reaching* for a toy or tool in a storage bin • *Pacing* tempo of movements to clean the room • *Coordinating* body movements to complete a job task • *Maintaining balance* while walking on an uneven surface or while showering • *Anticipating or adjusting posture and body position* in response to environmental circumstances, such as obstacles • *Manipulating* keys or lock to open the door
Sensory–perceptual skills	Actions or behaviors a client uses to locate, identify, and respond to sensations and to select, interpret, associate, organize, and remember sensory events based on discriminating experiences through a variety of sensations that include visual, auditory, proprioceptive, tactile, olfactory, gustatory, and vestibular.	• *Positioning the body* in the exact location for a safe jump • *Hearing and locating* the voice of your child in a crowd • *Visually* determining the correct size of a storage container for leftover soup • *Locating* keys by touch from many objects in a pocket or purse (i.e., *stereognosis*) • *Timing the appropriate moment* to cross the street safely by determining one's own position and speed relative to the speed of traffic • *Discerning* distinct flavors within foods or beverages
Emotional regulation skills	Actions or behaviors a client uses to identify, manage, and express feelings while engaging in activities or interacting with others	• *Responding* to the feelings of others by acknowledgment or showing support • *Persisting* in a task despite frustrations • *Controlling* anger toward others and reducing aggressive acts • *Recovering* from a hurt or disappointment without lashing out at others • *Displaying* the emotions that are appropriate for the situation • *Utilizing* relaxation strategies to cope with stressful events
Cognitive skills	Actions or behaviors a client uses to plan and manage the performance of an activity	• *Judging* the importance or appropriateness of clothes for the circumstance • *Selecting* tools and supplies needed to clean the bathroom • *Sequencing* tasks needed for a school project • *Organizing* activities within the time required to meet a deadline • *Prioritizing* steps and *identifying* solutions to access transportation • *Creating* different activities with friends that are fun, novel, and enjoyable • *Multitasking*—doing more than one thing at a time, necessary for tasks such as work, driving, and household management

TABLE 4. PERFORMANCE SKILLS

(Continued)

Skill	Definition	Examples
Communication and social skills	Actions or behaviors a person uses to communicate and interact with others in an interactive environment (Fisher, 2006)	• *Looking* where someone else is pointing or gazing • *Gesturing* to emphasize intentions • *Maintaining* acceptable physical space during conversation • *Initiating and answering* questions with relevant information • *Taking turns* during an interchange with another person verbally and physically • *Acknowledging* another person's perspective during an interchange

motor skills of gripping and manipulating objects and the cognitive skills of initiating and sequencing the steps of the activity. The observed skills are supported by underlying body functions related to movement and cognition and by the environmental context of the bank. Proficient occupational performance observed in playing a game of tennis or playing the piano requires multiple sets of performance skills.

Further resources informing occupational therapy practice related to performance skills include Fisher (2006); Bloom, Krathwohl, and Masia (1984); Harrow (1972); and Chapparo and Ranka (1997). Detailed information about the way that skills are used in occupational therapy practice also may be found in the literature on specific theories such as sensory integration theory (Ayres, 1972, 2005) and motor learning and motor control theory (Shumway-Cook & Wollacott, 2007).

Performance Patterns

Performance patterns refer to **habits, routines, roles,** and **rituals** used in the process of engaging in occupations or activities. *Habits* refer to specific, automatic behaviors that can be useful, dominating, or impoverished (Clark, 2000; Neistadt & Crepeau, 1998), whereas *routines* are established sequences of occupations or activities that provide a structure for daily life. Routines also can be

health promoting or damaging (Fiese et al., 2002; Segal, 2004). *Roles* are sets of behaviors expected by society, shaped by culture, and may be further conceptualized and defined by the client. Roles can provide guidance in selecting occupations or can lead to stereotyping and restricted engagement patterns. Jackson (1998a, 1998b) cautioned that describing people by their roles can be limiting and can promote segmented rather than

> "...only occupational therapy practitioners focus this process toward the end-goal of supporting health and participation in life through engagement in occupations."

enfolded occupations. When considering roles within occupational therapy, occupational therapy practitioners are concerned with the way clients construct their occupations to fulfill their perceived roles and identity and reinforce their

"Occupational therapy practitioners apply theory, evidence, knowledge, and skills regarding the therapeutic use of occupations to positively affect the client's health, well-being, and life satisfaction."

values and beliefs. *Rituals* are symbolic actions with spiritual, cultural, or social meaning that contribute to the client's identity and reinforce the client's values and beliefs (Fiese et al., 2002; Segal, 2004). Habits, routines, roles, and rituals can support or hinder occupational performance.

People, organizations, and populations demonstrate performance patterns in daily life. They develop over time and are influenced by all other aspects of the domain. When practitioners consider the client's patterns of performance, they are better able to understand the frequency and manner in which performance skills and occupations are integrated into the client's life. While a client may have the ability or capacity for skilled performance, if he or she does not embed those skills in a productive set of engagement patterns, health and participation may be negatively affected. For example, a client who has the skills and resources to engage in appropriate grooming, bathing, and meal preparation but does not embed them into a consistent

routine, may struggle with poor nutrition and social isolation. Tables 5a, 5b, and 5c provide examples of performance patterns for persons, organizations, and populations.

Context and Environment

A client's engagement in occupation takes place within a social and physical environment situated within context. In the literature, the terms *environment* and *context* often are used interchangeably. In the *Framework,* both terms are used to reflect the importance of considering the wide variety of interrelated conditions both internal and external to the client that influence performance.

The term **environment** refers to the external physical and social environments that surround the client and in which the client's daily life occupations occur. **Physical environment** refers to the natural and built nonhuman environment and the objects in them. The **social environment** is constructed by the presence, relationships, and expectations of persons, groups, and organizations with whom the client has contact.

The term *context* refers to a variety of interrelated conditions that are within and surrounding the client. These interrelated contexts often are less tangible than physical and social environments but nonetheless exert a strong influence on performance. Contexts, as described in the *Framework,* are **cultural, personal, temporal,** and **virtual.** *Cultural context* includes customs, beliefs, activity patterns, behavior standards, and expectations accepted by the society of which the client is a member. *Personal context* refers to demographic features of the individual such as age, gender, socioeconomic status, and educational level that are not part of a health condition (WHO, 2001). *Temporal context* includes stages of life, time of day or year, duration, rhythm of activity, or history. *Virtual context* refers to interactions in simulated, real-time, or near-time situ-

TABLE 5A. PERFORMANCE PATTERNS—PERSON

Patterns of behavior related to an individual's or significant other's daily life activities that are habitual or routine.

	Examples
HABITS—"Automatic behavior that is integrated into more complex patterns that enable people to function on a day-to-day basis" (Neistadt & Crepeau, 1998, p. 869). Habits can be useful, dominating, or impoverished and either support or interfere with performance in areas of occupation.	– Automatically puts car keys in the same place. – Spontaneously looks both ways before crossing the street – Repeatedly rocks back and forth when asked to initiate a task – Repeatedly activates and deactivates the alarm system before entering the home – Maintains the exact distance between all hangers when hanging clothes in a closet
ROUTINES—Patterns of behavior that are observable, regular, repetitive, and that provide structure for daily life. They can be satisfying, promoting, or damaging. Routines require momentary time commitment and are embedded in cultural and ecological contexts (Fiese et al., 2002; Segal, 2004).	– Follows the morning sequence to complete toileting, bathing, hygiene, and dressing – Follows the sequence of steps involved in meal preparation
RITUALS—Symbolic actions with spiritual, cultural, or social meaning, contributing to the client's identity and reinforcing values and beliefs. Rituals have a strong affective component and represent a collection of events (Fiese et al., 2002; Segal, 2004).	– Uses the inherited antique hairbrush and brushes her hair with 100 strokes nightly as her mother had done – Prepares the holiday meals with favorite or traditional *accoutrements*, using designated dishware – Kisses a sacred book before opening the pages to read
ROLES—A set of behaviors expected by society, shaped by culture, and may be further conceptualized and defined by the client.	– Mother of an adolescent with developmental disabilities – Student with learning disability studying computer technology – Corporate executive returning to work after experiencing a stroke

Note. Information for "Habits" section of this table adapted from Dunn (2000b).

TABLE 5B. PERFORMANCE PATTERNS—ORGANIZATION

Patterns of behavior related to the daily functioning of an organization.

	Examples
ROUTINES—Patterns of behavior that are observable, regular, repetitive, and that provide structure for daily life. They can be satisfying, promoting, or damaging. Routines require momentary time commitment and are embedded in cultural and ecological contexts (Fiese et al., 2002; Segal, 2004).	– Holds regularly scheduled meetings for staff, directors, executive boards – Follows documentation practices for annual reports, timecards, and strategic plans – Turns in documentation on a scheduled basis – Follows the chain of command – Follows safety and security routines (e.g., signing in/out, using pass codes) – Maintains dress codes (e.g., casual Fridays) – Socializes during breaks, lunch, at the water cooler – Follows beginning or ending routines (e.g., opening/closing the facility) – Offers activities to meet performance expectations or standards

(Continued)

TABLE 5B. PERFORMANCE PATTERNS—ORGANIZATION

(Continued)

	Examples
RITUALS—Symbolic actions that have meaning, contributing to the organization's identity and reinforcing values and beliefs (adapted from Fiese et al., 2002; Segal, 2004).	– Holds holiday parties, company picnics – Conducts induction, recognition, and retirement ceremonies – Organizes annual retreats or conferences – Maintains fundraising activities for organization to support local charities
ROLES—A set of behaviors by the organization expected by society, shaped by culture, and may be further conceptualized and defined by the client.	– Nonprofit organization provides housing for persons living with mental illness – Humanitarian organization distributes food and clothing donations to refugees – University educates and provides service to the surrounding community

Note. In this document, habits are addressed only in Table 5A (Person).

TABLE 5C. PERFORMANCE PATTERNS—POPULATION

Patterns of behavior related to a population.

	Examples
ROUTINES—Patterns of behavior that are observable, regular, repetitive, and that provide structure for daily life. They can be satisfying, promoting, or damaging. Routines require momentary time commitment and are embedded in cultural and ecological contexts (Fiese et al., 2002; Segal, 2004).	– Follows health practices, such as scheduled immunizations for children and yearly health screenings for adults – Follows business practices, such as provision of services for the disadvantaged populations (e.g., loans to underrepresented groups) – Follows legislative procedures, such as those associated with IDEA and Medicare – Follows social customs for greeting
RITUALS—Rituals are shared social actions with traditional, emotional, purposive, and technological meaning, contributing to values and beliefs within the population.	– Holds cultural celebrations – Has parades or demonstrations – Shows national affiliations/allegiances – Follows religious, spiritual, and cultural practices, such as touching the mezuzah or using holy water when leaving/entering, praying to Mecca
ROLES	– SEE DESCRIPTION OF THESE AREAS FOR INDIVIDUALS WITHIN THE POPULATION

Note. In this document, habits are addressed only in Table 5A (Person).

TABLE 6. CONTEXTS AND ENVIRONMENTS

Context and *environment* (including cultural, personal, temporal, virtual, physical, and social) refers to a variety of interrelated conditions within and surrounding the client that influence performance.

The term *context* refers to a variety of interrelated conditions that are within and surrounding the client. Contexts include cultural, personal, temporal, and virtual. The term *environment* refers to the external physical and social environments that surround the client and in which the client's daily life occupations occur.

Context and Environment	Definition	Examples
Cultural	Customs, beliefs, activity patterns, behavior standards, and expectations accepted by the society of which the client is a member. Includes ethnicity and values as well as political aspects, such as laws that affect access to resources and affirm personal rights. Also includes opportunities for education, employment, and economic support.	*Person:* Shaking hands when being introduced *Organization:* Employees marking the end of the work week with casual dress on Friday *Population:* Celebrating Independence Day
Personal	"[F]eatures of the individual that are not part of a health condition or health status" (WHO, 2001, p. 17). Personal context includes age, gender, socioeconomic status, and educational status. Can also include organizational levels (e.g., volunteers and employees) and population levels (e.g., members of society).	*Person:* Twenty-five-year-old unemployed man with a high school diploma *Organization:* Volunteers working in a homeless shelter *Population:* Teenage women who are pregnant or new mothers
Temporal	"Location of occupational performance in time" (Neistadt & Crepeau, 1998, p. 292). The experience of time as shaped by engagement in occupations. The temporal aspects of occupation "which contribute to the patterns of daily occupations" are "the rhythm…tempo…synchronization…duration…and sequence" (Larson & Zemke, 2004, p. 82; Zemke, 2004, p. 610). Includes stages of life, time of day or year, duration, rhythm of activity, or history.	*Person:* A person retired from work for 10 years *Organization:* Annual fundraising campaign *Population:* Engaging in siestas or high teas
Virtual	Environment in which communication occurs by means of airways or computers and an absence of physical contact. Includes simulated or real-time or near-time existence of an environment via chat rooms, email, video-conferencing, radio transmissions.	*Person:* Text message to a friend *Organization:* Video conference, telephone conference call, instant message, interactive white boards among all the members *Population:* Virtual community of gamers
Physical	Natural and built nonhuman environment and the objects in them: • Natural environment includes geographic terrain, sensory qualities of environment, plants and animals • Built environment and objects includes buildings, furniture, tools or devices.	*Person:* Individual's house, apartment *Organization:* Office building, factory *Population:* Transportation system
Social	Is constructed by presence, relationships, and expectations of persons, organizations, populations. • Availability and expectations of significant individuals, such as spouse, friends, and caregivers • Relationships with individuals, groups, or organizations • Relationships with systems (e.g., political, legal, economic, institutional) that are influential in establishing norms, role expectations, and social routines.	*Person:* Friends, colleagues *Organization:* Advisory board *Population:* City government

---

EVALUATION

Occupational profile—The initial step in the evaluation process that provides an understanding of the client's occupational history and experiences, patterns of daily living, interests, values, and needs. The client's problems and concerns about performing occupations and daily life activities are identified, and the client's priorities are determined.

Analysis of occupational performance—The step in the evaluation process during which the client's assets, problems, or potential problems are more specifically identified. Actual performance is often observed in context to identify what supports performance and what hinders performance. Performance skills, performance patterns, context or contexts, activity demands, and client factors are all considered, but only selected aspects may be specifically assessed. Targeted outcomes are identified.

INTERVENTION

Intervention plan—A plan that will guide actions taken and that is developed in collaboration with the client. It is based on selected theories, frames of reference, and evidence. Outcomes to be targeted are confirmed.

Intervention implementation—Ongoing actions taken to influence and support improved client performance. Interventions are directed at identified outcomes. Client's response is monitored and documented.

Intervention review—A review of the implementation plan and process as well as its progress toward targeted outcomes.

OUTCOMES (Supporting Health and Participation in Life Through Engagement in Occupation)

Outcomes—Determination of success in reaching desired targeted outcomes. Outcome assessment information is used to plan future actions with the client and to evaluate the service program (i.e., program evaluation).

Figure 5. Process of Service Delivery.
The process of service delivery is applied within the profession's domain to support the client's health and participation.

ations absent of physical contact. Some contexts are external to the client (e.g., virtual), some are internal to the client (e.g., personal), and some may have both external features and internalized beliefs and values (e.g., cultural).

Clients' engagement in occupations evolves within their social and physical environments and reflects their interdependence with these environments. Cultural contexts often influence how occupations are chosen, prioritized, and organized. Contexts and environments affect a client's accessibility to occupations and influence the quality of performance and satisfaction with performance. A client who has difficulty performing effectively in one environment or context may be successful when the environment or context is changed. The context within which the engagement in occupations occurs is unique for each client. Contexts and environments are interrelated both with each other and all other aspects of the domain (see Table 6 for a description of the different kinds of contexts and environments).

Process of Occupational Therapy

Overview

This second section of the *Occupational Therapy Practice Framework* describes the process that outlines the way in which occupational therapy practitioners operationalize their expertise to provide services to clients (see Figure 5). This process includes evaluation, intervention, and outcome monitoring; occurs within the purview of the domain; and involves collaboration among the occupational therapist, occupational therapy assistant, and the client. Occupational therapy practitioners are required to maintain appropriate credentials and abide by ethical standards, existing laws, and regulatory requirements for each step of the occupational therapy process.

Many professions use the process of evaluating, intervening, and targeting intervention **outcomes.** However, only occupational therapy practitioners focus this process toward the end-goal of supporting health and participation in life through engagement in occupations. Occupational therapy practitioners also use occupations as a method of intervention implementation by engaging clients throughout the process in occupations that are therapeutically selected. The profession's use of occupation as both means and end is a unique application of the process (Trombly, 1995).

Although for the purpose of organization the *Framework* describes the process in a linear manner, in reality, the process does not occur in a sequenced, step-by-step fashion (see Table 7). Instead, it is fluid and dynamic, allowing occupational therapy practitioners to operate with an ongoing focus on outcomes while continually reflecting on and changing an overall plan to accommodate new developments and insights along the way.

Occupational therapy involves facilitating interactions among the client, the environments or contexts, and the activities or occupations in order to help the client reach the desired outcomes that support health and participation in life. Occupational therapy practitioners apply theory, evidence, knowledge, and skills regarding the therapeutic use of occupations to positively affect the client's health, well-being, and life satisfaction.

The broader definition of *client* included in this document is indicative of the profession's increasing involvement in providing services not only to a person but also to organizations and populations. Regardless of whether the client is a person, organization, or population, the client's wants, needs, occupational risks, and problems are evaluated, and information is gathered, synthesized, and framed from an occupational perspective. This perspective is based on the theories, knowledge, and skills generated and used by the profession and informed by available evidence. Client concerns are viewed relative to problems or risks in occupational performance.

Occupational therapy practitioners develop a collaborative relationship with clients in order to understand their experiences and desires for intervention, as noted in Figure 2. The collaborative approach, which is used throughout the process, honors the contributions of the client and the occupational therapy practitioner. Clients bring knowledge about their life experiences and their **hopes** and dreams for the future. They identify and share their needs and priorities. Occupational therapy practitioners bring their knowledge about how engagement in occupation affects health and performance. This information is coupled with the practitioner's **clinical reasoning** and theoretical perspectives to critically observe, analyze, describe, and interpret human performance. Occupational therapy practitioners also apply knowledge and skills to reduce the effects of disease, disability, and deprivation and to promote health and well-being. Together, practitioners and clients identify and prioritize the focus of the intervention plan. This collaboration may include family, significant others, community members, and stakeholders who affect or are affected by the client's engagement in occupation, health, and participation.

Rarely is an individual the exclusive focus of the intervention. For example, the needs of an at-risk infant may be the initial impetus for intervention, but the concerns and priorities of the parent, the extended family, and funding agencies also are considered. Similarly, services addressing independent-living skills for adults coping with serious and persistent mental illness may involve the needs and expectations of state and local services agencies as well as business groups.

Throughout the process, the occupational therapy practitioner is engaged continually in clinical reasoning about the client's engagement in occupation. Clinical reasoning enables the occupational therapy practitioner to (1) identify

TABLE 7. OPERATIONALIZING THE OCCUPATIONAL THERAPY PROCESS

Evaluation		Intervention			Outcomes
					Supporting Health and Participation in Life through Engagement in Occupation
Occupational Profile ⟷	*Analysis of Occupational Performance*	*Intervention Plan*	*Intervention Implementation*	*Intervention Review*	

Identify
• Who is the client?
• Why is the client seeking services?
• What occupations and activities are successful or are causing problems?
• What contexts and environments support or inhibit desired outcomes?
• What is the client's occupational history?
• What are the client's priorities and targeted outcomes?
	• Synthesize information from the occupational profile.
	• Observe client's performance in desired occupation/activity.
	• Note the effectiveness of performance skills and patterns and select assessments to identify factors (context or contexts, activity demands, client factors) that may be influencing performance skills and patterns.
	• Interpret assessment data to identify facilitators and barriers to performance.
	• Develop and refine hypotheses about client's occupational performance strengths and weaknesses.
	• Collaborate with client to create goals that address targeted outcomes.
	• Delineate areas for intervention based on best practice and evidence.
		• Develop plan that includes
		  –Objective and measurable goals with time frame,
		  –Occupational therapy intervention approach based on theory and evidence, and
		  –Mechanisms for service delivery.
		• Consider discharge needs and plan.
		• Select outcome measures.
		• Make recommendation or referral to others as needed.
			• Determine types of occupational therapy interventions to be used and carry them out.
			• Monitor client's response according to ongoing assessment and reassessment.
				• Reevaluate plan relative to achieving targeted outcomes.
				• Modify plan as needed.
				• Determine need for continuation, discontinuation, or referral.
					• Focus on outcomes as they relate to supporting health and participation in life through engagement in occupation.
					• Select outcome measures.
					• Measure and use outcomes.

⟵———— Continue to renegotiate intervention plans and targeted outcomes. ————⟶

⟵———— Ongoing interaction among evaluation, intervention, and outcomes occurs throughout the process. ————⟶

204

the multiple demands, skills, and potential meanings of the activity and (2) gain a deeper understanding of the interrelationships between aspects of the domain that affect performance and those that will support client-centered interventions and outcomes.

Evaluation

The **evaluation** process begins with an evaluation conducted by the occupational therapist and is focused on finding out what the client wants and needs to do, determining what the client can do and has done, and identifying those factors that act as supports or barriers to health and participation. Evaluation often occurs both formally and informally during all interactions with the client. The type and focus of the evaluation differs depending on the practice setting.

The evaluation consists of the **occupational profile** and **analysis of occupational performance.** The *occupational profile* includes information about the client and the client's needs, problems, and concerns about performance in areas of occupation. The *analysis of occupational performance* focuses on collecting and interpreting information using **assessment** tools designed to observe, measure, and inquire about factors that support or hinder occupational performance. Although the ways occupational therapists collect client information are described separately and sequentially in the *Framework,* the exact manner is influenced by the client needs and the practice setting. Information related to the occupational profile is gathered throughout the occupational therapy process.

The occupational therapist's knowledge and skills, as well as theoretical principles and available evidence, guide his or her clinical reasoning for the selection and application of various theories and frames of reference throughout the evaluation process. Concurrently, the occupational therapist's

knowledge and skills in these areas influence the information that is collected during the evaluation. Knowledge and evidence about occupational performance problems and diagnostic conditions are used to guide information gathering and synthesis of information for interpretation and intervention planning. The occupational therapist's skilled interpretation of assessment results relative to the whole evaluation leads to a clear delineation of the strengths and limitations affecting the client's occupational performance. The occupational therapy assistant contributes to the evaluation process based on established competencies and under the supervision of an occupational therapist.

Occupational Profile

An *occupational profile* is defined as a summary of information that describes the client's occupational history and experiences, patterns of daily living, **interests,** values, and needs. Because the profile is designed to gain an understanding of the client's perspective and background, its format varies depending on whether the client is a person, organization, or population. Using a **client-centered approach,** the occupational therapy practitioner gathers information to understand what is currently important and meaningful to the client. The profile includes inquiry related to what the client wants and needs to do in the present or future as well as past experiences and interests that may assist in identifying strengths and limitations. Refinement of the information collected during the occupational profile subsequently refines the intervention plan and identified outcomes.

During the process of collecting this information, the client's priorities and desired outcomes that will lead to engagement in occupation for improved health are identified. Clients identify occupations that give meaning to their lives and select the **goals** and priorities important to them. Valuing and respecting the client's collaboration in the therapeutic process helps foster client involvement and more efficiently guide interventions.

The process and timing of completing the occupational profile varies depending on the circumstances. Occupational therapy practitioners may gather information formally and informally in one session or over a longer period while working with the client. Obtaining information through both formal interview and casual conversation helps establish a therapeutic relationship with the client. Ideally, the information obtained during the development of the occupational profile leads to a more client-centered approach in the evaluation, intervention planning, and intervention implementation stages.

Specifically, the information collected answers the following questions:

- Who is the client (person, including family, caregivers, and significant others; population; or organization)?
- Why is the client seeking services, and what are the client's current concerns relative to engaging in occupations and in daily life activities?
- What areas of occupation are successful, and what areas are causing problems or risks (see Table 1)?
- What contexts and environments support or inhibit participation and engagement in desired occupations?
- What is the client's occupational history (i.e., life experiences, values, interests, previous patterns of engagement in occupations and in daily life activities, the meanings associated with them)?
- What are the client's priorities and desired outcomes?

Once the profile data are collected and documented, the occupational therapist reviews the information; identifies the client's strengths, limitations, and needs; and develops a working hypothe-sis regarding possible reasons for identified problems and concerns. The occupational therapy assistant contributes to this process. The information from the occupational therapy profile often guides the selection of outcome measures. If an organization or population is the identified client, the strengths and needs are those that affect the collective entity rather than the individual.

Analysis of Occupational Performance

Occupational performance is the accomplishment of the selected occupation resulting from the dynamic transaction among the client, the context and environment, and the activity. Evaluation of occupational performance involves one or more of the following:

- Synthesizing information from the occupational profile to focus on specific areas of occupation and contexts that need to be addressed;
- Observing the client's performance during activities relevant to desired occupations, noting effectiveness of the performance skills and performance patterns;
- Selecting and using specific assessments to measure performance skills and performance patterns, as appropriate;
- Selecting assessments, as needed, to identify and measure more specifically contexts or environments, activity demands, and client factors influencing performance skills and performance patterns;
- Interpreting the assessment data to identify what supports performance and what hinders performance;
- Developing and refining hypotheses about the client's occupational performance strengths and limitations;
- Creating goals in collaboration with the client that address the desired outcomes;
- Determining procedures to measure the outcomes of intervention; and

• Delineating a potential intervention approach or approaches based on best practices and available evidence.

Multiple methods often are used during the evaluation process to assess the client, the context, the occupation or activity, and the occupational performance. Methods may include an interview with the client and significant others, observation of performance and context, record review, and direct assessment of specific aspects of performance. Formal and informal, structured and unstructured, and standardized criterion or norm-referenced assessment tools can be used. Standardized assessments are preferred, when appropriate, to provide objective data about the various aspects of the domain influencing engagement and performance. "Obtaining reliable and valid information [through the use of standard assessments] provides a high level of support that can justify the need for occupational therapy services" (Gutman, Mortera, Hinojosa, & Kramer, 2007, p. 121).

Activity analysis is an important process used by occupational therapy practitioners to understand the demands that a specific desired activity places on a client. "Activity analysis addresses the typical demands of an activity, the range of skills involved in its performance, and the various cultural meanings that might be ascribed to it" (Crepeau, 2003, p. 192). When activity analysis is completed and the demands of a specific activity that the client wants and needs to do are understood, the client's specific skills and abilities are then compared with the selected activity's demands.

> Occupation-based activity analysis places the person [client] in the foreground. It takes into account the particular person's [client's] interests, goals, abilities, and contexts, as well as the demands of the activity itself. These considerations shape the practitioner's efforts to help the…person [client] reach his/her goals through carefully designed evaluation and intervention. (Crepeau, 2003, p. 193)

Examining the environments and contexts in which occupational performance can or does occur provides insights into overarching, underlying, and embedded influences on engagement. The external environments and context (e.g., physical and social environment, virtual context) provide resources that support or inhibit the client's performance (e.g., doorway widths as part of the physical environment that allow for wheelchair passage, presence or absence of a caregiver as part of the social environment, access to a computer to communicate with others as part of the virtual context). Different environments (e.g., community, institution, home) provide different supports and resources for service delivery (e.g., assessment of an infant or toddler in the hospital without the primary caregivers present yields different results than while at home with a parent).

The client's personal context affects service delivery by influencing personal beliefs, perceptions, and expectations. The cultural context exists within small groups of related individuals, such as a nuclear family, and within larger groups of people, such as populations of a country or ethnic group. The expectations, beliefs, and customs of various cultures can affect a client's **identity** and activity choices and need to be considered when determining how and when services may be delivered. Note that in Figure 2, context and environment are depicted as surrounding and underlying the process.

Analyzing occupational performance requires an understanding of the complex and dynamic interaction among performance skills, performance patterns, contexts and environments, activity demands, and client factors. Occupational therapy practitioners attend to each aspect and gauge the influence of each aspect on the others—individually and collectively. By understanding how these aspects dynamically influence each other, occupational therapists can better evaluate how they contribute to the client's performance-related concerns, and how they

"Supporting health and participation in life through engagement in occupation is the broad, overarching outcome of the occupational therapy intervention process."

potentially contribute to interventions that support occupational performance. When working with an organization or population, occupational therapy practitioners consider the collective occupational performance abilities of the respective members.

Intervention

The **intervention** process consists of the skilled actions taken by occupational therapy practitioners in collaboration with the client to facilitate engagement in occupation related to health and participation. Occupational therapy practitioners use the information about the client gathered during the evaluation and from theoretical principles to direct occupation-centered interventions. Intervention is provided then to assist the client in reaching a state of physical, mental, and social well-being; to identify and realize aspirations; to satisfy needs; and to change or cope with the environment. A variety of types of occupational therapy interventions are discussed in Table 8.

Intervention is intended to be health-promoting. *Health promotion* is "the process of enabling people to increase control over, and to improve, their health" (WHO, 1986). Wilcock (2006) states

[F]ollowing an occupation-focused health promotion approach to well-being embraces a belief that the potential range of what people can do, be, and strive to become is the primary concern and that health is a by-product. A varied and full occupational lifestyle will coincidentally maintain and improve health and well-being if it enables people to be creative and adventurous physically, mentally, and socially. (p. 315)

Interventions vary depending on the client—person, organization, or population—and the context of service delivery (Moyers & Dale, 2007). The actual term used for clients receiving occupational therapy varies among practice settings and delivery models. For example, when working in a hospital, the person might be referred to as a *patient,* and in a school, the client might be a *student, teacher, parent,* or *administrator.* When providing services to an organization, the client may be called the *consumer.* When serving a population, the client may be specific entities, such as disability groups, veterans who are homeless, or refugees.

The term *person* includes others who also may help or be served indirectly, such as caregiver, teacher, parent, employer, or spouse. When addressing the person or a small group of persons who support or care for the client in need of services (e.g., caregiver, teacher, partner, employer, spouse), the practitioners address the interaction among client factors, performance skills, performance patterns, contexts and environments, and activity demands that influence occupational performance within those occupations the person needs and wants to do. The intervention focus is on modifying the environment/contexts and activity demands or patterns, promoting health, establishing or restoring and maintaining occupational performance, and preventing further disability and occupational performance problems.

Interventions provided to *organizations* are designed to affect the organization to more efficiently and effectively meet the needs of the clients or

TABLE 8. TYPES OF OCCUPATIONAL THERAPY INTERVENTIONS

THERAPEUTIC USE OF SELF—An occupational therapy practitioner's planned use of his or her personality, insights, perceptions, and judgments as part of the therapeutic process (adapted from Punwar & Peloquin, 2000, p. 285).

THERAPEUTIC USE OF OCCUPATIONS AND ACTIVITIES[a]—Occupations and activities selected for specific clients that meet therapeutic goals. To use occupations/activities therapeutically, context or contexts, activity demands, and client factors all should be considered in relation to the client's therapeutic goals. Use of assistive technologies, application of universal-design principles, and environmental modifications support the ability of clients to engage in their occupations.

Occupation-based intervention	*Purpose:* Client engages in client-directed occupations that match identified goals. *Examples:* • Completes morning dressing and hygiene using adaptive devices • Purchases groceries and prepares a meal • Utilizes the transportation system • Applies for a job • .Plays on playground and community recreation equipment • Participates in a community festival • Establishes a pattern of self-care and relaxation activities in preparation for sleep
Purposeful activity	*Purpose:* Client engages in specifically selected activities that allow the client to develop skills that enhance occupational engagement. *Examples:* • Practices how to select clothing and manipulate clothing fasteners • Practices safe ways to get in and out of a bathtub • Practices how to prepare a food list and rehearses how to use cooking appliances • Practices how to use a map and transportation schedule • Rehearses how to write answers on an application form • .Practices how to get on and off playground and recreation equipment • Role plays when to greet people and initiates conversation • Practices how to use adaptive switches to operate home environmental control system
Preparatory methods	*Purpose:* Practitioner selects directed methods and techniques that prepare the client for occupational performance. Used in preparation for or concurrently with purposeful and occupation-based activities. *Examples:* • Provides sensory enrichment to promote alertness • Administers physical agent modalities to prepare muscles for movement • Provides instruction in visual imagery and rhythmic breathing to promote rest and relaxation • Issues orthotics/splints to provide support and facilitate movement • Suggests a home-based conditioning regimen using Pilates and yoga • Provides hand-strengthening exercises using therapy putty and theraband • Provides instruction in assertiveness to prepare for self-advocacy

(Continued)

TABLE 8. TYPES OF OCCUPATIONAL THERAPY INTERVENTIONS

(Continued)

CONSULTATION PROCESS—A type of intervention in which occupational therapy practitioners use their knowledge and expertise to collaborate with the client. The collaborative process involves identifying the problem, creating possible solutions, trying solutions, and altering them as necessary for greater effectiveness. When providing consultation, the practitioner is not directly responsible for the outcome of the intervention (Dunn, 2000a, p. 113).

Person	• Advises a family about architectural options • Advises family how to create pre-sleep nighttime routines for their children
Organization	• Recommends work pattern modifications and ergonomically designed workstations for a company • Recommends disaster evacuation strategies for a residential community related to accessibility and reduced environmental barriers
Population	• Advises senior citizens on older driver initiatives

EDUCATION PROCESS—An intervention process that involves imparting knowledge and information about occupation, health, and participation and that does not result in the actual performance of the occupation/activity.

Person	• Instructs a classroom teacher on sensory regulation strategies
Organization	• Teaches staff at a homeless shelter how to structure daily living, play, and leisure activities for shelter members
Population	• Instructs town officials about the value of and strategies for making walking and biking paths accessible for all community members

ADVOCACY—Efforts directed toward promoting occupational justice and empowering clients to seek and obtain resources to fully participate in their daily life occupations.

Person	• Collaborates with a person to procure reasonable accommodations at worksite
Organization	• Serves on policy board of an organization to procure supportive housing accommodations for persons with disabilities
Population	• Collaborates with adults with serious mental illness to raise public awareness of the impact of this stigma • Collaborates with and educates federal funding sources for the disabled population to include cancer patients prior to their full remission

[a]Information adapted from Pedretti and Early (2001).

consumers and stakeholders. Practitioners address features of the organization or agency such as its mission, values, organizational culture and structure, policies and procedures, and built and natural environments. Practitioners evaluate how each of these features either supports or inhibits the overall performance of individuals within the organization. For example, to enable the staff at a skilled-nursing facility to provide better services, an occupational therapy practitioner may recommend the walls in each hallway be painted a different color, enabling residents to more easily locate their rooms.

Interventions provided to *populations* are directed to all the members of the group collectively rather than individualized to specific people within the group. Practitioners direct their interventions toward current or potential health problems and disabling conditions within the population and community. Their goal is to enhance the health of all people within the population by addressing services and supports within the community that can be implemented to improve the population's performance. The intervention focus often is on health promotion activities, self-management educational services, and environmental modification. For instance, the occupational therapy practitioner may design developmentally based day care programs run by college student volunteers for homeless shelters catering to families in a large metropolitan area. Practitioners may work with a wide variety of populations experiencing difficulty in accessing and engaging in health occupations due to conditions such as poverty, homelessness, and discrimination.

The intervention process is divided into three steps: (1) intervention plan, (2) intervention implementation, and (3) intervention review. During the intervention process, information from the evaluation is integrated with theory, practice models, frames of reference, and evidence. This information guides the clinical reasoning of the occupa-

tional therapist and the occupational therapy assistant in the development, implementation, and review of the intervention plan.

Intervention Plan

The intervention plan directs the actions of the occupational therapist and occupational therapy assistant. It describes the selected occupational therapy approaches and types of interventions for reaching the client's identified outcomes. The intervention plan is developed collaboratively with the client and is based on the client's goals and priorities. Depending on whether the client is a person, organization, or population, others such as family members, significant others, board members, service providers, and community groups also may collaborate in the development of the plan.

The design of the intervention plan is directed by the

- Client's goals, values, beliefs, and occupational needs;
- Client's health and well-being;
- Client's performance skills and performance patterns;
- Collective influence of the context, environment, activity demands, and client factors on the client;
- Context of service delivery in which the intervention is provided (e.g., caregiver expectations, organization's purpose, payer's requirements, applicable regulations); and
- Best available evidence.

The selection and design of the intervention plan and goals are directed toward addressing the client's current and potential problems related to engagement in occupations or activities.

Intervention planning includes the following steps:

1. *Developing the plan.* The occupational therapist develops the plan with the client, and the

occupational therapy assistant contributes to the plan's development. The plan includes

- Objective and measurable goals with a time-frame
- Occupational therapy **intervention approach** or approaches (see Table 9)
  - Create or promote
  - Establish or restore
  - Maintain
  - Modify
  - Prevent.
- Mechanisms for service delivery
  - People providing the intervention
  - Types of interventions
  - Frequency and duration of service.

2. *Considering potential discharge needs and plans*
3. *Selecting outcome measures*
4. *Making recommendation or referral to others as needed.*

Intervention Implementation

Intervention implementation is the process of putting the plan into action. It involves the skilled process of altering factors in the client, activity, and context and environment for the purpose of effecting positive change in the client's desired engagement in occupation, health, and participation.

Interventions may focus on a single aspect of the domain, such as a specific performance pattern, or several aspects of the domain, such as performance patterns, performance skills, and context. Given that the factors are interrelated and influence one another in a continuous, dynamic process, occupational therapy practitioners expect that the client's ability to adapt, change, and develop in one area will affect other areas. Because of this dynamic interrelationship, assessment and intervention planning continue throughout the implementation process. Intervention implementation includes the following steps:

1. Determining and carrying out the type of occupational therapy intervention or interventions to be used (see Table 8)
   - Therapeutic use of self
   - Therapeutic use of occupations or activities
     - **Occupation-based interventions**
     - **Purposeful activity**
     - **Preparatory methods.**
   - **Consultation process**
   - **Education process**
   - **Advocacy.**
2. Monitoring the client's response to interventions based on ongoing assessment and reassessment of the client's progress toward goals.

Intervention Review

Intervention review is the continuous process of reevaluating and reviewing the intervention plan, the effectiveness of its delivery, and the progress toward outcomes. As during intervention planning, this process includes collaboration with the client based on his or her goals. Depending on whether the client is a person, organization, or population, various stakeholders, such as family members, significant others, board members, other service providers, and community groups, also may collaborate in the intervention review. **Re-evaluation** and review may lead to change in the intervention plan.

The intervention review includes the following steps:

1. Re-evaluating the plan and how it is implemented relative to achieving outcomes
2. Modifying the plan as needed
3. Determining the need for continuation or discontinuation of occupational therapy services and for referral to other services.

The intervention review may include program evaluations that critique the way that occupational therapy services are provided. This may include a review of client satisfaction and the client's perception of the benefits of receiving occupational ther-

TABLE 9. OCCUPATIONAL THERAPY INTERVENTION APPROACHES

Specific strategies selected to direct the process of intervention that are based on the client's desired outcome, evaluation data, and evidence.

Approach	Focus of Intervention	Examples
Create, promote (health promotion)[a]—An intervention approach that does not assume a disability is present or that any factors would interfere with performance. This approach is designed to provide enriched contextual and activity experiences that will enhance performance for all persons in the natural contexts of life (adapted from Dunn, McClain, Brown, & Youngstrom, 1998, p. 534).	**Performance skills**	• Create a parenting class to help first-time parents engage their children in developmentally appropriate play
	Performance patterns	• Promote effective handling of stress by creating time use routines with healthy clients
	Context or contexts or physical environments	• Promote a diversity of sensory play experiences by recommending a variety of equipment for playgrounds and other play areas
	Activity demands	• Serve food family style in the congregate dining area to increase the opportunities for socialization
	Client factors (body functions, body structures)	• Promote increased endurance by recommending year-round daily outdoor recess for all school children • Design a dance program for senior citizens that will enhance strength and flexibility
Establish, restore (remediation, restoration)[a]—An intervention approach designed to change client variables to establish a skill or ability that has not yet developed or to restore a skill or ability that has been impaired (adapted from Dunn et al., 1998, p. 533).	**Performance skills**	• Provide adjustable desk chairs to improve client sitting posture • Work with senior community centers to offer driving educational programs targeted at improving driving skills for persons ages 65 or older
	Performance patterns	• Collaborate with clients to help them establish morning routines needed to arrive at school or work on time • Provide classes in fatigue management for cancer patients and their families • Collaborate with clients to help them establish healthy sleep–wake patterns • Develop walking programs at the local mall for employees and community members
	Client factors (body functions, body structures)	• Support daily physical education classes for entire population of children in a school aimed at improving physical strength and endurance • Collaborate with schools and businesses to establish universal-design models in their buildings, classrooms, and so forth • Gradually increase time required to complete a computer game to increase client's attention span

(Continued)

TABLE 9. OCCUPATIONAL THERAPY INTERVENTION APPROACHES

(Continued)

Approach	Focus of Intervention	Examples
Maintain—An intervention approach designed to provide the supports that will allow clients to preserve the performance capabilities they have regained, that continue to meet their occupational needs, or both. The assumption is that, without continued maintenance intervention, performance would decrease, occupational needs would not be met, or both, thereby affecting health and quality of life.	Performance skills	• Maintain the ability of the client to organize tools by providing a tool outline painted on a pegboard • Develop a refresher safety program for industrial organizations to remind workers of need to continue to use safety skills on the job • Provide a program for community-dwelling older adults to maintain motor and praxis skills
	Performance patterns	• Enable client to maintain appropriate medication schedule by providing a timer to aid with memory • Establish occupational performance patterns to maintain a healthy lifestyle after significant weight loss
	Context or contexts or physical environments	• Maintain safe and independent access for persons with low vision by recommending increased hallway lighting • During a natural disaster, work with facilities identified as "shelters" to provide play and leisure activities for displaced people to allow a constructive outlet and semblance of normalcy • Incorporate principles of universal design in homes to allow people to age in place
	Activity demands	• Maintain independent gardening for persons with arthritic hands by recommending tools with modified grips, long-handled tools, seating alternatives, raised gardens, and so forth
	Client factors (body functions, body structures)	• Provide multisensory activities in which nursing-home residents may participate to maintain alertness • Provide hand-based thumb splint for client use during periods of stressful or prolonged intensive activity to maintain pain-free joints
Modify (compensation, adaptation)[a]—An intervention approach directed at "finding ways to revise the current context or activity demands to support performance in the natural setting, [including] compensatory techniques, [such as]...enhancing some features to provide cues or reducing other features to reduce distractibility" (Dunn et al., 1998, p. 533).	Performance patterns	• Provide a visual schedule to help a student follow routines and transition easily between activities at home and school • Simplify task sequence to help a person with cognitive issues complete a morning self-care routine
	Context or contexts or physical environments	• Assist a family in determining requirements for building a ramp at home for a family member who is returning home after physical rehabilitation • Consult with builders in designing homes that will allow families the ability to provide living space for aging parents (e.g., bedroom and full bath on the main floor of a multilevel dwelling) • Modify the number of people in a room to decrease client's distractibility

TABLE 9. OCCUPATIONAL THERAPY INTERVENTION APPROACHES

(Continued)

Approach	Focus of Intervention	Examples
	Activity demands	• Adapt writing surface used in classroom by fourth grader by adding adjustable incline board • Assist a patient with a terminal illness and his or her family in modifying tasks to maintain engagement • Consult with school teams on placement of switches to increase students' access to computers, augmentative communication devices, environmental devices, and so forth • Provide a seat at the assembly station to allow a client with decreased standing tolerance to be able to continue to perform
Prevent (disability prevention)[a]—An intervention approach designed to address clients with or without a disability who are at risk for occupational performance problems. This approach is designed to prevent the occurrence or evolution of barriers to performance in context. Interventions may be directed at client, context, or activity variables (adapted from Dunn et al., 1998, p. 534).	**Performance skills**	• Prevent poor posture when sitting for prolonged periods by providing a chair with proper back support
	Performance patterns	• Aid in the prevention of illicit chemical substance use by introducing self-initiated routine strategies that support drug-free behavior
	Context or contexts or physical environments	• Prevent social isolation of employees by promoting participation in after-work group activities • Reduce risk of falls by modifying the environment and removing known hazards in the home (e.g., throw rugs)
	Activity demands	• Prevent back injury by providing instruction in proper lifting techniques
	Client factors (body functions, body structures)	• Prevent repetitive stress injury by suggesting that clients wear a wrist support splint when typing • Consultation with hotel chain to provide an ergonomics educational program designed to prevent back injuries in housekeepers

[a]Parallel language used in Moyers and Dale (2007, p. 34).

apy services (adapted from Maciejewski, Kawiecki, & Rockwood, 1997). Examples may include (1) a letter of thanks from the family of a child with spinal bifida (person); (2) a request for additional occupational therapy services at a homeless shelter for their clients (organizations); and (3) procurement of funds to implement support groups for caregivers of people with Alzheimer's disease throughout the United States (populations).

Outcomes

Supporting health and participation in life through engagement in occupation is the broad, overarching outcome of the occupational therapy intervention process. This outcome statement acknowledges the profession's belief that active engagement in occupation promotes, facilitates, and maintains health and participation. *Outcomes* are defined as important dimensions of health, attributed to interventions, and include the ability to function, health perceptions, and satisfaction with care (adapted from Request for Planning Ideas, 2001). Outcomes are the end-result of the occupational therapy process and describe what occupational therapy intervention can achieve with clients.

The three interrelated concepts included in the profession's overarching outcome are defined as
1. *Health*—"[A] positive concept emphasizing social and personal resources, as well as physical capacities" (WHO, 1986).
2. *Participation*—That is, "involvement in a life situation" (WHO, 2001, p. 10). Participation naturally occurs when clients are actively involved in carrying out occupations or daily life activities they find purposeful and meaningful in desired contexts. More specific outcomes of occupational therapy intervention (see Table 10) are multidimensional and support the end-result of participation.
3. *Engagement in occupation*—The commitment made to performance in occupations as the

result of choice, motivation, and meaning and includes objective and subjective aspects of carrying out activities meaningful and purposeful to the individual person, organization, or population. Occupational therapy intervention focuses on creating or facilitating opportunities to engage in these occupations.

To determine the client's success in achieving health and participation in life through engagement in occupation, occupational therapy practitioners assess observable outcomes. This assessment takes into consideration the hypothesized relationships among various aspects of occupational performance. For example, a client's improved ability to embed performance skills into a routine (performance pattern) and improved strength or range of motion (body functions) enables engagement in managing a home (IADL).

Implicit in any outcome assessment used by occupational therapy practitioners are the client's beliefs systems and underlying assumptions regarding their desired occupational performance. The assessment tools and the variables measured often become the operational definition for the outcome. Therefore, occupational therapy practitioners select outcome assessments pertinent to the needs and desires of clients, congruent with the practitioner's theoretical model of practice, based on knowledge of the psychometric properties of standardized measures or the rationale and protocols of non-standardized measures and the available evidence. In addition, the client's perception of success in engaging in desired occupations is vital to any outcomes assessment. As a point of comparison and in collaboration with the client, the occupational therapist may revisit the occupational profile to assess change.

The benefits of occupational therapy are multifaceted and may occur in all aspects of the domain of concern. Supporting health and participation in life through engagement in occupation is the broad outcome of intervention. Clients' improved performance of occupations, perceived happiness, self-efficacy, and hopefulness about their life and abilities are valuable outcomes. For example, parents whose children received occupational therapy valued understanding their child's' behaviors in new ways and had greater perceived efficacy about their parenting (Cohn, 2001; Cohn, Miller, & Tickle-Degnan, 2000). Interventions designed for caregivers who provide care for people with dementia improve the quality of life for both the care recipient and the caregiver. Caregivers who received intervention reported fewer declines in the occupational performance of care recipients and less need for help and enhanced mastery and skill, self-efficacy, and well-being for themselves (Gitlin & Corcoran, 2005; Gitlin, Corcoran, Winter, Boyce, & Hauck, 2001; Gitlin et al., 2003).

Outcomes for people may include subjective impressions related to goals such as an improved outlook, confidence, hope, playfulness, self-efficacy, sustainability of valued occupations, resilience, or perceived well-being. Outcomes also may include measurable increments of progress in factors related to occupational performance such as skin integrity, amount of sleep, endurance, desire, initiation, balance, visual–motor skills, and at the participation level, activity participation and community re-integration. Outcomes for organizations may include increased workplace morale, productivity, reduced injuries, and improved worker satisfaction. Outcomes for populations may include health promotion, social justice, and access to services. The definitions and connotations of outcomes are specific to clients, groups, and organizations as well as to payers and regulators. Specific outcomes as well as documentation of those outcomes vary by practice setting and are influenced by the particular stakeholders in each setting.

The focus on outcomes is interwoven throughout the process of occupational therapy. The occupational therapist and client collaborate during the evaluation to identify the client's initial desired outcomes related to engagement in valued occupations or daily life activities. During intervention implementation and re-evaluation, the client and therapist and, when appropriate, the occupational therapy assistant, may modify desired outcomes to accommodate changing needs, contexts, and performance abilities. As further analysis of occupational performance and the development of the intervention plan occur, the occupational therapist and client may redefine the desired outcomes.

Implementation of the outcomes process includes the following steps:

1. Selecting types of outcomes and measures, including but not limited to **occupational performance, adaptation, health and wellness, participation, prevention, self-advocacy, quality of life, and occupational justice** (see Table 10).
   - Selecting outcome measures early in the intervention process (see "Evaluation" above)
   - Selecting outcome measures that are valid, reliable, and appropriately sensitive to change in the client's occupational performance and are consistent with the outcomes
   - Selecting outcome measures or instruments for a particular client that are congruent with client goals
   - Selecting outcome measures that are based on their actual or purported ability to predict future outcomes.
2. Using outcomes to measure progress and adjust goals and interventions
   - Comparing progress toward goal achievement to outcomes throughout the intervention process
   - Assessing outcome use and results to make decisions about the future direction of intervention (e.g., continue intervention, modify intervention, discontinue intervention, provide follow-up, refer to other services).

TABLE 10. TYPES OF OUTCOMES

The examples listed specify how the broad outcome of engagement in occupation may be operationalized. The examples are not intended to be all-inclusive.

Outcome	Description
Occupational performance	The act of doing and accomplishing a selected activity or occupation that results from the dynamic transaction among the client, the context, and the activity. Improving or enabling skills and patterns in occupational performance leads to engagement in occupations or activities (adapted in part from Law et al., 1996, p. 16). • *Improvement*—Used when a performance limitation is present. These outcomes document increased occupational performance for the person, organization, or population. Outcome examples may include (1) the ability of a child with autism to play interactively with a peer (person); (2) the ability of an older adult to return to the home from a skilled-nursing facility (person); (3) decreased incidence of back strain in nursing personnel as a result of an in-service education program in body mechanics for carrying out job duties that require bending, lifting, and so forth (organizations); and (d) construction of accessible playground facilities for all children in local city parks (populations). • *Enhancement*—Used when a performance limitation is not currently present. These outcomes document the development of performance skills and performance patterns that augment existing performance or prevent potential problems from developing in life occupations. Outcome examples may include (1) increased confidence and competence of teenage mothers to parent their children as a result of structured social groups and child development classes (person); (2) increased membership of the local senior citizen center as a result of diverse social wellness and exercise programs (organization); (3) increased ability by school staff to address and manage school-age youth violence as a result of conflict resolution training to address "bullying" (organizations); and (4) increased opportunities for seniors to participate in community activities due to ride share programs (populations).
Adaptation	A change in response approach that the client makes when encountering an occupational challenge. "This change is implemented when the [client's] customary response approaches are found inadequate for producing some degree of mastery over the challenge" (adapted from Schultz & Schkade, 1997, p. 474). Examples of adaptation outcomes include (1) clients modifying their behaviors to earn privileges at an adolescent treatment facility (person); (2) a company redesigning the daily schedule to allow for an even workflow and to decrease times of high stress (organizations); and (3) a community making available accessible public transportation and erecting public and "reserved" benches for older adults to socialize and rest (populations).
Health and wellness	Health is a resource for everyday life, not the objective of living. For individuals, it is a state of physical, mental, and social well-being, as well as a positive concept emphasizing social and personal resources and physical capacities (WHO, 1986). Health of organizations and populations includes these individual aspects but also includes social responsibility of members to society as a whole. *Wellness* is "[a]n active process through which individuals [organizations or populations] become aware of and make choices toward a more successful existence" (Hettler, 1984, p. 1170). Wellness is more than a lack of disease symptoms; it is a state of mental and physical balance and fitness (adapted from *Taber's Cyclopedic Medical Dictionary*, 1997, p. 2110). Outcome examples may include (1) participation in community outings by a client with schizophrenia in a group home (person); (2) implementation of a company-wide program to identify problems and solutions for balance among work, leisure, and family life (organizations); and (3) decreased incidence of childhood obesity (populations).
Participation	Engagement in desired occupations in ways that are personally satisfying and congruent with expectations within the culture.

TABLE 10. TYPES OF OUTCOMES

(Continued)

Outcome	Description
Prevention	"[H]ealth promotion is equally and essentially concerned with creating the conditions necessary for health at individual, structural, social, and environmental levels through an understanding of the determinants of health: peace, shelter, education, food, income, a stable ecosystem, sustainable resources, social justice, and equity" (Kronenberg, Algado, & Pollard, 2005, p. 441). Occupational therapy promotes a healthy lifestyle at the individual, group, organizational, community (societal), and governmental or policy level (adapted from Brownson & Scaffa, 2001). Outcome examples may include (1) appropriate seating and play area for a child with orthopedic impairments (person); (2) implementation of a program of leisure and educational activities for a drop-in center for adults with severe mental illness (organizations); and (3) access to occupational therapy services in underserved areas regardless cultural or ethnic backgrounds (populations).
Quality of life	The dynamic appraisal of the client's life satisfaction (perceptions of progress toward one's goals), hope (the real or perceived belief that one can move toward a goal through selected pathways), self-concept (the composite of beliefs and feelings about oneself), health and functioning (including health status, self-care capabilities, and socioeconomic factors, e.g., vocation, education, income; adapted from Radomski, 1995; Zhan, 1992). Outcomes may include (1) full and active participation of a deaf child from a hearing family during a recreational activity (person); (2) residents being able to prepare for outings and travel independently as a result of independent-living skills training for care providers of a group (organization); and (3) formation of a lobby to support opportunities for social networking, advocacy activities, and sharing scientific information for stroke survivors and their families (population).
Role competence	The ability to effectively meet the demands of roles in which the client engages.
Self-advocacy	Actively promoting or supporting oneself or others (individuals, organizations, or populations); requires an understanding of strengths and needs, identification of goals, knowledge of legal rights and responsibilities, and communicating these aspects to others (adapted from Dawson, 2007). Outcomes may include (1) a student with a learning disability requesting and receiving reasonable accommodations such as textbooks on tape (person); (2) a grassroots employee committee requesting and procuring ergonomically designed keyboards for their computers at work (organization); and (3) people with disabilities advocating for universal design with all public and private construction (population).
Occupational justice	Access to and participation in the full range of meaningful and enriching occupations afforded to others. Includes opportunities for social inclusion and the resources to participate in occupations to satisfy personal, health, and societal needs (adapted from Townsend & Wilcock, 2004). Outcomes may include (1) people with intellectual disabilities serving on an advisory board to establish programs offered by a community recreation center (person); (2) workers who have enough of break time to have lunch with their young children at day care centers (organization); (3) people with persistent mental illness welcomed by community recreation center due to anti-stigma campaign (organization); and (4) alternative adapted housing options for older adult to "age in place" (populations).

Historical and Future Perspectives on the *Occupational Therapy Practice Framework*

The *Occupational Therapy Practice Framework* emerged out of the examination of documents related to *Uniform Terminology*. The first document was the *Occupational Therapy Product Output Reporting System and Uniform Terminology for Reporting Occupational Therapy Services* (AOTA, 1979). This original text created consistent terminology that could be used in official documents, practice, and education. The second edition of *Uniform Terminology for Occupational Therapy* (AOTA, 1989) was adopted by the AOTA Representative Assembly (RA) and published in 1989. The document focused on delineating and defining only the occupational performance areas and occupational performance components that are addressed in occupational therapy direct services. The last revision, *Uniform Terminology for Occupational Therapy—Third Edition* (UT–III; AOTA, 1994), was adopted by the RA in 1994 and was "expanded to reflect current practice and to incorporate contextual aspects of performance" (p. 1047). Each revision reflected changes in current practice and provided consistent terminology that could be used by the profession. Originally a document that responded to a federal requirement to develop a uniform reporting system, the text gradually shifted to describing and outlining the domain of concern of occupational therapy.

In the fall of 1998, the AOTA Commission on Practice (COP) embarked on the journey that culminated in the *Occupational Therapy Practice Framework: Domain and Process* (*Framework;* AOTA, 2002b). During that time, AOTA published *The Guide to Occupational Therapy Practice* (Moyers, 1999), which outlined many of the contemporary shifts of the day, and the COP careful-ly reviewed this document. In light of those changes and the feedback received during the review process of *UT–III,* the COP decided that practice needs had changed and that it was time to develop a different kind of document.

Because the *Framework* is an official AOTA document, it is reviewed on a 5-year cycle. During the review period, the COP collected feedback from membership, scholars, authors, and practitioners to determine the needed changes. Revisions ensued to maintain the integrity of the *Framework* and change only what was necessary. The revisions reflect the contributions of the current COP, refinement of the writing of the document, and emerging concepts and changes in occupational therapy. The rationale for specific changes is listed in Table 11.

The *Framework* is an evolving document and will undergo another review in 5 years, which again will examine the usefulness of the document and need for further refinements and change. The next iteration likely will change as the result of the profession's progress toward AOTA's 2017 *Centennial Vision* of "occupational therapy [as] a powerful, widely recognized, science-driven, and evidence-based profession with a globally connected and diverse workforce meeting society's occupational needs" (AOTA, 2007a).

Although the *Framework* represents the latest in the profession's evolution, it builds on a set of values that the profession of occupational therapy has held since its founding in 1917. This founding vision had at its center a profound belief in the value of therapeutic occupations as a way to remediate illness and maintain health (Slagle, 1924). It emphasized the importance of establishing a therapeutic relationship with each client and designing a treatment plan based on knowledge about the individual's environment, values, goals, and desires (Meyer, 1922). And it advocated for a scientific practice based on systematic observation

TABLE 11. SUMMARY OF SIGNIFICANT *FRAMEWORK* REVISIONS

Domain Area	Change	Intended Benefit	Rationale
Title	Supporting Health and Participation in Life Through Engagement in Occupation	Increase clarity of intent	Changing from the original title of Figure 1, Engagement in Occupation to Support Participation in Context or Contexts, emphasizes that the vehicle for occupational therapy to health and participation is engagement in occupation. Deleted "in context" to shorten the title, because it is discussed in the text and implied by the definition of occupation.
Spirituality	Move from Context to Client Factor	Reflect the way in which occupational therapy practitioners view and analyze meaning, values, and beliefs of a broad range of clients	More commonly, individuals consider spirituality residing within the client rather than as part of a context. Moreira-Almeida and Koenig (2006) discussed spirituality, religion, and personal beliefs as components of quality of life. Their definitions are included in the text.
Performance Skills	Broaden categories with more generic language	Provide language inclusive of a broad range of assessments and interventions as well as commonly used terms in the literature related to skills	Based on her work with the Assessment of Motor and Process Skills (AMPS), Fisher (2006) provides the most distinct categories and definitions of skill functions. An attempt is made in this revision to address critiques of the 2002 *Framework* that Fisher's categories are limited. To broaden skill categories to more generic and inclusive language, the COP considered at length the differences among *body functions, abilities, capacities, skills, levels of skills,* and *components of occupations.* In most articles, authors use terms related to skills interchangeably with *abilities* and *capacities,* confusing the issue. To add to the difficulty in providing readers with a list of performance skills, the proposed categories are not completely distinct from one another. Without creating an artificial distinction between categories, it is necessary to tolerate the overlap in these skill areas. For example, according to Filley (2001), "skill learning and acquisition of praxis may well be identical phenomena" (p. 89). Perception often is discussed in cognitive literature; social cognition implies a specific skill set, as do social–emotional skills; and sensory–motor skills are often considered together.
Rest and Sleep	Move from ADL to Area of Occupation	Highlight the importance of rest and sleep, especially as they relate to supporting or hindering engagement in other areas of occupation	Rest and sleep are two of the four main categories of occupation discussed by Adolf Meyer (1922). Unlike any other area of occupation, all people rest as a result of engaging in occupations and engage in sleep for multiple hours per day throughout their life span. Within the occupation of rest and sleep are activities such as preparing the self and environment for sleep, interactions with others who share the sleeping space, reading or listening to music to fall asleep, napping, dreaming, nighttime care of toileting needs, nighttime caregiving duties, and ensuring safety. Sleep significantly affects all other areas of occupation. Jonsson (2007) suggested that providing sleep prominence in the framework as an area of occupation will promote the consideration of lifestyle choices as an important aspect of participation and health.
Context	Change to context and environment	Allow use of broader language consistent with external audiences and existing occupational therapy theories	The terms *context* and *environment* are not the same but often are used interchangeably. In the general literature, environment is used more frequently. Occupational therapy theories often use environment rather than context. This change allows for a cross-walk between the two terms. In the narrative, context is used to include environment.

(Continued)

TABLE 11. SUMMARY OF SIGNIFICANT *FRAMEWORK* REVISIONS

(Continued)

Domain Area	Change	Intended Benefit	Rationale
Occupational justice	Include narrative about the importance of social justice specific to occupational therapy	Highlight the importance of occupational therapy values in the global community	The discussion of concepts of occupational justice encourages practitioners to examine the multiple contributors to engagement and social participation. Townsend and Wilcock (2004) are leaders in our understanding of this important concept. Gupta and Walloch (2006) provide a nice summary of this work.

Process Area	Change	Intended Benefit	Rationale
Client	Include person, organization, population	Broaden the scope of occupational therapy services and provides language consistent with advocacy and policy-making groups.	Consistent with *The Guide to Occupational Therapy Practice* (Moyers & Dale, 2007). Language in occupational therapy literature often is focused on the individual or person. This change highlights the way in which occupational therapy contributes to groups of persons, populations, and organizations, often in nontraditional practice arenas.
Clinical Reasoning	Identify the way in which the practitioner's view of the client is informed via knowledge, skills, and evidence	Highlight the importance of the practitioner's problem-solving skills in the interaction with the client	Clinical reasoning was expanded in the document to emphasize its importance throughout the occupational therapy process. Intrinsic to any interaction between the practitioner and the client is the critical thinking implicit within clinical-reasoning skills that inform and guide the intervention.
Activity Analysis Activity Synthesis	Include discussion about analyzing activities in and of themselves and in relation to the client	Highlight the importance of this critical skill that informs intervention	Occupational therapy practitioners have a high level of skill in identifying the demands of an activity and then synthesizing this information by comparing it with the client's needs and abilities to identify specific occupational performance difficulties.
Self-Advocacy	Include self-advocacy as an outcome	Provide focus on empowerment as a key feature in health and participation	When working with individuals, populations, or organizations, occupational therapy provides intervention, which promotes self-advocacy as a means toward improved health and participation.
Evidence-based practice	Emphasize the role of research in informing practice	Articulate the value of a science-driven profession	Occupational therapy is a profession founded on basic and applied science informing practice.

TABLE 11. SUMMARY OF SIGNIFICANT *FRAMEWORK* REVISIONS

(Continued)

Terminology	Change	Intended Benefit	Rationale
Transactive and interactive	Include the idea that areas of the domain are transactive and the client is interactive	Create distinction between the relationships of concepts within the domain and interactions between clients and practitioners	*Transactive* is used to describe the dynamic way in which the areas of the occupational therapy domain intersect. *Interactive* is the way in which clients and occupational therapy practitioners engage together or with others. Occupational therapy is therefore the interaction between practitioners and clients within one or more areas of the domain to meet the overarching objective of engagement in occupation to support health and participation.
Activity/ occupation and purposeful activity	Use occupation to include activity in the narrative	To increase readability of the document	Recognizing the work of scholars in the field, the authors acknowledge the differences in activity and occupation. However, this document does not engage in this debate. In the *Framework,* occupation is used to include activity. Activity is used specific to tasks considered in isolation of the client. Purposeful activity is used to describe a type of intervention determined by the therapist to be "purposeful" for achieving the goals of intervention, not in judging whether or not a client's chosen activity is purposeful or not.

Outcomes	Change	Intended Benefit	Rationale
Outcomes	Added occupational justice and self-advocacy to Table 10: Types of Outcomes	To acknowledge occupational therapy's commitment to occupational justice and self-determination for all people	Recognizing that an important outcome of occupational therapy intervention may be enabling all individuals to be able to meet basic needs and to have equal opportunities and life chances to reach toward his or her potential through engagement in diverse and meaningful occupation.

and treatment (Dunton, 1934). Paraphrased using today's lexicon, the founders proposed a vision that was occupation-based, client-centered, contextual, and evidence-based—the vision articulated in the *Framework* today.

Acknowledgments

The Commission on Practice (COP) expresses sincere appreciation to all those who participated in the development of the *Occupational Therapy Practice Framework: Domain and Process, 2nd Edition.* This new edition represents the combined efforts of numerous esteemed colleagues providing a collective description of the architecture of occupational therapy within which the ecology of the profession occurs. In addition to those named

below, the COP wishes to thank everyone who has contributed to the dialogue, feedback, and concepts presented in the document.

Sincere and heartfelt appreciation is extended to Wendy Schoen for all her support; to AOTA's past-president, Carolyn Baum, PhD, OTR/L, FAOTA, and current president Penelope A. Moyers Cleveland, EdD, OTR/L, BCMH, FAOTA, for their insights and direction; the Representative Assembly Coordinating Council (RACC) members, especially Brent Braveman, PhD, OTR/L, FAOTA, and Wendy Hildenbrand, MPH, OTR/L, FAOTA; to those providing significant content and reviews, including Ina Elfant Asher, MS, OTR/L; Kathleen Barker Schwartz, EdD, OTR/L, FAOTA; Mary Frances Baxter, PhD, OTR/L; Christine Beall, OTR/L; Stefanie

Bodison, MA, OTR/L; Sarah Burton, MS, OT/L; Denea S. Butts, OTD, OTR/L; Jane Case-Smith, EdD, OTR, BCP, FAOTA; Florence Clark, PhD, OTR/L, FAOTA; Gloria Frolek Clark, MS, OTR/L, FAOTA; Elizabeth Crepeau, PhD, OTR, FAOTA; Anne E. Dickerson, PhD, OTR/L, FAOTA; Winifred Dunn, PhD, OTR, FAOTA; Lisa Ann Fagan, MS, OTR/L; Anne G. Fisher, PhD, OTR, FAOTA; Naomi Gil, MSc, OT; Lou Ann Griswald, PhD, OTR, FAOTA; Sharon A. Gutman, PhD, OTR/L; Jim Hinojosa, PhD, OT, FAOTA; Hans Jonsson, PhD, OT(Reg); Paula Kramer, PhD, OTR/L, FAOTA; Patricia LaVesser, PhD, OTR/L; Donna Lucente-Surber, OTR/L; Stephen H. Luster, MS, OTR, CHT; Zoe Mailloux, MA, OTR/L, FAOTA; Jean McKinley-Vargas, MS, OTR/L; David Nelson, PhD, OTR/L, FAOTA; L. Diane Parham, PhD, OTR/L, FAOTA; Marta Pelczarski, OTR; Kathlyn L. Reed, PhD, OTR, FAOTA; Barbara Schell, PhD, OTR/L, FAOTA; Camille Skubik-Peplaski, MS, OTR/L, BCP; Virginia Carroll Stoffel, PhD, OT, BCMH, FAOTA; Marjorie Vogeley, OTR/L; and Naomi Weintraub, PhD, OTR.

Glossary

A

Activities of daily living (ADLs)

Activities oriented toward taking care of one's own body (adapted from Rogers & Holm, 1994, pp. 181–202). **ADL** also is referred to as *basic activities of daily living (BADL)* and *personal activities of daily living (PADL)*. These activities are "fundamental to living in a social world; they enable basic survival and well-being" (Christiansen & Hammecker, 2001, p. 156) (see Table 1 for definitions of terms).

Activity (Activities)

A class of human actions that are goal directed.

Activity analysis

"...addresses the typical demands of an activity, the range of skills involved in its performance, and the various cultural meanings that might be ascribed to it" (Crepeau, 2003, p. 192).

Activity demands

The aspects of an activity, which include the objects and their physical properties, space, social demands, sequencing or timing, required actions or skills, and required underlying body functions and body structures needed to carry out the activity (see Table 3).

Adaptation

The response approach the client makes encountering an occupational challenge. "This change is implemented when the individual's customary response approaches are found inadequate for producing some degree of mastery over the challenge" (Schultz & Schkade, 1997, p. 474).

Advocacy

The "pursuit of influencing outcomes—including public policy and resource allocation decisions within political, economic, and social systems and institutions—that directly affect people's lives" (Advocacy Institute, 2001, as cited in Goodman-Lavey & Dunbar, 2003, p. 422).

Analysis of occupational performance

Part of the evaluation process. Collecting information via assessment tools designed to observe, measure, and inquire about selected factors that support or hinder occupational performance.

Areas of occupations

Various kinds of life activities in which people engage, including the following categories: ADLs, IADLs, rest and sleep, education, work, play, leisure, and social participation (see Table 1).

Assessment

"Specific tools or instruments that are used during the evaluation process" (AOTA, 2005, p. 663).

B

Belief

Any cognitive content held as true by the client (Moyers & Dale, 2007).

Body functions

"The physiological functions of body systems (including psychological functions)" (WHO, 2001, p. 10) (see Table 2).

Body structures

"Anatomical parts of the body such as organs, limbs, and their components [that support body function]" (WHO, 2001, p. 10) (see Table 2).

C

Client

The entity that receives occupational therapy services. Clients may include (1) individuals and other persons relevant to the individual's life, including family, caregivers, teachers, employers, and others who also may help or be served indirectly; (2) organizations such as business, industries, or agencies; and (3) populations within a community (Moyers & Dale, 2007).

Client-centered approach

An orientation that honors the desires and priorities of clients in designing and implementing interventions (adapted from Dunn, 2000a, p. 4).

Client factors

Those factors residing within the client that may affect performance in areas of occupation. Client factors include values, beliefs, and spirituality; body functions; and body structures (see Table 2).

Clinical reasoning

"Complex multi-faceted cognitive process used by practitioners to plan, direct, perform, and reflect on intervention" (Crepeau et al., 2003, p. 1027).

Communication and social skills

Actions or behaviors a person uses to communicate and interact with others in an interactive environment (Fisher, 2006).

Cognitive skills

Actions or behaviors a client uses to plan and manage the performance of an activity.

Context

Refers to a variety of interrelated conditions within and surrounding the client that influence performance. Contexts include cultural, personal, temporal, and virtual (see Table 6).

Co-occupations

Activities that implicitly involve at least two people (Zemke & Clark, 1996).

Cultural (context)

"Customs, beliefs, activity patterns, behavior standards, and expectations accepted by the society of which the [client] is a member. Includes ethnicity and values as well as political aspects, such as laws that affect access to resources and affirm personal rights. Also includes opportunities for education, employment, and economic support" (AOTA, 1994, p. 1054).

D

Domain

A sphere of activity, concern, or function (*American Heritage Dictionary*, 2006).

E

Education

Includes learning activities needed when participating in an environment (see Table 1).

Emotional regulation skills

Actions or behaviors a client uses to identify, manage, and express feelings while engaging in activities or interacting with others.

Engagement

The act of sharing activities.

Environment

The external physical and social environment that surrounds the client and in which the client's daily life occupations occur (see Table 6).

Evaluation

"The process of obtaining and interpreting data necessary for intervention. This includes planning for and documenting the evaluation process and results" (AOTA, 2005, p. 663).

G

Goals

"The result or achievement toward which effort is directed; aim; end" (*Webster's Encyclopedic Unabridged Dictionary of the English Language*, 1994, p. 605).

H

Habits

"Automatic behavior that is integrated into more complex patterns that enable people to function on a day-to-day basis..." (Neistadt & Crepeau, 1998, p. 869). Habits can be useful, dominating, or impoverished and either support or interfere with performance in areas of occupation.

Health

Health is a resource for everyday life, not the objective of living. It is a state of complete physical, mental, and social well-being, as well as a positive concept emphasizing social and personal resources, as well as physical capacities (adapted from WHO, 1986).

Health promotion

"[T]he process of enabling people to increase control over, and to improve, their health. To reach a state of complete physical, mental, and social well-being, an individual or group must be able to identify and realize aspirations, to satisfy needs, and to change or cope with the environment" (WHO, 1986).

"[C]reating the conditions necessary for health at individual, structural, social, and environmental levels through an understanding of the determinants of health: peace, shelter, education, food, income, a stable ecosystem, sustainable resources, social justice, and equity" (Trentham & Cockburn, 2005, p. 441).

Hope

The real or perceived belief that one can move toward a goal through selected pathways (Lopez et al., 2004).

I

Identity

"A composite definition of the self and includes an interpersonal aspect…an aspect of possibility or potential (who we might become), and a values aspect (that suggests importance and provides a stable basis for choices and decisions)…. Identity can be viewed as the superordinate view of ourselves that includes both self-esteem and self-concept but also importantly reflects and is influenced by the larger social world in which we find ourselves" (Christiansen, 1999, pp. 548–549).

Independence

"A self-directed state of being characterized by an individual's ability to participate in necessary and preferred occupations in a satisfying manner irrespective of the amount or kind of external assistance desired or required

- Self-determination is essential to achieving and maintaining independence;
- An individual's independence is unrelated to whether he or she performs the activities related to an occupation himself or herself, performs the activities in an adapted or modified environment, makes use of various devices or alternative strategies, or oversees activity completion by others;
- Independence is defined by the individual's culture and values, support systems, and ability to direct his or her life; and
- An individual's independence should not be based on preestablished criteria, perception of outside observers, or how independence is accomplished" (AOTA, 2002a, p. 660).

Instrumental activities of daily living (IADLs)

Activities to support daily life within the home and community that often require more complex interactions than self-care used in ADL (see Table 1).

Interdependence

The "reliance that people have on each other as a natural consequence of group living" (Christiansen & Townsend, 2004, p. 277). "Interdependence engenders a spirit of social inclusion, mutual aid, and a moral commitment and responsibility to recognize and support difference" (p. 146).

Interests

"What one finds enjoyable or satisfying to do" (Kielhofner, 2002, p. 25).

Intervention

The process and skilled actions taken by occupational therapy practitioners in collaboration with the client to facilitate engagement in occupation related to health and participation. The intervention process includes the plan, implementation, and review (see Table 7).

Intervention approaches

Specific strategies selected to direct the process of interventions that are based on the client's desired outcome, evaluation date, and evidence (see Table 9).

L

Leisure

"A nonobligatory activity that is intrinsically motivated and engaged in during discretionary time, that is, time not committed to obligatory occupations such as work, self-care, or sleep" (Parham & Fazio, 1997, p. 250).

M

Motor and praxis skills
Motor

Actions or behaviors a client uses to move and physically interact with tasks, objects, contexts, and environments (adapted from Fisher, 2006). Includes planning, sequencing, and executing novel movements.

Also see Praxis.

O

Occupation

"Goal-directed pursuits that typically extend over time have meaning to the performance, and involve multiple tasks" (Christiansen et al., 2005, p. 548).

"Daily activities that reflect cultural values, provide structure to living, and meaning to individuals; these activities meet human needs for self-care, enjoyment, and participation in society" (Crepeau et al., 2003, p. 1031).

"Activities that people engage in throughout their daily lives to fulfill their time and give life meaning. Occupations involve mental abilities and skills and may or may not have an observable physical dimension" (Hinojosa & Kramer, 1997, p. 865).

"[A]ctivities...of everyday life, named, organized, and given value and meaning by individuals and a culture. Occupation is everything people do to occupy themselves, including looking after themselves...enjoying life...and contributing to the social and economic fabric of their communities" (Law et al., 1997, p. 32).

"A dynamic relationship among an occupational form, a person with a unique developmental structure, subjective meanings and purpose, and the resulting occupational performance" (Nelson & Jepson-Thomas, 2003, p. 90).

"[C]hunks of daily activity that can be named in the lexicon of the culture" (Zemke & Clark, 1996, p. vii).

Occupation-based intervention

A type of occupational therapy intervention—a client-centered intervention in which the occupational therapy practitioner and client collaboratively select and design activities that have specific relevance or meaning to the client and support the client's interests, need, health, and participation in daily life.

Occupational justice

"Justice related to opportunities and resources required for occupational participation sufficient to satisfy personal needs and full citizenship" (Christiansen & Townsend, 2004, p. 278). To experience meaning and enrichment in one's occupations; to participate in a range of occupations for health and social inclusion; to make choices and share decision-making power in daily life; and to receive equal privileges for diverse participation in occupations (Townsend & Wilcock, 2004).

Occupational performance

The act of doing and accomplishing a selected activity or occupation that results from the dynamic transaction among the client, the context, and the activity. Improving or enabling skills and patterns in occupational performance leads to engagement in occupations or activities (adapted in part from Law et al., 1996, p. 16).

Occupational profile
A summary of the client's occupational history, patterns of daily living, interests, values, and needs.

Occupational science
An interdisciplinary academic discipline in the social and behavioral sciences dedicated to the study of the form, the function, and the meaning of human occupations (Zemke & Clark, 1996).

Occupational therapy
The practice of occupational therapy means the therapeutic use of everyday life activities (occupations) with individuals or groups for the purpose of participation in roles and situations in home, school, workplace, community, and other settings. Occupational therapy services are provided for the purpose of promoting health and wellness and to those who have or are at risk for developing an illness, injury, disease, disorder, condition, impairment, disability, activity limitation, or participation restriction. Occupational therapy addresses the physical, cognitive, psychosocial, sensory, and other aspects of performance in a variety of contexts to support engagement in everyday life activities that affect health, well-being, and quality of life (AOTA, 2004a).

Organizations
Entities with a common purpose or enterprise such as businesses, industries, or agencies.

Outcomes
What occupational therapy actually achieves for the consumers of its services (adapted from Fuhrer, 1987). Change desired by the client that can focus on any area of the client's occupational performance (adapted from Kramer, McGonigel, & Kaufman, 1991).

P

Participation
"Involvement in a life situation" (WHO, 2001, p. 10).

Performance patterns
Patterns of behavior related to daily life activities that are habitual or routine. They can include habits, routines, rituals, and roles (see Table 5).

Performance skills
The abilities clients demonstrate in the actions they perform (see Table 4).

Persons
Individuals, including families, caregivers, teachers, employees, and relevant others.

Personal
"Features of the individual that are not part of a health condition or health status" (WHO, 2001, p. 17). Personal context includes age, gender, socioeconomic, and educational status. Can also include organizational levels (i.e., volunteers, employees) and population levels (i.e., members of a society).

Physical environment
The natural and built nonhuman environment and objects in them.

Play
"Any spontaneous or organized activity that provides enjoyment, entertainment, amusement, or diversion" (Parham & Fazio, 1997, p. 252) (see Table 1).

Populations
Large groups as a whole, such as refugees, homeless veterans, and people who need wheelchairs.

Praxis
Skilled purposeful movements (Heilman & Rothi, 1993). The ability to carry out sequential motor acts as part of an overall plan rather than individual acts (Liepmann, 1920). The ability to carry out learned

motor activity, including following through on a verbal command, visual spatial construction, ocular and oral–motor skills, imitation of a person or an object, and sequencing actions (Ayres, 1985; Filley, 2001). Organization of temporal sequences of actions within the spatial context; which form meaningful occupations (Blanche & Parham, 2002).
Also see Motor.

Preparatory methods

Methods and techniques that prepare the client for occupational performance. Used in preparation for or concurrently with purposeful and occupation-based activities.

Prevention

"[H]ealth promotion is equally and essentially concerned with creating the conditions necessary for health at individual, structural, social, and environmental levels through an understanding of the determinants of health: peace, shelter, education, food, income, a stable ecosystem, sustainable resources, social justice, and equity" (Kronenberg, Algado, & Pollard, 2005, p. 441).

Promoting a healthy lifestyle at the individual, group, organizational, community (societal), governmental/policy level (adapted from Brownson & Scaffa, 2001).

Process

A description of the way in which occupational therapy practitioners operationalize their expertise to provide services to clients. The process includes evaluation, intervention, and outcome monitoring; occurs within the purview of the domain; and involves collaboration among the occupational therapist, occupational therapy assistant, and the client.

Purposeful activity

A goal-directed behavior or activity within a therapeutically designed context that leads to an occupation or occupations. Specifically selected activities that allow the client to develop skills that enhance occupational engagement.

Q

Quality of life

A client's dynamic appraisal of life satisfactions (perceptions of progress toward identified goals), self-concept (the composite of beliefs and feelings about themselves), health and functioning (including health status, self-care capabilities), and socioeconomic factors (e.g., vocation, education, income) (adapted from Radomski, 1995; Zhan, 1992).

R

Re-evaluation

A reassessment of the client's performance and goals to determine the type and amount of change.

Rest

Quiet and effortless actions that interrupt physical and mental activity, resulting in a relaxed state (Nurit & Michel, 2003, p. 227).

Ritual

Symbolic actions with spiritual, cultural, or social meaning, contributing to the client's identity and reinforcing the client's values and beliefs (Fiese et al., 2002; Segal, 2004). Rituals are highly symbolic, with a strong affective component and representative of a collection of events.

Roles

Roles are sets of behaviors expected by society, shaped by culture, and may be further conceptualized and defined by the client.

Routines

Patterns of behavior that are observable, regular, repetitive, and that provide structure for daily life. They can be satisfying, promoting, or damaging. Routines require momentary time commitment and are embedded in cultural and ecological contexts (Fiese et al., 2002; Segal, 2004).

S

Self-advocacy

Understanding your strengths and needs, identifying your personal goals, knowing your legal rights and responsibilities, and communicating these to others (Dawson, 2007).

Sensory–perceptual skills

Actions or behaviors a client uses to locate, identify, and respond to sensations and to select, interpret, associate, organize, and remember sensory events via sensations that include visual, auditory, proprioceptive, tactile, olfactory, gustatory, and vestibular sensations.

Sleep

"A natural periodic state of rest for the mind and body, in which the eyes usually close and consciousness is completely or partially lost, so that there is a decrease in bodily movement and responsiveness to external stimuli. During sleep the brain in humans and other mammals undergoes a characteristic cycle of brain-wave activity that includes intervals of dreaming" (*The Free Dictionary,* 2007) (see Table 1).

A series of activities resulting in going to sleep, staying asleep, and ensuring health and safety through participation in sleep involving engagement with the physical and social environments.

Social environment

Is constructed by the presence, relationships, and expectations of persons, organizations, and populations.

Social justice

"Ethical distribution and sharing of resources, rights, and responsibilities between people, recognizing their equal worth as citizens. [It recognizes] 'their equal right to be able to meet basic needs, the need to spread opportunities and life chances as widely as possible, and finally the requirement that we reduce and where possible eliminate unjustified inequalities'" (Commission on Social Justice, 1994, p. 1).

"The promotion of social and economic change to increase individual, community, and political awareness, resources, and opportunity for health and well-being" (Wilcock, 2006, p. 344).

Social participation

"Organized patterns of behavior that are characteristic and expected of an individual in a given position within a social system" (Mosey, 1996, p. 340) (see Table 1).

Spirituality

"[T]he personal quest for understanding answers to ultimate questions about life, about meaning, and about relationship with the sacred or transcendent, which may (or may not) lead to or arise from the development of religious rituals and the formation of community" (Moreira-Almeida & Koenig, 2006, p. 844).

T

Temporal

"Location of occupational performance in time" (Neistadt & Crepeau, 1998, p. 292). The experience of time as shaped by engagement in occupations. The temporal aspects of occupations "which contribute to the patterns of daily occupations" are "the rhythm...tempo...synchronization...duration...and sequence" (Larson & Zemke, 2004, p. 82; Zemke, 2004, p. 610). It includes stages of life, time of day, duration, rhythm of activity, or history.

Transactional

A process that involves two or more individuals or elements that reciprocally and continually influence and affect one another through the ongoing relationship (Dickie, Cutchin, & Humphry, 2006).

V

Values

Principles, standards, or qualities considered worthwhile or desirable by the client who holds them (Moyers & Dale, 2007).

Virtual

Environment in which communication occurs by means of airways or computers and an absence of physical contact. Includes simulated or real-time or near-time existence of an environment, such as chat rooms, email, video conferencing, and radio transmissions.

W

Wellness

"An active process through which individuals become aware of and make choices toward a more successful existence" (Hettler, 1984, p. 1117). Wellness is more than a lack of disease symptoms. It is a state of mental and physical balance and fitness (adapted from *Taber's Cyclopedic Medical Dictionary*, 1997, p. 2110).

Work

"Activities needed for engaging in remunerative employment or volunteer activities" (Mosey, 1996, p. 341) (see Table 1).

References

American Heritage Dictionary of the English Language (4th ed.). (2006). Boston: Houghton-Mifflin.

American Occupational Therapy Association. (1979). *Occupational therapy product output reporting system and uniform terminology for reporting occupational therapy services.* (Available from American Occupational Therapy Association, 4720 Montgomery Lane, PO Box 31220, Bethesda, MD 20824-1220)

American Occupational Therapy Association. (1989). *Uniform terminology for occupational therapy* (2nd ed.). (Available from American Occupational Therapy Association, 4720 Montgomery Lane, PO Box 31220, Bethesda, MD 20824-1220)

American Occupational Therapy Association. (1994). Uniform terminology for occupational therapy (3rd ed.). *American Journal of Occupational Therapy, 48,* 1047–1054.

American Occupational Therapy Association. (2002a). Broadening the construct of independence [Position Paper]. *American Journal of Occupational Therapy, 56,* 660.

American Occupational Therapy Association. (2002b). Occupational therapy practice framework: Domain and process. *American Journal of Occupational Therapy, 56,* 609–639.

American Occupational Therapy Association. (2004a). *Definition of occupational therapy practice for the AOTA Model Practice Act.* Bethesda, MD: Author. (Available from the State Affairs Group, 4720 Montgomery Lane, PO Box 31220, Bethesda, MD 20824–1220)

American Occupational Therapy Association. (2004b). Guidelines for supervision, roles, and responsibilities during the delivery of occupational therapy services. *American Journal of Occupational Therapy, 58,* 663–667.

American Occupational Therapy Association. (2004c). Occupational therapy's commitment to nondiscrimination and inclusion (edited 2004). *American Journal of Occupational Therapy, 58,* 666.

American Occupational Therapy Association. (2005). Standards of practice for occupational therapy. *American Journal of Occupational Therapy, 59,* 663–665.

American Occupational Therapy Association. (2006). Policy 1.44: Categories of occupational therapy personnel. In *Policy manual* (2007 ed., pp. 33–34). Bethesda, MD: Author.

American Occupational Therapy Association. (2007a). AOTA Centennial Vision and executive summary. *American Journal of Occupational Therapy, 61,* 613–614.

American Occupational Therapy Association. (2007b). Specialized knowledge and skills in feeding, eating, and swallowing for occupational therapy practice. *American Journal of Occupational Therapy, 61,* 686–700.

Ayres, A. J. (1972). *Sensory integration and learning disorders.* Los Angeles: Western Psychological Services.

Ayres, A. J. (1985). *Developmental dyspraxia and adult onset apraxia.* Torrance, CA: Sensory Integration International.

Ayres, A. J. (2005). *Sensory integration and the child.* Los Angeles: Western Psychological Services.

Baum, C. M., Bass-Haugen, J., & Christiansen, C. H. (2005). Person–environment–occupation–performance: A model for planning interventions for individuals and organizations. In C. H. Christiansen, C. M. Baum, & J. Bass-Haugen (Eds.), *Occupational therapy: Performance, participation, and well-being* (3rd ed., pp. 373–392). Thorofare, NJ: Slack.

Bergen, D. (Ed.). (1988). *Play as a medium for learning and development: A handbook of theory and practice.* Portsmouth, NH: Heinemann.

Blanche, E. I., & Parham, L. D. (2002). Praxis and organization of behavior in time and space. In S. Smith Roley, E. I. Blanche, & R. C. Schaaf (Eds.), *Understanding the nature of sensory integration with diverse populations* (pp. 183–200). San Antonio, TX: Therapy Skill Builders.

Bloom, B. S., Krathwohl, D. R., & Masia, B. B. (1984). *Taxonomy of educational objectives: The classification of educational goals.* New York: Longman.

Brownson, C. A., & Scaffa, M. E. (2001). Occupational therapy in the promotion of health and the prevention of disease and disability. *American Journal of Occupational Therapy, 55,* 656–660.

Calvert, G., Spence, C., & Stein, B. E. (Eds.). (2004). *The handbook of multisensory processes.* Cambridge, MA: MIT Press.

Chapparo, C., & Ranka, J. (1997). The perceive, recall, plan, perform (PRPP) system of task analysis. In C. Chapparo & J. Ranka (Eds.), *Occupational performance model* (Australian Monograph 1, pp. 189–197). Sydney: Occupational Performance Network.

Christiansen, C. H. (1999). Defining lives: Occupation as identity—An essay on competence, coherence, and the creation of meaning [1999 Eleanor Clarke Slagle Lecture]. *American Journal of Occupational Therapy, 53,* 547–558.

Christiansen, C. H., & Baum, M. C. (Eds.). (1997). *Occupational therapy: Enabling function and well-being.* Thorofare, NJ: Slack.

Christiansen, C., Baum, M. C., & Bass-Haugen, J. (Eds.). (2005). *Occupational therapy: Performance, participation, and well-being.* Thorofare, NJ: Slack.

Christiansen, C. H., & Hammecker, C. L. (2001). Self care. In B. R. Bonder & M. B. Wagner (Eds.), *Functional performance in older adults* (pp. 155–175). Philadelphia: F. A. Davis.

Christiansen, C. H., & Townsend, E. A. (Eds.). (2004). *Introduction to occupation: The art and science of living.* Upper Saddle River, NJ: Prentice Hall.

Clark, F. A. (2000). The concept of habit and routine: A preliminary theoretical synthesis. *Occupational Therapy Journal of Research, 20,* 123S–137S.

Cohn, E. S. (2001). Parent perspectives of occupational therapy using a sensory integration approach. *American Journal of Occupational Therapy, 55,* 285–294.

Cohn, E. S., Miller, L. J., & Tickle-Degnan, L. (2000). Parental hopes for therapy outcomes: Children with sensory modulation disorders. *American Journal of Occupational Therapy, 54,* 36–43.

Commission on Social Justice. (1994). *Social justice: Strategies for national renewal. The report of the Commission on Social Justice.* London: Vintage.

Crepeau, E. (2003). Analyzing occupation and activity: A way of thinking about occupational performance. In E. Crepeau, E. Cohn, & B. Schell (Eds.), *Willard and Spackman's occupational therapy* (10th ed., pp. 189–198). Philadelphia: Lippincott Williams & Wilkins.

Crepeau, E., Cohn, E., & Schell, B. (Eds.). (2003). *Willard and Spackman's occupational therapy.* Philadelphia: Lippincott Williams & Wilkins.

Dawson, J. (2007). *Self-advocacy: A valuable skill for your teenager.* Retrieved January 20, 2007, from www.schwablearning.org

Dickie, V., Cutchin, M. P., & Humphry, R. (2006). Occupation as transactional experience: A critique of individualism in occupational science. *Journal of Occupational Science, 13,* 83–93.

Dunlea, A. (1996). An opportunity for co-adaptation: The experience of mothers and their infants who are blind. In R. Zemke & F. Clark (Eds.), *Occupational science: The evolving discipline* (pp. 227–342). Philadelphia: F. A. Davis.

Dunn, W. (2000a). *Best practice in occupational therapy in community service with children and families.* Thorofare, NJ: Slack.

Dunn, W. (2000b, Fall). Habit: What's the brain got to do with it? *Occupational Therapy Journal of Research, 20*(Suppl. 1), 6S–20S.

Dunn, W., McClain, L. H., Brown, C., & Youngstrom, M. J. (1998). The ecology of human performance. In M. E. Neistadt & E. B. Crepeau (Eds.), *Willard and Spackman's occupational therapy* (9th ed., pp. 525–535). Philadelphia: Lippincott Williams & Wilkins.

Dunton, W. R. (1934). The need for and value of research in occupational therapy. *Occupational Therapy and Rehabilitation, 13,* 325–328.

Esdaile, S. A., & Olson J. A. (2004). *Mothering occupations: Challenge, agency, and participation.* Philadelphia: F. A. Davis.

Fiese, B. H., Tomcho, T. J., Douglas, M., Josephs, K., Poltrock, S., & Baker, T. (2002). A review of 50 years of research on naturally occurring family routines and rituals: Cause for celebration? *Journal of Family Psychology, 16,* 381–390.

Filley, C. M. (2001). *Neurobehavioral anatomy.* Boulder: University Press of Colorado.

Fisher, A. (2006). Overview of performance skills and client factors. In H. Pendleton & W. Schultz-Krohn (Eds.), *Pedretti's occupational therapy: Practice skills for physical dysfunction* (pp. 372–402). St. Louis: Mosby/Elsevier.

Foucault, M. (1973). *The birth of the clinic: An archaeology of medical perception.* New York: Pantheon Books.

Fuhrer, M. J. (Ed.). (1987). *Rehabilitation outcomes analysis and measurement.* Baltimore: Brookes.

Gitlin, L. N., & Corcoran, M. A. (2005). *Occupational therapy and dementia care: The Home Environmental Skill-Building Program for individuals and families.* Bethesda, MD: AOTA Press.

Gitlin, L. N., Corcoran, M. A., Winter, L., Boyce, A., & Hauck, W. W. (2001). A randomized controlled trial of a home environmental intervention to enhance self-efficacy and reduce upset in family caregivers of persons with dementia. *The Gerontologist, 41,* 15–30.

Gitlin, L. N., Winter, L., Corcoran, M., Dennis, M., Schinfeld, S., & Hauck, W. (2003). Effects of the Home Environmental Skill-Building Program on the caregiver–care recipient dyad: Six-month outcomes from the Philadelphia REACH initiative. *The Gerontologist, 43,* 532–546.

Goodman-Lavey, M., & Dunbar, S. (2003). Federal legislative advocacy. In G. McCormack, E. Jaffe, & M. Goodman-Lavey (Eds.), *The occupational therapy manager* (4th ed., pp. 421–438). Bethesda, MD: AOTA Press.

Gupta, J., & Walloch, C. (2006). Process of infusing social justice into the practice framework: A case study. *OT Practice, 11*(15), CE1–CE8.

Gutman, S. A., Mortera, M. H., Hinojosa, J., & Kramer, P. (2007). Revision of the occupational therapy practice framework. *American Journal of Occupational Therapy, 61,* 119–126.

Hakansson, C., Dahlin-Ivanoff, S., & Sonn, U. (2006). Achieving balance in everyday life. *Journal of Occupational Science, 13,* 74–82.

Harrow, A. J. (1972). *A taxonomy of the psychomotor domain: A guide for developing behavioral objectives.* New York: McKay.

Heilman, K. M., & Rothi, L. J. G. (1993). *Clinical neuropsychology* (3rd ed.). New York: Oxford University Press.

Hettler, W. (1984). Wellness—The lifetime goal of a university experience. In J. D. Matarazzo, S. M. Weiss, J. A. Herd, N. E. Miller, & S. M. Weiss (Eds.), *Behavioral health: A handbook of health enhancement and disease prevention* (p. 1117). New York: Wiley.

Hinojosa, J., & Kramer, P. (1997). Fundamental concepts of occupational therapy: Occupation, purposeful activity, and function [Statement]. *American Journal of Occupational Therapy, 51,* 864–866.

Jackson, J. (1998a). Contemporary criticisms of role theory. *Journal of Occupational Science, 5*(2), 49–55.

Jackson, J. (1998b). Is there a place for role theory in occupational science? *Journal of Occupational Science 5*(2), 56–65.

Jonsson, H. (2007). *Towards a new direction in the conceptualization and categorization of occupation* [Wilma West Lecture, Occupational Science Symposium]. Los Angeles: University of Southern California, Occupational Science and Occupational Therapy.

Kielhofner, G. (2002). Motives, patterns, and performance of occupation: Basic concepts. In G. Kielhofner (Ed.), *A model of human occupation: Theory and application* (3rd ed., pp. 13–27). Philadelphia: Lippincott Williams & Wilkins.

Kramer, S., McGonigel, M., & Kaufmann, R. (1991). Developing the IFSP: Outcomes, strategies, activities, and services. In M. McGonigel, R. Kaufmann, & B. Johnson (Eds.), *Guidelines and recommended practices for the individualized family service plan* (2nd ed., pp. 41–49). Bethesda, MD: Association for the Care of Children's Health.

Kronenberg, F., Algado, S. S., & Pollard, N. (2005). *Occupational therapy without borders: Learning from the spirit of survivors.* Philadelphia: Elsevier/Churchill Livingstone.

Larson, E., & Zemke, R. (2004). Shaping the temporal patterns of our lives: The social coordination of occupation. *Journal of Occupational Science, 10,* 80–89.

Law, M., Baum, M. C., & Dunn, W. (2005). *Measuring occupational performance: Supporting best practice in occupational therapy* (2nd ed.). Thorofare, NJ: Slack.

Law, M., Cooper, B., Strong, S., Stewart, D., Rigby, P., & Letts, L. (1996). Person–environment–occupation model: A transactive approach to occupational performance. *Canadian Journal of Occupational Therapy, 63,* 9–23.

Law, M., Polatajko, H., Baptiste, W., & Townsend, E. (1997). Core concepts of occupational therapy. In E. Townsend (Ed.), *Enabling occupation: An occupational therapy perspective* (pp. 29–56). Ottawa, ON: Canadian Association of Occupational Therapists.

Liepmann, H. (1920). Apraxie. *Ergebnisse der Gesamten Medizin, 1,* 516–543.

Lopez, S. J., Snyder, C. R., Magyar-Moe, J., Edwards, L. M., Pedrotti, J. T., Janowski, K., et al. (2004). Strategies for accentuating hope. In P. A. Linley & S. Joseph (Eds.), *Positive psychology in practice* (pp. 388–404). Hoboken, NJ: John Wiley & Sons.

Maciejewski, M., Kawiecki, J., & Rockwood, T. (1997). Satisfaction. In R. L. Kane (Ed.), *Understanding health care outcomes research* (pp. 67–89). Gaithersburg, MD: Aspen.

Meyer, A. (1922). The philosophy of occupational therapy. *Archives of Occupational Therapy, 1,* 1–10.

Moreira-Almeida, A., & Koenig, H. G. (2006). Retaining the meaning of the words religiousness and spirituality: A commentary on the WHOQOL SRPB group's "A cross-cultural study of spirituality, religion, and personal beliefs as components of quality of life" (62:6, 2005, pp. 1486–1497). *Social Science and Medicine, 63,* 843–845.

Mosey, A. C. (1996). *Applied scientific inquiry in the health professions: An epistemological orientation* (2nd ed.). Bethesda, MD: American Occupational Therapy Association.

Moyers, P. A. (1999). The guide to occupational therapy practice. *American Journal of Occupational Therapy, 53,* 247–322.

Moyers, P. A., & Dale, L. M. (2007). *The guide to occupational therapy practice* (2nd ed.). Bethesda, MD: AOTA Press.

Neistadt, M. E., & Crepeau, E. B. (Eds.). (1998). *Willard and Spackman's occupational therapy* (9th ed.). Philadelphia: Lippincott Williams & Wilkins.

Nelson, D., & Jepson-Thomas, J. (2003). Occupational form, occupational performance, and a conceptual framework for therapeutic occupation. In P. Kramer, J. Hinojosa, & C. Brasic Royeen (Eds.), *Perspectives in human occupation: Participation in life* (pp. 87–155). Philadelphia: Lippincott Williams & Wilkins.

Nurit, W., & Michel, A. B. (2003). Rest: A qualitative exploration of the phenomenon. *Occupational Therapy International, 10,* 227–238.

Olsen, J. A. (2004). Mothering co-occupations in caring for infants and young children. In S. A. Esdaile & J. A. Olson (Eds.), *Mothering occupations* (pp. 28–51). Philadelphia: F. A. Davis.

Parham, L. D., & Fazio, L. S. (Eds.). (1997). *Play in occupational therapy for children.* St. Louis, MO: Mosby.

Pedretti, L. W., & Early, M. B. (2001). Occupational performance and model of practice for physical dysfunction. In L. W. Pedretti & M. B. Early (Eds.), *Occupational therapy practice skills for physical dysfunction* (pp. 7–9). St. Louis, MO: Mosby.

Pierce, D. (2001). Untangling occupation and activity. *American Journal of Occupational Therapy, 55,* 138–146.

Punwar, A. J., & Peloquin, S. M. (2000). *Occupational therapy principles and practice* (3rd ed.). Philadelphia: Lippincott Williams & Wilkins.

Radomski, M. V. (1995). There is more to life than putting on your pants. *American Journal of Occupational Therapy, 49,* 487–490.

Reed, K. L. (2005). An annotated history of the concepts used in occupational therapy. In C. H. Christiansen, M. C. Baum, & J. Bass-Haugen (Eds.), *Occupational therapy: Performance, participation, and well-being* (3rd ed., pp. 567–626). Thorofare, NJ: Slack.

Request for Planning Ideas for the Development of the Children's Health Outcomes Initiative, 66 Fed. Reg. 11296 (2001).

Rogers, J. C., & Holm, M. B. (1994). Assessment of self-care. In B. R. Bonder & M. B. Wagner (Eds.), *Functional performance in older adults* (pp. 181–202). Philadelphia: F. A. Davis.

Rogers, J. C., & Holm, M. B. (2008). The occupational therapy process: Evaluation and intervention. In E. B. Crepeau, E. S. Cohn, & B. A. B. Schell (Eds.), *Willard and Spackman's occupational therapy* (11th ed., pp. 478–518). Baltimore: Lippincott Williams & Wilkins.

Schell, B. A. B., Cohn, E. S., & Crepeau, E. B. (2008). Overview of personal factors affecting performance. In E. B. Crepeau, E. S. Cohn, & B. A. B. Schell (Eds.), *Willard and Spackman's occupational therapy* (11th ed., pp. 650–657). Baltimore: Lippincott Williams & Wilkins.

Schultz, S., & Schkade, J. (1997). Adaptation. In C. Christiansen & M. C. Baum (Eds.), *Occupational therapy: Enabling function and well-being* (p. 474). Thorofare, NJ: Slack.

Segal, R. (2004). Family routines and rituals: A context for occupational therapy interventions. *American Journal of Occupational Therapy, 58,* 499–508.

Shumway-Cook, A., & Wollacott, M. H. (2007). *Motor control: Translating research into clinical practice* (3rd ed.). Philadelphia: Lippincott Williams & Wilkins.

Slagle, E. C. (1924). A year's development of occupational therapy in New York state hospitals. *Modern Hospital, 22*(1), 98–104.

Sleep. (2007). *The free dictionary.* Retrieved June 1, 2007, from http://freedictionary.org

Taber's cyclopedic medical dictionary. (1997). Philadelphia: F. A. Davis.

Townsend, E. A., & Wilcock, A. A. (2004). Occupational justice. In C. H. Christiansen & E. A. Townsend (Eds.), *Introduction to occupation: The art and science of living* (pp. 243–273). Upper Saddle River, NJ: Prentice Hall.

Trentham, B., & Cockburn, L. (2005). Participating in action research: Creating new knowledge and opportunities for occupational engagement. In F. Kronenberg, S. S. Algado, & N. Pollard (Eds.), *Occupational therapy without borders: Learning from the spirit of survivors* (pp. 440–453). Philadelphia: Elsevier/Churchill Livingstone.

Trombly, C. (1995). Occupation: Purposefulness and meaningfulness as therapeutic mechanism. *American Journal of Occupational Therapy, 49,* 960–972.

Uniform Data System for Medical Rehabilitation. (1996). *Guide for the uniform data set for medical rehabilitation (including the FIM instrument).* Buffalo, NY: Author.

Weber, M. (1978). *Economy and society: An outline of interpretive sociology* (G. Roth & C. Wittich, Eds.; E. Fischoff et al., Trans.). Berkeley: University of California Press.

Webster's encyclopedic unabridged dictionary of the English language. (1994). Avenel, NJ: Gramercy Books.

Wilcock, A. A. (2006). *An occupational perspective of health* (2nd ed.). Thorofare, NJ: Slack.

Wilcock, A. A., & Townsend, E. A. (2008). Occupational justice. In E. B. Crepeau, E. S. Cohn, & B. B. Schell (Eds.), *Willard and Spackman's occupational therapy* (11th ed., pp. 192–199). Baltimore: Lippincott Williams & Wilkins.

World Health Organization. (1986, November 21). *The Ottawa Charter for Health Promotion.* First International Conference on Health Promotion, Ottawa. Retrieved February 4, 2008, from http://www.who.int/healthpromotion/conferences/previous/ottawa/en/print.html

World Health Organization. (2001). *International classification of functioning, disability, and health (ICF).* Geneva: Author.

Zemke, R. (2004). Time, space, and the kaleidoscopes of occupation [Eleanor Clarke Slagle Lecture]. *American Journal of Occupational Therapy, 58,* 608–620.

Zemke R., & Clark, F. (1996). *Occupational science: An evolving discipline.* Philadelphia: F. A. Davis.

Zhan, L. (1992). Quality of life: Conceptual and measurement issues. *Journal of Advanced Nursing, 17,* 795–800.

Bibliography

Accreditation Council for Occupational Therapy Education. (2007a). Accreditation standards for a doctoral-degree-level educational program for the occupational therapist. *American Journal of Occupational Therapy, 61,* 641–651.

Accreditation Council for Occupational Therapy Education. (2007b). Accreditation standards for an educational program for the occupational therapy assistant. *American Journal of Occupational Therapy, 61,* 662–671.

Accreditation Council for Occupational Therapy Education. (2007c). Accreditation standards for a master's-degree-level educational program for the occupational therapist. *American Journal of Occupational Therapy, 61,* 652–661.

American Occupational Therapy Association. (1995). Occupation: A position paper. *American Journal of Occupational Therapy, 49,* 1015–1018.

Baum, M. C. (1999, November). *At the core of our profession: Occupation-based practice* [Overhead presentation]. Presented at the AOTA Practice Conference, Reno, Nevada.

Blanche, E. I. (1999). *Play and process: The experience of play in the life of the adult.* Ann Arbor: University of Michigan.

Blount, M. L., Blount, W., & Hinojosa, J (2004). Perspectives. In J. Hinojosa & M. L. Blount (Eds.), *The texture of life: Purposeful activities in occupational therapy* (2nd ed., pp. 17–38). Bethesda, MD: AOTA Press.

Borg, B., & Bruce, M. (1991). Assessing psychological performance factors. In C. H. Christiansen & C. M. Baum (Eds.), *Occupational therapy: Overcoming human performance deficits* (pp. 538–586). Thorofare, NJ: Slack.

Borst, M. J., & Nelson, D. L. (1993). Use of uniform terminology by occupational therapists. *American Journal of Occupational Therapy, 47,* 611–618.

Buckley, K. A., & Poole, S. E. (2004). Activity analysis. In J. Hinojosa & M. L. Blount (Eds.), *The texture of life: Purposeful activities in occupational ther-*

apy (2nd ed., pp. 69–114). Bethesda, MD: AOTA Press.

Canadian Association of Occupational Therapists. (1997). *Enabling occupation: An occupational therapy perspective.* Ottawa, ON: CAOT Publications ACE.

Christiansen, C. H. (1997). Acknowledging a spiritual dimension in occupational therapy practice. *American Journal of Occupational Therapy, 51,* 169–172.

Christiansen, C. H., & Matuska, K. M. (2004). The importance of everyday activities. In C. H. Christiansen & K. M. Matuska (Eds.), *Ways of living: Adaptive strategies for special needs* (3rd ed., pp. 1–20). Bethesda, MD: AOTA Press.

Clark, F. A., Parham, D., Carlson, M. C., Frank, G., Jackson, J., Pierce, D., et al. (1991). Occupational science: Academic innovation in the service of occupational therapy's future. *American Journal of Occupational Therapy, 45,* 300–310.

Clark, F. A., Wood, W., & Larson, E. (1998). Occupational science: Occupational therapy's legacy for the 21st century. In M. E. Neistadt & E. B. Crepeau (Eds.), *Willard and Spackman's occupational therapy* (9th ed., pp. 13–21). Philadelphia: Lippincott Williams & Wilkins.

Culler, K. H. (1993). Occupational therapy performance areas: Home and family management. In H. L. Hopkins & H. D. Smith (Eds.), *Willard and Spackman's occupational therapy* (8th ed., pp. 207–269). Philadelphia: Lippincott Williams & Wilkins.

Dunn, W., Brown, C., & McGuigan, A. (1994). The ecology of human performance: A framework for considering the effect of context. *American Journal of Occupational Therapy, 48,* 595–607.

Gardner, H. (1999). *Intelligence reframed: Multiple intelligences for the 21st century.* New York: Basic Books.

Hill, J. (1993). Occupational therapy performance areas. In H. L. Hopkins & H. D. Smith (Eds.), *Willard and Spackman's occupational therapy* (8th ed., pp. 191–268). Philadelphia: Lippincott.

Hinojosa, J., & Blount, M. L. (2004). Purposeful activities within the context of occupational therapy. In J. Hinojosa & M. L. Blount (Eds.), *The texture of life: Purposeful activities in occupational ther-*

apy (2nd ed., pp. 1–16). Bethesda, MD: AOTA Press.

Holm, M. B., Rogers, J. C., & Stone, R. G. (1998). Treatment of performance contexts. In M. E. Neistadt & E. B. Crepeau (Eds.), *Willard and Spackman's occupational therapy* (9th ed., pp. 471–517). Philadelphia: Lippincott Williams & Wilkins.

Horsburgh, M. (1997). Towards an inclusive spirituality: Wholeness, interdependence, and waiting. *Disability and Rehabilitation, 19,* 398–406.

Intagliata, S. (1993). Rehabilitation centers. In H. L. Hopkins & H. D. Smith (Eds.), *Willard and Spackman's occupational therapy* (8th ed., pp. 784–789). Philadelphia: Lippincott.

Kane, R. L. (1997). Approaching the outcomes question. In R. L. Kane (Ed.), *Understanding health care outcomes research* (pp. 1–15). Gaithersburg, MD: Aspen.

Kielhofner, G. (1992). *Conceptual foundations of occupational therapy.* Philadelphia: F. A. Davis.

Kielhofner, G. (2002). Habituation: Patterns of daily occupation. In G. Kielhofner (Ed.), *Model of human occupation: Theory and application* (3rd ed., pp. 63–80). Philadelphia: Lippincott Williams & Wilkins.

Law, M. (1991). The environment: A focus for occupational therapy. *Canadian Journal of Occupational Therapy, 58,* 171–179.

Law, M. (1993). Evaluating activities of daily living: Directions for the future. *American Journal of Occupational Therapy, 47,* 233–237.

Law, M. (1998). Assessment in client-centered occupational therapy. In M. Law (Ed.), *Client-centered occupational therapy* (pp. 89–106). Thorofare, NJ: Slack.

Lifson, L. E., & Simon, R. I. (Eds.). (1998). *The mental health practitioner and the law: A comprehensive handbook.* Cambridge, MA: Harvard University Press.

Llorens, L. (1993). Activity analysis: Agreement between participants and observers on perceived factors and occupation components. *Occupational Therapy Journal of Research, 13,* 198–211.

Ludwig, F. M. (1993). Anne Cronin Mosey. In R. J. Miller & K. F. Walker (Eds.), *Perspectives on theory for the practice of occupational therapy* (pp. 41–63). Gaithersburg, MD: Aspen.

Mosey, A. C. (1981). Legitimate tools of occupational therapy. In A. Mosey (Ed.), *Occupational therapy: Configuration of a profession* (pp. 89–118). New York: Raven.

Mosey, A. C. (1986). *Psychosocial components of occupational therapy.* New York: Raven.

Nelson, D. L. (1988). Occupation: Form and performance. *American Journal of Occupational Therapy, 42,* 633–641.

Pierce, D. (1999, September). Putting occupation to work in occupational therapy curricula. *Education Special Interest Section Quarterly, 9*(3), 1–4.

Pollock, N., & McColl, M. A. (1998). Assessments in client-centered occupational therapy. In M. Law (Ed.), *Client-centered occupational therapy* (pp. 89–105). Thorofare, NJ: Slack.

Reed, K., & Sanderson, S. (1999). *Concepts of occupational therapy* (4th ed.). Philadelphia: Lippincott Williams & Wilkins.

Schell, B. B. (1998). Clinical reasoning: The basis of practice. In M. E. Neistadt & E. B. Crepeau (Eds.), *Willard and Spackman's occupational therapy* (9th ed., pp. 90–100). Philadelphia: Lippincott Williams & Wilkins.

Scherer, M. J., & Cushman, L. A. (1997). A functional approach to psychological and psychosocial factors and their assessment in rehabilitation. In S. S. Dittmar & G. E. Gresham (Eds.), *Functional assessment and outcomes measurement for the rehabilitation health professional* (pp. 57–67). Gaithersburg, MD: Aspen.

Urbanowski, R., & Vargo, J. (1994). Spirituality, daily practice, and the occupational performance model. *Canadian Journal of Occupational Therapy, 61,* 88–94.

Watson, D. E., & Wilson, S. A. (2003). *Task analysis: An individual and population approach* (2nd ed.). Bethesda, MD: AOTA Press.

Yerxa, E. J. (1980). Occupational therapy's role in creating a future climate of caring. *American Journal of Occupational Therapy, 34,* 529–534.

Authors

THE COMMISSION ON PRACTICE:

Susanne Smith Roley, MS, OTR/L, FAOTA,
Chairperson, 2005–2008

Janet V. DeLany, DEd, OTR/L, FAOTA,
Chairperson-Elect, 2007–2008

Cynthia J. Barrows, MS, OTR/L

Susan Brownrigg, OTR/L

DeLana Honaker, PhD, OTR/L, BCP

Deanna Iris Sava, MS, OTR/L

Vibeke Talley, OTR/L

Kristi Voelkerding, BS, COTA/L, ATP

Deborah Ann Amini, MEd, OTR/L, CHT,
SIS Liaison

Emily Smith, MOT, *ASD Liaison*

Pamela Toto, MS, OTR/L, BCG, FAOTA,
Immediate-Past SIS Liaison

Sarah King, MOT, OTR, *Immediate-Past
ASD Liaison*

Deborah Lieberman, MHSA, OTR/L, FAOTA,
AOTA Headquarters Liaison

With contributions from

M. Carolyn Baum, PhD, OTR/L, FAOTA

Ellen S. Cohn, ScD, OTR/L, FAOTA

Penelope A. Moyers Cleveland, EdD, OTR/L,
BCMH, FAOTA

Mary Jane Youngstrom, MS, OTR, FAOTA

for

THE COMMISSION ON PRACTICE

Susanne Smith Roley MS, OTR/L, FAOTA,
Chairperson

Adopted by the Representative Assembly 2008C5.

This document replaces the 2002 *Occupational
Therapy Practice Framework: Domain and Process.*

Specialized Knowledge and Skills Papers

Specialized Knowledge and Skills in Adult Vestibular Rehabilitation for Occupational Therapy Practice

Introduction

People with impairments of the vestibular system often have subtle problems that have profound ramifications for their ability to engage in daily life tasks and activities at home and to participate in society outside the home. Vestibular impairment often restricts an individual's ability to participate in everyday occupations, affecting not only that individual but also significant others, including family members, friends, coworkers, and caregivers. Occupational therapy facilitates increased independence in daily life tasks and participation in work and social occupations. For these reasons, occupational therapy is an appropriate intervention for clients needing vestibular rehabilitation to decrease symptoms and increase independence in all aspects of their lives. Thus, vestibular rehabilitation is within the scope of practice for occupational therapists and occupational therapy assistants[1] who have specialized knowledge and skills in this area. This document provides an understanding of the essential knowledge and skills needed by practitioners working with individuals with vestibular impairments and will be of interest to payers, practitioners, or consumers who wish to know more about occupational therapy practice using vestibular rehabilitation techniques.

People with vestibular disorders may present with symptoms including vertigo, oscillopsia, nausea, disequilibrium, spatial disorientation, visual motion sensitivity, decreased dynamic visual acuity, decreased concentration, and decreased skill in dual task performance. Spatial orientation deficits and disequilibrium may be manifested as head and body tilt while sitting or standing, perception of tilt while sitting or standing, veering or drifting to the side while walking or steering a vehicle, or a sense of not knowing which way is up. These problems may result in fear of falling. These symptoms may affect occupational performance and can result in social withdrawal and depression. For example, visual motion sensitivity may cause disequilibrium, vertigo, nausea, and disorientation, leading to slower or more awkward performance of self-care skills, decreased participation in social activities, and decreased ability to perform home management tasks outside of the home, such as grocery shopping. Vertigo, disequilibrium, and other symptoms may interfere with job skills as they cause difficulty standing, reaching, walking, turning the head to scan the environment, or making social gestures with the head such as nodding.

Definition

The term *vestibular rehabilitation* refers to intervention to decrease symptoms and increase independence, safety, and participation in people with specific disorders of the peripheral vestibular apparatus, the central vestibular pathways, and age-related disequilibrium. Interventions include, but are not limited to, exercise and activity programs to reduce vertigo and oscillopsia, repositioning interventions for positional vertigo, exercises and activities to improve standing and walking balance during activities, and safety

---

[1]*Occupational therapists* are responsible for all aspects of occupational therapy service delivery and are accountable for the safety and effectiveness of the occupational therapy service delivery process. *Occupational therapy assistants* deliver occupational therapy services under the supervision of and in partnership with an occupational therapist (AOTA, 2004).

training at home and at work. A client receiving occupational therapy including vestibular rehabilitation techniques may also receive occupational therapy using other interventions. For example, a client with a head injury may also receive perceptual, motor, or life skills training.

Vestibular rehabilitation is used to treat the sequelae of specific medical conditions, and provides an alternative or adjunct to pharmacologic and surgical intervention by the physician. Clients who receive vestibular rehabilitation have specific medical conditions that can be demonstrated with objective diagnostic tests or otherwise medically determined. Most people who are referred for vestibular rehabilitation are adults. They have a wide variety of health conditions including, but not limited to, benign paroxysmal positional vertigo (BPPV); acute, chronic, and recurrent labyrinthitis; vestibular neuronitis; some autoimmune disorders; postconcussion vertigo; postoperative vertigo; Ménierè's disease; bilateral vestibular weakness or total vestibular loss due to ototoxicity; presbystasis or disequilibrium of aging; some cases of strokes, some cases of multiple sclerosis, some cases of Parkinson's disease, some Parkinsonian syndromes, and some cases of migraine.

Although the focus of this document is on adult vestibular rehabilitation, we note that the same or similar vestibular impairments may occur in children. The literature has few papers on the efficacy of vestibular rehabilitation in children. These disorders are difficult to diagnose because children may not be able to describe their symptoms and because, for technical reasons, young children cannot always be tested with standard objective diagnostic tests. Vestibular disorders that occur in childhood that may respond to vestibular rehabilitation include childhood paroxysmal vertigo, which may be related to migraine; BPPV; labyrinthitis; vestibular neuronitis; bilateral impairment due to ototoxicity; some autoimmune disorders; and congenital malformations of the inner ear. In pediatric vestibular rehabilitation, treatment activities must be age appropriate.

Knowledge and Skills for Entry-Level and Advanced Practitioners

Clients with vestibular disorders have a complex combination of physiological and psychological problems. The effects of vestibular impairments are subtle and pervasive. Many people with these problems are not able to describe the sensations they have or the motions that elicit vertigo or disequilibrium. Therefore, rehabilitation of most individuals with vestibular impairments requires skills beyond entry-level competence. The specialized nature of this intervention requires specific, advanced-level knowledge. Intervention may require specific techniques that focus directly on the vestibular impairment. Advanced skills build on earlier competencies in knowledge, performance, critical reasoning, interpersonal abilities, and ethical reasoning and additional competencies developed during independent study of the literature, continuing education coursework, and additional practice.

An in-depth understanding of the structure and function of the vestibular system, visual/vestibular/proprioceptive interactions, and the principles of motor control is essential when providing vestibular rehabilitation. Occupational therapy entry-level education provides a foundation in functional anatomy, neuroscience, and motor control that assists the practitioner in understanding the types of complex problems experienced by clients with vestibular impairments. Practitioners need further training, however, to address the subtle problems of clients with these disorders. Advanced-level skills are necessary for evaluation of the deficits and specific manipulations that alter vestibular function. This knowledge and these skills are not provided to occupational therapists at the entry level. Appendix 1 outlines the basic science knowledge necessary for advanced practice.

Occupational therapists use knowledge of vestibular system anatomy and physiology when determining underlying problems that affect occupational performance. An individual's central nervous system uses information about head movement to help control four classes of behavior: (a) postural reflexes for control of balance, (b) vestibulo-ocular reflexes to stabilize gaze so the individual can see clearly, (c) coding of spatial coordinates for object orientation and navigation, and (d) some autonomic responses to prepare for "fight-or-flight" behavior. Appendix 2 outlines the applied science knowledge necessary for advanced practice.

The occupational therapist must be highly skilled at evaluating the consequences of subtle vestibular deficits, such as balance disturbances due to head movements while sitting, standing, walking, reaching, and performing transfers between positions. Understanding the potential impact of vestibular impairment on participation in healthy occupations requires knowledge of the effect of vestibular impairment on the life of the person. See Appendices 3–8 for specific examples of how vestibular impairments impact performance in occupation (AOTA, 2002).

Refined skills in activity analysis are essential for evaluation of and intervention planning for these clients. The occupational therapist uses knowledge of body structure and function in conjunction with observation and activity analysis when evaluating subtle decrements in performance during typical daily activities. At the entry level, occupational therapists and occupational therapy assistants are familiar with the location of the vestibular labyrinth and know that the symptoms of vestibular disorders include vertigo, poor balance, and fear of falling. Their use of the occupational profile helps to determine which tasks elicit those symptoms. They are able to determine if clients would benefit from adaptive safety equipment; to recommend equipment appropriate for the home; and to educate clients about other safety concerns, such as appropriate clothing and shoes. They also are able to evaluate many activities of daily living directly to determine if training is needed and provide training when necessary. Appendix 9 outlines the essential evaluation skills for the advanced practitioner. Appendix 10 outlines specific information on intervention using vestibular rehabilitation methods.

Occupation therapy practitioners who do vestibular rehabilitation may seek reimbursement through Medicare and other third-party payers. Examples of possible Current Procedural Technology (CPT) codes include, but are not limited to, codes for neuromuscular reeducation of movement, balance, coordination, and/or posture for sitting and/or standing activities (97112); manual therapy (97140); and therapeutic activities to improve functional performance (97530) (American Medical Association, 2006).

The occupational therapist assumes the ultimate responsibility for the delivery of occupational therapy services, including evaluation of the person and development of the intervention plan. The advanced occupational therapist may delegate certain selected interventions to an entry-level occupational therapist or to an occupational therapy assistant who has demonstrated service competency in those interventions. All practitioners should know when and how to refer clients to other health professionals when needed, including but not limited to: specialty physicians, certified driving rehabilitation specialists, psychologists, physical therapists, audiologists, and social workers.

Brief Review of the Research Literature

Vestibular rehabilitation in occupational therapy practice is supported by the literature, although considerable research remains to be done. This section is not an exhaustive review of the research but gives an overview of the research on vestibular impairment and vestibular rehabilitation that is relevant to occupational therapy. Suggested readings not cited here are listed in the "Additional Reading" list.

In the first paper describing the use of exercises for vertigo, Cawthorne (1944) indicated that some patients with postconcussion vertigo are rendered "helpless and immobile," preceding later work by occupational therapists and their collaborators showing that patients with disorders that cause vertigo have significantly reduced independence in activities of daily living (Cohen, 1992; Cohen, Ewell, & Jenkins, 1995; Cohen & Jerabek, 1999; Cohen & Kimball, 2000; Cohen, Kimball, & Adams, 2000; Cohen, Wells, Kimball, & Owsley, 2003; Farber, 1989; Morris, 1991).

In Cooksey's first paper describing vestibular rehabilitation exercises (Cooksey, 1945), he mentioned the need for teamwork by rehabilitation staff, including occupational therapists. Cooksey specifically noted the role of occupational therapy in the early resumption of purposeful activity. In his 1946 paper, Cooksey indicated that purposeful activity should be incorporated into the daily exercise program for these patients. Structured, purposeful activity is an effective treatment modality for reducing vertigo, improving balance, and increasing independence in activities of daily living (Cohen, Kane-Wineland, Miller, & Hatfield, 1995; Cohen, Miller, Kane-Wineland, & Hatfield, 1995). Vertigo habituation exercises are also effective in decreasing symptoms, improving spatial orientation skills, and increasing independence and ability to perform purposeful activity that involves repetitive head movements (Cohen & Kimball, 2002, 2003, 2004b, 2004c). Thus, exercises and purposeful activities may be components of a successful rehabilitation program for many patients with vertigo. For a critical review of more recent studies on vertigo habituation treatments and other issues, see Cohen's 2006 review paper.

A series of studies has shown that patients with vestibular disorders also have high rates of anxiety and other psychosocial problems (Eagger, Luxon, Davies, Coelho, & Ron, 1992; Yardley & Hallam, 1996; Yardley, Luxon, & Haacke, 1994; Yardley & Putman, 1992). Many of these kinds of problems might be appropriate for intervention by occupational therapists, combining our understanding of physical and psychosocial disorders.

Patients with benign paroxysmal positional vertigo are best treated with passive maneuvers of the head that are thought to reposition otoconial particles that have become displaced from one compartment to another. Occupational therapists and their collaborators have been in the forefront of investigators showing that these repositioning maneuvers are effective treatments (Cohen & Jerabek, 1999; Cohen Kimball, 2004a, 2005; Macias, Lambert, Massingale, Ellensohn, & Fritz, 2000; Steenerson & Cronin, 1996; Steenerson, Cronin, & Marbach, 2005).

Appendixes

The following Appendixes outline the basic knowledge needed to understand and treat vestibular disorders, the effects of vestibular disorders on occupational performance, and the types of interventions occupational therapists use. The appendices are not exhaustive. Further knowledge of specific conditions may be needed in some circumstances, particularly when clients have more than one diagnosis or health condition. Also, by the nature of growth in clinical skills, the division between entry-level and advanced knowledge is somewhat fluid as the practitioner learns more and advances in clinical knowledge and skill. Furthermore, the knowledge base listed here is not absolute. Research in basic and applied science continues to expand the available knowledge base. Therefore, practitioners continue to read the literature, attend continuing education courses, and otherwise engage in activities to maintain and improve their knowledge and understanding of intervention in this area, to support their evidence-based practice.

Vestibular disorders decrease the ability to be independent in many activities of daily living. In general, tasks that require rapid or repeated head movements, tasks that require good postural control, especially while standing or walking, and tasks that require good spatial orientation may be affected. Clients who have fallen or who are at risk for falls may severely restrict their movements and may actually increase their risk of falling as a result. These people often cease participation in exercise programs for strengthening, cardiovascular conditioning, weight loss, or bone health. In a few rare instances, avoiding motions or positions that elicit vertigo may even mean delaying necessary surgical procedures due to potential discomfort during postoperative bed rest.

Clients with vestibular impairments often require more time to complete routine self-care skills. They may need to adapt the environment for safety or change the way in which they perform some tasks (e.g., to sit rather than stand or to hold an object for safety while standing). They may need to reduce the amount

Appendix 1. Basic Science Knowledge for Vestibular Rehabilitation

Detailed knowledge of the structure of the ear and vestibular labyrinth, including semicircular canals, otoliths, and vestibular nerve

Detailed knowledge of the physiology of the vestibular labyrinth, including basic understanding of the inertial mechanisms of the semicircular canals and otoliths

Understanding of central vestibular projections, including vestibular nuclei, vestibulocerebellar projections, vestibulospinal projections, vestibulo-ocular projections, and vestibulocortical projections

Understanding of multisensory interactions, including visual, vestibular, haptic, and proprioceptive

Understanding of vestibulo-autonomic interactions

Manifestations of the vestibular influence on postural control (e.g., vestibulopostural responses)

Manifestations of vestibuloocular control (e.g., vestibuloocular reflex)

Understanding of other eye movements and oculomotor responses: saccades, smooth pursuit, optokinetic responses, fixation/suppression, and interaction of vestibulo-ocular reflex with other eye movements

Manifestations of vestibular influence on spatial orientation: vertical orientation and path integration

Manifestations of vestibulo-autonomic responses

Appendix 2. Applied Science Knowledge for Vestibular Rehabilitation

Familiarity with symptoms of vestibular disorders: vertigo and oscillopsia, balance deficits, path integration impairments, autonomic signs, cognitive problems, psychosocial problems, hearing loss, and auditory/perceptual illusions on rare occasions

Familiarity with principles of objective diagnostic tests: low-frequency sinusoidal tests of the vestibuloocular reflex, bithermal caloric tests, vestibular-evoked myogenic potentials, Dix-Hallpike and side-lying tests, and computerized dynamic posturography. Advanced practitioners should be familiar with the standard techniques for recording eye movements, including electrooculography/electronystagmography and infrared videooculography. Advanced practitioners should also be familiar with related oculomotor tests and auditory screening tests.

Familiarity with peripheral vestibular disorders: Labyrinthitis/vestibular neuronitis; acute, self-limiting, recurrent, and chronic benign paroxysmal positional vertigo, Ménierè's disease, perilymph fistula, acoustic neuroma, Tullio's phenomenon, ototoxicity, and other causes of bilateral vestibular impairment

Familiarity with central vestibular disorders: presbystasis, cerebellopontine angle tumor, Arnold Chiari malformation, medulloblastoma, migraine, multiple sclerosis, Parkinson's disease and the Parkinsonian syndromes, lateral medullary syndrome and other cerebrovascular accidents, traumatic brain injury, and vertebrobasilar insufficiency

Familiarity with systemic disorders: diabetes, autoimmune disorders, especially those causing connective tissue disorders

Understanding of relevant physician subspecialties: otology/neurotology and otoneurology

Understanding of cognitive strategies and problems in dual- and multitask performance

of extraneous stimulation in the environment during task performance since divided attention becomes more difficult, so they may require reduced noise, less visual clutter, or fewer tasks requiring simultaneous attention. Therefore, they may become less efficient when performing tasks.

Many clients deliberately constrain their lives, becoming less active within and outside the home. So, they may abandon activities that they consider to be nonessential and reduce their participation in essential tasks. Many people stop driving or drive only within their neighborhoods and avoid highway driving. They may even change jobs to reduce travel or to avoid other job-related requirements that elicit vertigo or disequilibrium. Many people with vestibular disorders stop socializing or attending worship services because they are embarrassed by their ataxic gaits and do not want to give the appearance of intoxication. Some clients, who have vertigo when they bow during required prayers or who are unable to kneel while praying, may feel spiritually bereft. These problems can affect relationships with family, friends, and coworkers. Even the most understanding spouses may become upset when intimate sexual activity is interrupted by vertigo, quiet time together while taking a walk is made unpleasant due to repeated stumbling or drifting back and forth, and the affected individual may no longer be able to participate in shared sports or other exercise activities. See Appendixes 3–8 for further examples.

Specific evaluation and intervention skills are used in vestibular rehabilitation. The occupational therapy practitioner who works in this specialty must be familiar with the evaluation skills in Appendix 9 and the intervention skills in Appendix 10.

Appendix 3. Examples of Impact on Activities of Daily Living

Eating: Leaning across a table to pass something

Bathing: Bending to reach the legs, feet, perineal area, closing eyes to wash hair

Toileting: Bending to wipe, bending to pull garments up or down, maintaining balance while standing to urinate (males), twisting to reach toilet paper if behind toilet

Transferring: Sit-to-stand transfers from toilet, other seats

Grooming and hygiene: Bending the head forward to groom hair or brush teeth

Taking medication: Bending the head back to swallow medication

Sexual activity: Being in the superior position and weight shifting or moving the head rapidly; stability on water bed or other positioning furniture

Sleep: Head movements during sleep, changing sleeping positions, or maintaining the head in certain positions during sleep will elicit vertigo and cause waking, possibly nausea, and disequilibrium while groggy

Instrumental Activities of Daily Living

Meal preparation, cleaning, other home management skills: Bending down, looking into high or low cabinets or shelves, and tasks that require repetitive head movements may all elicit symptoms. Task performance may be compromised or the task may be abandoned altogether.

Gardening, yard work: Tasks may be performed less efficiently or abandoned; falls may occur on uneven ground.

Vehicle care: Car washing and changing oil and filters may be difficult or impossible.

Child, elder, and pet care: Tasks that involve picking up and carrying loads, bending rapidly, performing or assisting in transfers, diaper changing, cleaning up messes on floor

Community mobility: Driving will be more difficult, especially under conditions of reduced visibility, and may be abandoned or performed only for limited errands.

Shopping: Navigating stores, carrying packages, bending to pick up items, scanning shelves for items will be more difficult and may be abandoned.

Safety: Ascending/descending fire escapes and stairs, dim areas with only emergency lighting

Play, leisure, social participation, religious activities: Visual motion sensitivity, difficulty kneeling, navigating in crowds, vertigo elicited by repetitive head movements or bending the head down; activities and rituals may be severely restricted or abandoned.

Work, either paid employment or volunteer jobs: Symptoms elicited by a wide range of tasks will cause reduced efficiency and sometimes total inability to perform some jobs, depending on task demands.

Appendix 4. Examples of Performance Skills Affected by Vestibular Impairments

Posture: Standing balance is impaired in most people with vestibular impairments. People may tilt the head and/or body off the vertical. They may have difficulty attaining and maintaining upright standing. This skill is particularly difficult when visual cues are absent or decreased. Static head and trunk posture while seated are sometimes impaired; dynamic sitting balance may also be impaired.

Mobility: Mobility skills are manifested as veering toward one side while walking, ataxic gait, and falling or stumbling, particularly on uneven surfaces. Load compensation skills are impaired. Clients may need to use light touch to improve orientation and stability.

Coordination: Dual-task performance skill is decreased.

Energy: Routine tasks take more energy than usual, and endurance is decreased.

Appendix 5. Examples of Performance Patterns Affected by Vestibular Impairments

Habits: Skill components of habits may be disrupted, and performance efficiency may be reduced, increasing the cognitive load and increasing the difficulty of performing habitual skills that were previously easy to perform (e.g., basic activities of daily living may have to be performed with modifications).

Routines: Due to effects on performance skills, routines are less efficient and may need to be changed or abandoned altogether (e.g., hair washing may require supervision for safety and may take too long in the morning before work, so the client's morning and evening routines may be changed).

Roles: Some roles may be reduced or even abandoned, with consequent detrimental economic and psychosocial effects (e.g., clients with Ménierè's disease may have to leave their jobs).

Appendix 6. Examples of Context Affected by Vestibular Impairments

Physical: The physical environment may require modifications for safety (e.g., installing bathroom grab bars), or the home environment may require significant change (e.g., removing throw rugs, changing lighting patterns).

Social: Misunderstanding of symptoms and problems by family, friends, and significant others may lead to hard feelings, reduced participation in socialization, changes in preferred social environments. These problems may occur due to decreased self-confidence, fear of falling, and a history of falls.

Spiritual: Falls, vertigo, decreased concentration, and decreased ability in dual task performance, which all lead to decreased performance in vocational and vocational activities and decreased participation in the community, can cause decreased sense of self-worth, self-doubt, and decreased joy in life.

Virtual: Visual motion sensitivity may lead to avoidance of virtual environments.

Appendix 7. Examples of Activity Demands Affected by Vestibular Impairments

Timing: Tasks may take longer than before.

Space demands: Lighting, flooring, and support surfaces may have to be changed.

Social demands: Reduced social interaction per task may be required due to reduced tolerance for auditory and visual noise.

Required bodily functions: Reduced function of vestibulo-ocular reflex, vestibulospinal reflex, and reduced spatial orientation skills all affect functional performance.

Appendix 8. Examples of Client Factors Affected by Vestibular Impairments

Mental functions: Reduced attention skills, reduced ability for dual task performance

Sensory functions: Reduced vestibular function, sometimes reduced auditory function

Neuromuscular functions: Reduced postural control, reduced dynamic visual acuity, impaired gait

Vestibular labyrinth: In some instances, structural abnormalities in the physical labyrinth may be present, but these features cannot be observed; they may only be inferred.

Appendix 9. Occupational Therapy Evaluation Skills for Vestibular Rehabilitation

Detailed occupational and health histories relevant to symptoms

Objective clinical tests involving the vestibuloocular reflex head thrusts, Dix-Hallpike and sidelying maneuvers, and other tests of positional vertigo in lateral and anterior canals

Tests of path integration skill

Oculomotor tests: saccades, pursuit, optokinetic nystagmus, vergence, visual/vestibuloocular reflex interaction, evaluation of spontaneous nystagmus

Standardized and nonstandardized tests of standing and walking balance, including Clinical Test of Sensory Organization on Balance, Functional Reach, Berg Balance Scale, Get Up and Go/Timed Up and Go, Dynamic Gait Index, expert observation of other gait and balance skills including stair climbing, subtle gait deficits, and weight-shifting deficits

Qualitative self-evaluations of ADL independence: Activities-Specific Balance Confidence scale, Dizziness Handicap Inventory, and Vestibular Disorders Activities of Daily Living scale

Tests of dynamic visual acuity and oscillopsia

Measures to evaluate vertigo: head shaking, repetitive activities

Cognitive and psychosocial assessments: qualitative assessments and self-report on scales

Evaluation of independence in activities of daily living, including subtle changes and problems

Home, work, and driving safety

Appendix 10. Occupational Therapy Intervention Skills for Vestibular Rehabilitation

Repositioning treatments for benign paroxysmal positional vertigo, including canalith repositioning, liberatory maneuvers, log-rolling maneuvers, Brandt Daroff exercises, other repositioning exercises and activities

Vertigo habituation exercises and activity programs

Gaze stabilization exercises and activities, including eye–head coordination tasks

Balance therapy: exercises and activities for "static" standing, weight shifting, and balance control; exercises and activities for "dynamic" balance control during translation through space, leading to independence in dual task performance and safety during obstacle avoidance tasks

Home and work safety, including environmental modifications for lighting, flooring, modification of work area

Training in mobility skills on the bed; transfers to and from the floor, in the home, and in the external environment for falls prevention (e.g., use of a ladder, elevator, escalator, stairs, opening door, transfers to and from automobile, and functional mobility through visually challenging environments and environments with challenging support surfaces)

Knowledge of community and online resources for patient information

Patient education about condition, symptoms

Specific to Ménierè's disease patients: in coordination with nursing, work on meal-planning skills if dietary restriction is recommended by the physician

In coordination with audiology, for patients with hearing loss, recommend communication and functional devices for telephone, alarm clock, and other devices for which sound is important; recommendations for modification of work and other tasks, as needed, for hearing loss

Recommendation of assistive devices for balance and safety during standing, walking, carrying objects, and other activities of daily living

Task modification to reduce cognitive load during dual- and multitask performance; dual-task performance training

Glossary

Benign paroxysmal positional vertigo
A common disorder of the vestibular system characterized by vertigo elicited by head movements in the pitch plane and characterized by a positive response on the Dix–Hallpike maneuver.

Disequilibrium
Poor balance.

Labyrinthitis
Inflammation or disease of the vestibular labyrinth of the inner ear.

Ménière's disease
A disorder of the inner ear affecting both the auditory and vestibular systems. It is characterized by sensorineural hearing loss on at least one occasion, two or more spontaneous episodes of vertigo lasting at least 20 minutes, and tinnitus or aural fullness in the affected ear. Nystagmus is present during an attack (Committee on Hearing and Equilibrium, American Academy of Otolaryngology—Head and Neck Surgery, 1995).

Neurotologist
An otolaryngologist who specializes in ear and inner-ear disorders, including vestibular disorders.

Nystagmus
A stereotyped combination of repetitive slow- and fast-phase eye movements. The slow phase, usually difficult to observe with the naked eye, represents compensatory vestibulo-ocular or optokinetic responses; the fast phase represents rapid saccades that reset the position of the globe in the eye socket.

Optokinetic responses
Conjugate eye movements used to follow a full-field moving visual stimulus (i.e., when the entire visual scene moves around the person).

Oscillopsia
The illusion of object motion during head movement.

Otolaryngologist
A physician who specializes in ear, nose, and throat disorders.

Otoneurologist
A neurologist who specializes in vestibular and auditory disorders.

Presbystasis
Disequilibrium of aging. This diagnosis excludes known causes of balance problems, such as central neurologic conditions, peripheral vestibular impairments, or peripheral neuropathies that affect the lower extremities (e.g., diabetic neuropathies).

Pursuit
Also known as *smooth pursuit*. Conjugate eye movements are used to follow a discrete moving visual stimulus.

Saccades
Conjugate eye movements in which the eyes move for one of three reasons: (1) as the quick phase of nystagmus, to reset the position of the globe in the eye socket; (2) for gaze error correction (i.e., to catch up with a visual stimulus that is moving too fast for pursuit movements); and (3) volitional movements to look around a stationary visual environment. Saccades are the only volitional eye movements that we are able to generate. (You are using saccades to read this page.)

Spatial orientation
Awareness of one's position relative to gravity and the environment.

Vergence
Disconjugate eye movements used to make the eyes move toward or away from each other, in order to focus on an object.

Vertigo
The illusion of self-motion (e.g., spinning or falling).

Vestibular rehabilitation
The use of activities and exercise to treat vertigo, balance problems, functional limitations, and disability caused by impairments in the vestibular system.

Vestibular system
The sensory system with receptors in the vestibular labyrinth of the inner ear. It detects head motion and contributes to control of posture, eye movements, and spatial orientation. The brain pathways include the vestibular portion of Cranial Nerve VIII; the vestibular nuclei; the parts of the cerebellum that receive and process vestibular signals; the projections from the vestibular nuclei that descend in the spinal cord via the vestibulospinal tracts; the projections from the vestibular nuclei that ascend in the medial longitudinal fasciculus to Cranial Nerves III, IV, and VI to control the vestibulo-ocular reflex; and the smaller projections that ascend from the vestibular nuclei to the thalamus and related nuclei with further small projections to the vestibular cortex.

References

American Medical Association. (2006). *Current procedural terminology* (2006 ed.). Chicago: Author.

American Occupational Therapy Association. (2002). Occupational therapy practice framework: Domain and process. *American Journal of Occupational Therapy, 56,* 609–639.

American Occupational Therapy Association. (2004). Guidelines for supervision, roles, and responsibilities during the delivery of occupational therapy services. *American Journal of Occupational Therapy, 58,* 663–667.

Cawthorne, T. (1944). The physiological basis for head exercises. *Journal of the Chartered Society of Physiotherapy, 29,* 106–107.

Cohen, H. (1992). Vestibular rehabilitation reduces functional disability. *Otolaryngology—Head and Neck Surgery, 107,* 638–643.

Cohen, H. S. (2006). Disability and rehabilitation in the dizzy patient. *Current Opinion in Neurology, 19,* 49–54.

Cohen, H., Ewell, L. R., & Jenkins, H. A. (1995). Disability in Ménière's disease. *Archives of Otolaryngology, 121,* 29–33.

Cohen, H. S., & Jerabek, J. (1999). Effectiveness of liberatory maneuvers for benign paroxysmal positional vertigo of the posterior canal. *Laryngoscope, 109,* 584–590.

Cohen, H., Kane-Wineland, M., Miller, L. V., & Hatfield, C. L. (1995). Occupation and visual/vestibular interaction in vestibular rehabilitation. *Otolaryngology—Head and Neck Surgery, 112,* 526–532.

Cohen, H. S., & Kimball, K. T. (2000). Development of the Vestibular Disorders Activities of Daily Living Scale. *Archives of Otolaryngology, 126,* 881–887.

Cohen, H. S., & Kimball, K. T. (2002). Improvements in path integration after vestibular rehabilitation. *Journal of Vestibular Research, 12,* 47–51.

Cohen, H. S., & Kimball, K. T. (2003). Increased independence and decreased vertigo after vestibular rehabilitation. *Otolaryngology—Head and Neck Surgery, 128,* 560–566.

Cohen, H. S., & Kimball, K. T. (2004a). Treatment variations on the Epley maneuver for benign paroxysmal positional vertigo. *American Journal of Otolaryngology, 25,* 33–37.

Cohen, H. S., & Kimball, K. T. (2004b). Changes in a repetitive head movement task after vestibular rehabilitation. *Clinical Rehabilitation, 18,* 125–131.

Cohen, H. S., & Kimball, K. T. (2004c). Decreased ataxia and improved balance after vestibular rehabilitation. *Otolaryngology—Head and Neck Surgery, 130,* 418–425.

Cohen, H. S., & Kimball, K. T. (2005). Effectiveness of treatments for benign paroxysmal positional vertigo of the posterior canal. *Otology and Neurotology, 26,* 1034–1040.

Cohen, H. S., Kimball, K. T., & Adams, A. (2000). Application of the Vestibular Disorders Activities of Daily Living Scale. *Laryngoscope, 110,* 1204–1209.

Cohen, H., Miller, L. V., Kane-Wineland, M., & Hatfield, C. L. (1995). Case Report—Vestibular rehabilitation with graded occupations. *American Journal of Occupational Therapy, 49,* 362–367.

Cohen, H. S., Wells, J., Kimball, K. T., & Owsley, C. (2003). Driving disability in dizziness. *Journal of Safety Research, 34*(4), 361–369.

Committee on Hearing and Equilibrium, American Academy of Otolaryngology—Head and Neck Surgery. (1995). Guidelines for the diagnosis and evaluation of therapy in Ménierè's disease. *Otolaryngology—Head and Neck Surgery, 113,* 181–185.

Cooksey, F. S. (1945). Physical medicine. *Practitioner, 155,* 300–305.

Cooksey, F. S. (1946). Rehabilitation in vestibular injuries. *Proceedings of the Royal Society of Medicine, 39,* 273–278.

Eagger, S., Luxon, L. M., Davies, R. A., Coelho, A., & Ron, M. A. (1992). Psychiatric morbidity in clients with peripheral vestibular disorder: A clinical and neuro-otological study. *Journal of Neurology, Neurosurgery, and Psychiatry, 55,* 383–387.

Farber, S. D. (1989). Living with Ménière's disease: An occupational therapist's perspective. *American Journal of Occupational Therapy, 43,* 341–343.

Macias, J. D., Lambert, K. M., Massingale, S., Ellensohn, A., & Fritz, J. A. (2000). Variables affecting treatment in benign paroxysmal positional vertigo. *Laryngoscope, 110,* 1921–1924.

Morris, P. A. (1991). A habituation approach to treating vertigo in occupational therapy. *American Journal of Occupational Therapy, 45,* 556–558.

Steenerson, R. L., & Cronin, G. W. (1996). Comparison of the canalith repositioning procedure and vestibular habituation training in forty patients with benign paroxysmal positional vertigo. *Otolaryngology—Head and Neck Surgery, 1214,* 61–64.

Steenerson, R. L., Cronin, G. W., & Marbach, P. M. (2005). Effectiveness of treatment techniques in 932 cases of benign paroxysmal positional vertigo. *Laryngoscope, 115,* 226–231.

Yardley, L., & Hallam, R. S. (1996). Psychosocial aspects of balance and gait disorders. In A. M. Bronstein, T. Brandt, & M. Woollacott (Eds.), *Clinical disorders of balance, posture and gait* (pp. 251–267). London: Arnold.

Yardley, L., Luxon, L. M., & Haacke, N. P. (1994). A longitudinal study of symptoms, anxiety, and subjective well-being in clients with vertigo. *Clinical Otolaryngology and Allied Sciences, 19,* 109–116.

Yardley, L., & Putman, J. (1992). Quantitative analysis of factors contributing to handicap and distress in vertiginous clients: A questionnaire study. *Clinical Otolaryngology and Allied Sciences, 17,* 231–236.

Additional Reading

Aw, S. T., Halmagyi, G. M., Black, R. A., Curthoys, I. S., Yavor, R. A., & Todd, M. J. (1999). Head impulses reveal loss of individual semicircular canal function. *Journal of Vestibular Research, 9,* 173–180.

Baloh, R. W., Furman, J. M. R., Halmagyi, M., & Allum, J. H. J. (1995). Recent advances in clinical neurotology. *Journal of Vestibular Research, 5,* 231–252.

Baloh, R. W., & Halmagyi, G. M. (Eds.). (1996). *Disorders of the vestibular system.* New York: Oxford University Press.

Baloh, R. W., & Honrubia, V. (1990). *Clinical neurophysiology of the vestibular system* (2nd ed.). Philadelphia: F. A. Davis.

Black, R. A., Halmagyi, G. M., Thurtell, M. J., Todd, M. J., & Curthoys, I. S. (2005). The active head-impulse test in unilateral peripheral vestibulopathy. *Annals of Neurology, 62,* 290–293.

Brandt, T. (1998). *Vertigo: Its multisensory syndromes.* Berlin: Springer-Verlag.

Brandt, T., Steddin, S., & Daroff, R. B. (1994). Therapy for benign paroxysmal positioning vertigo, revisited. *Neurology, 44,* 796–800.

Bronstein, A. M., Brandt, T., & Woollacott, M. (Eds.). (1996). *Clinical disorders of balance, posture and gait.* London: Arnold/Hodder Headline PLC.

Campbell, A. J., Robertson, M. C., La Grow, S. J., Kerse, N. M., Sanderson, G. F., Jacobs, R. J., et al. (2005, October). Randomised controlled trial of prevention of falls in people aged 75 with severe visual impairment: The VIP trial. *British Medical Journal, 331*(7520), 817. Retrieved March 21, 2006, from http://bmj.bmjjournals.com/cgi/reprint_abr/331/7520/817

Cawthorne, T. (1946). Vestibular injuries. *Proceedings of the Royal Society of Medicine, 39,* 270–273.

Chronister, K. M. (2003). Divided attention: The role that cognition plays in fall prevention programs has been overlooked. *Rehab Management, 16,* 30, 32–33.

Chronister, K. (2004). Cognition: The missing link in fall-prevention programs. *Rehab Management, 9,* 11–14.

Clemson, L., Cumming, R. G., Kendig, H., Swann, M., Heard, R., & Taylor, K. (2004). The effectiveness of a community-based program for reducing the incidence of falls in the elderly: A randomized trial. *Journal of the American Geriatric Society, 52,* 1487–1494.

Cohen, H. (1994). Vestibular rehabilitation improves daily life function. *American Journal of Occupational Therapy, 48,* 919–925.

Cohen, H. (1998). *Special senses 2: The vestibular system. Neuroscience for rehabilitation.* Philadelphia: Lippincott Williams & Wilkins.

Cohen, H. S. (2000). Vertigo and balance disorders: Vestibular rehabilitation. *Occupational Therapy Practice, 5,* 14–18.

Cohen, H. S. (2004). Vestibular rehabilitation and stroke. In G. Gillen & A. Burkhardt (Eds.), *Stroke rehabilitation: A function-based approach* (2nd ed., pp. 164–171). St. Louis, MO: Mosby.

Cohen, H. S. (in press). Disability in vestibular disorders. In S. J. Herdman (Ed.), *Vestibular rehabilitation* (3rd ed). Philadelphia: F. A. Davis.

Cohen, H., Blatchly, C. A., & Gombash, L. L. (1993). A study of the clinical test of sensory interaction and balance. *Physical Therapy, 73,* 346–351.

Cohen, H., Friedman, E. M., Lai, D., Duncan, N., Pellicer, M., & Sulek, M. (1997). Balance in children with otitis media with effusion. *International Journal of Pediatric Oto-Rhino-Laryngology, 42,* 107–115.

Cohen, H. S., & Gavia, J. A. (1998). A task for assessing vertigo elicited by repetitive head movements. *American Journal of Occupational Therapy, 52,* 644–649.

Cohen, H., Heaton, L. G., Congdon, S. L., & Jenkins, H. A. (1996). Changes in sensory organization test scores with age. *Age and Ageing, 25,* 39–44.

Cohen, H. S., Kimball, K. T., & Stewart, M. G. (2004). Benign paroxysmal positional vertigo and co-morbid conditions. *ORL—Journal of Oto-Rhino-Laryngology and Related Specialties, 66,* 11–15.

Cohen, H., Rubin, A. M., & Gombash, L. L. (1991). The team approach to intervention of the dizzy client. *Archives of Physical Medicine and Rehabilitation, 73,* 703–708.

Colebatch, J. G. (2001). Vestibular evoked potentials. *Current Opinion in Neurology, 14,* 21–26.

Colebatch, J. G., Halmagyi, G. M., & Skuse, N. F. (1994). Myogenic potentials generated by a click-evoked vestibulocollic reflex. *Journal of Neurology, Neurosurgery, and Psychiatry, 57,* 190–107.

Cronin, G. W. (1990). Vestibular rehab enhances patient's quality of life. *Advance for Occupational Therapists, 6*(43), 2.

Crowe, T. K., Deitz, J. C., Richardson, P. K., & Atwater, S. W. (1990). Interrater reliability of the Pediatric Clinical Test of Sensory Interaction for Balance. *Physical and Occupational Therapy in Pediatrics, 10,* 1–27.

Cumming, R. G., Thomas, M., Szonyi, G., Frampton, G., Salkeld, G., & Clemson, L. (2001). Adherence to occupational therapist recommendations for home modifications for falls prevention. *American Journal of Occupational Therapy, 55,* 641–648.

Davison, J., Bond, J., Dawson, P., Steen, I. N., & Kenny, R. A. (2005). Patients with recurrent falls attending accident and emergency benefit from multifactorial intervention—A randomized controlled trial. *Age and Ageing, 34,* 162–168.

De la Meilleure, G., Dehaene, I., Depondt, M., Damman, W., Crevits, L., & Vanhooren, G. (1996). Benign paroxysmal positional vertigo of the horizontal canal. *Journal of Neurology, Neurosurgery, and Psychiatry, 60,* 68–71.

Dix, M. R. (1974). Intervention of vertigo. *Physiotherapy, 60,* 380–384.

Dix, M. R. (1976). The physiological basis and practical value of head exercises in the intervention of vertigo. *Practitioner, 217,* 919–924.

Dix, M. R. (1984). Rehabilitation of vertigo. In M. R. Dix & J. D. Hood (Eds.), *Vertigo* (pp. 467–479). Chichester, NY: Wiley.

Fife, T. D., Tusa, R. J., Furman, J. M., Zee, D. S., Frohman, E., Baloh, R. W., et al. (2000). Assessment: Vestibular testing techniques in adults and children. Report of the Therapeutics and Technology Assessment Subcommittee of the American Academy of Neurology. *Neurology, 55,* 1431–1441.

Gottshall, K., Gray, N., & Drake, A. I. (2005). A unique collaboration of female medical providers within the United States Armed Forces: Rehabilitation of a marine with post-concussive vestibulopathy. *Work, 24,* 381–386.

Halmagyi, G. M., & Curthoys, I. A. (1988). A clinical sign of canal paresis. *Archives of Neurology, 45,* 737–739.

Hecker, H. C., Haug, C. O., & Herndon, J. W. (1974). Intervention of the vertiginous client using Cawthorne's vestibular exercises. *Laryngoscope, 84,* 2065–2072.

Hillman, E. J., Bloomberg, J. J., McDonald, V. P., & Cohen, H. S. (1999). Dynamic visual acuity while walking in normal and labyrinthine-deficient clients. *Journal of Vestibular Research, 9,* 49–57.

Honrubia, V., Bell, T. S., Harris, M. R., Baloh, R. W., & Fisher, L. M. (1996). Quantitative evaluation of dizziness characteristics and impact on quality of life. *American Journal of Otology, 17,* 595–602.

Horak, F. B., Shumway-Cook, A., Crowe, T. K., & Black, F. O. (1988). Vestibular function and motor proficiency of children with impaired hearing, or with learning disability and motor impairments. *Developmental Medicine and Child Neurology, 30,* 64–79.

Jacobson, G. P., & Newman, C. W. (1990). The development of the Dizziness Handicap Inventory. *Archives of Otolaryngology, 116,* 424–427.

Jacobson, G. P., Newman, C. W., & Kartush, J. M. (1993). *Handbook of balance function testing.* St. Louis, MO: Mosby/YearBook.

Konnur, M. K. (2000). Vertigo and vestibular rehabilitation. *Postgraduate Medicine, 46,* 222–223.

McCabe, B. F. (1970). Labyrinthine exercises in the intervention of diseases characterized by vertigo: Their physiologic basis and methodology. *Laryngoscope, 80,* 1429–1433.

Medeiros, I. R. T., Bittar, R. S. M., Pedalini, E. B., Lorenzi, M. C., Formigoni, L. G., et al. (2005). Vestibular rehabilitation therapy in children. *Otology and Neurotology, 26,* 699–703.

Myers, A. M., Powell, L. E., Maki, B. E., Holliday, P. J., Brawley, L. R., & Sherk, W. (1996). Psychological indicators of balance confidence: Relationship to actual and perceived abilities. *Journal of Gerontology: Medical Science, 51A,* M37–M43.

Norré, M. E., & De Weerdt, W. (1979). Vestibular habituation training: Technique and first results—Preliminary report. *Acta Oto-Rhino-Laryngologica Belgica, 33,* 347–364.

Parnes, L. S., & Sindwani, R. (1997). Impact of vestibular disorders on fitness to drive: A consensus of the American Neurotology Society. *American Journal of Otology, 18,* 79–85.

Rine, R. M., Braswell, J., Fisher, D., Joyce, K., Kalar, K., & Shaffer, M. (2004). Improvement of motor development and postural control following intervention in children with sensorineural hearing loss and vestibular impairment. *International Journal of Pediatric Oto-Rhino-Laryngology, 68,* 1141–1148.

Sherlock, J. (1996). Getting into balance. *Rehab Management, 9,* 33–38.

Shumway-Cook, A., & Horak, F. B. (1986). Assessing the influence of sensory interaction on balance. *Physical Therapy, 66,* 1548–1550.

Shumway-Cook, A., & Horak, F. B. (1989). Vestibular rehabilitation: An exercise approach to managing symptoms of vestibular dysfunction. *Seminars in Hearing, 10,* 196–208.

Sindwani, R., & Parnes, L. S. (1997). Reporting of vestibular clients who are unfit to drive: Survey of Canadian otolaryngologists. *Journal of Otolaryngology, 26,* 104–111.

Steultjens, E. M. J., Dekker, J., Bouter, L. M., Jellma, S., Bakker, E. B., & van den Ende, C. H. M. (2004). Occupational therapy for community dwelling elderly people: A systematic review. *Age and Ageing, 33,* 453–460.

Uneri, A., & Turkdogan, D. (2003). Evaluation of vestibular functions in children with vertigo attacks. *Archives of Disease in Childhood, 88*, 510–511.

Whitney, S. L., Poole, J. L., & Cass, S. P. (1998). A review of balance instruments for older adults. *American Journal of Occupational Therapy, 52*, 666–671.

Wilson, V. J., & Melvill Jones, G. (1979). *Mammalian vestibular physiology.* New York: Plenum.

Wilson, V. J., & Melvill Jones, G. (1985). *Adaptive mechanisms of gaze control.* New York: Plenum.

Yardley, L. (1994). Prediction of handicap and emotional distress in clients with recurrent vertigo: Symptoms, coping strategies, control beliefs, and reciprocal causation. *Social Science and Medicine, 39*, 573–581.

Yardley, L., Burgneau, J., Nazareth, I., & Luxon, L. (1998). Neuro-otological and psychiatric abnormalities in a community sample of people with dizziness: A blind, controlled investigation. *Journal of Neurology, Neurosurgery and Psychiatry, 65*, 679–684.

Other Information Resources

American Academy of Otolaryngology—Head and Neck Surgery
One Prince Street
Alexandria, VA 22314-3357
703-836-4444
www.entnet.org
This group is the professional organization for otolaryngologists, including neurotologists. To find a neurotologist in your area, see the "Find an ENT" link. See also useful patient information brochures.

Anatomical Chart Company
Lippincott Williams & Wilkins
www.lww.com/anatomicalchart/
They produce good charts and three-dimensional models of the vestibular labyrinth.

Journal of Vestibular Research
Eye and Ear Institute
203 Lothrop Street, Suite 500
Pittsburgh, PA 15213
e-mail: jvr@upmc.edu
Web address: www.jvr-web.org
This journal specializes in publishing research on basic and clinical vestibular sciences, including research on vestibular rehabilitation and balance disorders.

National Institute on Deafness and Other Communication Disorders (NIDCD)
National Institutes of Health
31 Center Drive, MSC 2320
Bethesda, MD 20892-2320
800-241-1044
www.nidcd.nih.gov
The NIH funds much of the biomedical and biobehavioral research in this country. The NIDCD, an institute of the NIH, funds research on balance and vestibular function, including research on vestibular rehabilitation. See their Web page for free patient information brochures and a tutorial for patients with balance problems.

Vestibular Disorders Association
PO Box 4467
Portland OR 97208
Telephone: 800-837-8428
Telephone in Oregon: 503-229-7705
e-mail: veda@vestibular.org
Web address: www.vestibular.org
This patient advocacy group has useful information for patients about a variety of vestibular disorders. They also maintain a resource list of health care professionals who specialize in care of people with vestibular disorders.

Authors
Helen S. Cohen, EdD, OTR, FAOTA, *Chairperson*
Ann Burkhardt, OTD, OTR/L, BCN, FAOTA
Gaye W. Cronin, OTD, OTR
Mary Jo McGuire, MS, OTR, FAOTA

for

The Commission on Practice
Susanne Smith Roley, MS, OTR/L, FAOTA, *Chairperson*

Adopted by the Representative Assembly 2006C405

This replaces the 2000 document "Specialized Knowledge and Skills in Adult Vestibular Rehabilitation for Occupational Therapy Practice" (*American Journal of Occupational Therapy, 55*, 661–665).

Specialized Knowledge and Skills in Feeding, Eating, and Swallowing for Occupational Therapy Practice

Introduction

Occupational therapy's long-standing expertise in activities of daily living includes involvement in the feeding, eating, and swallowing performance of individuals across the life span (American Occupational Therapy Association [AOTA], 2002). Both occupational therapists and occupational therapy assistants[1] provide essential services in the comprehensive management of feeding, eating, and swallowing problems. These problems can be wide ranging and may include physical difficulty (e.g., bringing food to the mouth), processing food in the mouth (e.g., motor or sensory deficits), dysphagia, psychosocially based eating disorders (e.g., food obsessions, maladaptive eating habits), dysfunction related to cognitive impairments (e.g., understanding nutrition or food preparation), surgical intervention, and neurological impairments, as well as positioning problems that affect feeding, eating, and swallowing. Interventions focused on occupations of daily living include facilitating an individual's ability to participate in feeding and eating activities that are valued and meaningful to that person, such as learning to eat independently, joining friends for lunch, or feeding a child. Occupational therapists and occupational therapy assistants possess the education, experience, knowledge, and skills necessary in the evaluation and intervention of feeding, eating, and swallowing problems. Physical, cognitive, social, emotional, and cultural elements of feeding, eating, and swallowing are considered in evaluation and intervention.

The purpose of this document is to describe the knowledge and skills that are necessary for occupational therapists and occupational therapy assistants to provide comprehensive feeding, eating, and swallowing management and services. It provides information on occupational therapists' and occupational therapy assistants' roles in feeding, eating, and swallowing; outlines advanced-level knowledge and skills; and defines feeding-, eating-, and swallowing-related terms.

Occupational Therapy's Role in Feeding, Eating, and Swallowing Management

Feeding, Eating, and Swallowing

Feeding and eating occur within the social environment and often include family members and caregivers as part of the process. Thus, when occupational therapy practitioners address feeding, eating, and swallowing concerns, the collaboration with and involvement of family members and caregivers as well as other professionals is paramount.

Feeding, eating, and swallowing are complex activities that require effective, coordinated function of the motor, sensory, and cognitive systems. In recent years, the complexity of occupational therapy services to address these issues has grown. Feeding, eating, and swallowing services now are often provided to clients who have complicated, specialized problems and who may be medically fragile. In addition, new

---

[1]*Occupational therapists* are responsible for all aspects of occupational therapy service delivery and are accountable for the safety and effectiveness of the occupational therapy service delivery process. *Occupational therapy assistants* deliver occupational therapy services under the supervision of and in partnership with an occupational therapist (AOTA, 2004).

technologies are increasingly available for evaluation and intervention of swallowing or dysphagia management. Thus, in a variety of situations, occupational therapists and occupational therapy assistants demonstrate baseline knowledge in feeding, eating, and swallowing and may provide advanced-level knowledge and skills in the field of dysphagia management.

Feeding, eating, and swallowing are interdependent activities, and definitions of each term overlap in literature sources. For purposes of this paper, broad definitions are noted. *Feeding* is the term used to describe "the process of setting up, arranging, and bringing food [or fluid] from the plate or cup to the mouth; sometimes called self-feeding" (AOTA, 2006a). *Eating* is defined as "the ability to keep and manipulate food or fluid in the mouth and swallow it; eating and swallowing are often used interchangeably" (AOTA, 2006a). Feeding and eating, essential to human functioning for nourishment of the body, is a form of social interaction and is involved in many facets of a person's culture—from leisure to professional activities. *Swallowing* involves a complicated act in which food, fluid, medication, or saliva is moved from the mouth through the pharynx and esophagus into the stomach (AOTA, 2006a). Thus, feeding, eating, and swallowing are strongly influenced by psychosocial, cultural, and environmental factors. As part of the evaluation and intervention process, occupational therapists and occupational therapy assistants under the supervision of an occupational therapist consider comprehensive management of feeding, eating, and swallowing problems; adaptive feeding equipment ranging from modified utensils to sophisticated feeding equipment (e.g., the Winsford Feeder); the physical and sensory difficulty of bringing food, liquid, or medication to the mouth; sensory processing issues in the mouth (e.g., oral defensiveness); management of mechanical devices for feeding; dysphagia; psychosocially based eating disorders (e.g., anorexia, bulimia); behaviorally based eating disorders (e.g., selective eating); dysfunction related to cognitive impairments, neurological impairments, or surgical intervention; and positioning problems that affect feeding, eating, and swallowing.

Feeding, eating, and swallowing are within the domain and scope of practice for occupational therapy. Occupational therapists and occupational therapy assistants have the knowledge and skills necessary to take a lead role in the evaluation and intervention of feeding, eating, and swallowing problems. Further, occupational therapists have the entry-level knowledge and skills to evaluate oral and pharyngeal swallowing function.

Occupational Therapy Services

Occupational therapy practitioners[2] use their knowledge and skills to provide services over a broad range of ages, medical conditions, and social or cultural situations. For many clients, feeding, eating, and swallowing issues are quite complex. For instance, in populations with complicated feeding problems such as post-surgical cancer patients, patients in intensive care units, or young infants, the interplay of medical and developmental factors is complex and requires advanced-level knowledge to provide safe and effective service. As foundational skills in understanding impairments in feeding, eating, and swallowing, occupational therapists and occupational therapy assistants receive education in the structure and function of the human body, including the biological and physical sciences (e.g., anatomy, physiology, neuroanatomy, kinesiology), human development throughout the life span, and human behavior, including the behavioral and social sciences (Accreditation Council for Occupational Therapy Education, 2006). They develop clinical-reasoning skills to consider the interplay of physical, cognitive, environmental, and sociocultural factors in providing effective services for feeding, eating, and swallowing dysfunction.

As part of therapeutic services, occupational therapists are trained to conduct comprehensive evaluations, which include selecting, administering, and interpreting assessment measures. They also develop specific intervention plans and provide therapeutic interventions.

---

[2]When the term *occupational therapy practitioner* is used in this document, it refers to both occupational therapists and occupational therapy assistants (AOTA, 2006b).

The occupational therapist assumes the ultimate responsibility for the delivery of occupational therapy services. Occupational therapy assistants are trained to provide services under the supervision of and in collaboration with an occupational therapist (AOTA, 2004). During the evaluation process, occupational therapy assistants may gather data and administer selected assessment tools or measures for which they have demonstrated competence.

During intervention, both occupational therapists and occupational therapy assistants select, administer, and adapt activities that support the intervention plan developed by the occupational therapist. Practitioners must always adhere to state and agency regulatory laws when providing services across these continua of care. Reimbursement for services may be available through various sources, including legislation (e.g., Individuals With Disabilities Education Act, Medicare), private insurance, Medicaid, and private pay. Information on specific entry-level knowledge and skills occupational therapists and occupational therapy assistants should have to serve clients with feeding, eating, and swallowing dysfunction can be found in Appendix A.

For both occupational therapists and occupational therapy assistants, the progression from entry-level knowledge and skills to advanced-level knowledge and skills is individualized. Although practitioners exit their academic program with the basic knowledge and skills to provide occupational therapy services to clients with feeding, eating, and swallowing dysfunction, over time they may develop additional individualized expertise such as in the area of dysphagia. Occupational therapy practitioners ensure advanced competence in feeding, eating, and swallowing by maintaining and documenting competence in practice, education, and research and by participating in professional development, educational activities, and critical examination of available evidence (AOTA, 2005a). In addition, higher level knowledge, skills, and clinical reasoning are developed through experience.

The practitioner's acquisition of advanced-level knowledge and skills as related to intervention with people with feeding, eating, and swallowing difficulties is individualized; thus, a practitioner may possess differing levels of expertise in a wide variety of skill areas and populations served by occupational therapy. For example, an occupational therapist with advanced-level skills in feeding with premature infants may possess only entry-level skills in assessing swallowing function in a client who has had a cerebral vascular accident resulting in hemiplegic weakness. It is the ethical responsibility of occupational therapists and occupational therapy assistants to ensure that they are competent in the services they provide and that they continually seek out new knowledge and techniques that apply to their clinical practice (AOTA, 2005a).

Supervision Considerations

The amount of supervision provided to an occupational therapist or occupational therapy assistant in the area of feeding, eating, and swallowing should directly relate to their training and experience and state practice acts. Occupational therapy assistants and entry-level occupational therapists should seek supervision and mentoring from a more experienced occupational therapist or an occupational therapist with advanced knowledge and skills in feeding, eating, and swallowing. The occupational therapist and occupational therapy assistant also may supervise other nonlicensed health care aides providing feeding and eating assistance to clients (AOTA, 2004). Most state practice acts mandate the frequency and duration for supervision for entry-level occupational therapists, occupational therapy assistants, and nonlicensed health care aides. The occupational therapist has the primary role in evaluation and intervention planning; the occupational therapy assistant collaborates with the occupational therapist in the provision of specific interventions (AOTA, 2004, 2005b). Occupational therapy assistants who hold an AOTA specialty certification in feeding, eating, and swallowing may have a more active role in collaborating in the evaluation process and in making intervention decisions. However, it is implicit that these tasks are carried out under the supervision of an occupational therapist. The supervising occupational therapist must be experienced in feeding, eating, and swallowing disorders or seek consultation from an occupational therapist who has such experience.

Knowledge and Skills

The progression from entry-level knowledge and skills to advanced-level knowledge and skills is individualized for each occupational therapist and occupational therapy assistant. Although practitioners exit their academic program with the basic knowledge and skills to provide occupational therapy services to clients with feeding, eating, and swallowing dysfunction, over time they may develop additional individualized expertise, such as in the area of dysphagia. Entry-level knowledge and skills for both occupational therapists and occupational therapy assistants, as supported by the 2006 Standards (Accreditation Council of Occupational Therapy Education, 2006), are delineated in Appendix A. The advanced-level knowledge and skills necessary to provide a continuum of services in the area of feeding, eating, and swallowing are delineated in Appendix B. These advanced-level skills build on existing knowledge, performance skills, critical reasoning, interpersonal abilities, and ethical reasoning.

Appendix A.
Entry-Level Knowledge and Skills Assessment

Occupational Therapists and Occupational Therapy Assistants Will Have Entry-Level Knowledge and Skills to Assess:

Context	Occupational Therapist	Occupational Therapy Assistant *(Based on the Establishment of Service Competency and Supervision by an Occupational Therapist)*
Cultural components that affect feeding: utensils, food types, meanings/symbolism of food, mealtime practices and rituals, dietary restrictions	✓	✓
Attitudes and values of client, family or caregivers, and friends toward feeding and mealtime	✓	✓
Settings where feeding/eating take place	✓	✓
Social opportunities during mealtime that support or interfere with social interaction	✓	✓
Aspects of the client's developmental status/life phase that support or interfere with eating/feeding	✓	—
Effect of medical condition/disability status on feeding performance	✓	—
Factors in the environment that support or interfere with feeding/eating (e.g., foods, seating, time, feeders)	✓	—
Pre-Oral Phase		
Role of appetite and hunger sensation	✓	✓
Tactile and proprioceptive qualities of food and equipment in both the hands and the mouth	✓	✓
Ability to see/locate food/drink/utensils	✓	✓
Ability to appreciate smell—pleasant/noxious	✓	✓
Need for use of auditory cues (verbal cues, utensils hitting plate)	✓	✓
Ability to achieve a position of proximal postural control that allows upper-extremity and oral function for eating	✓	✓
Nature of communication during feeding/mealtime	✓	✓
Feeding experience as satisfactory to self	✓	✓

✓ = able to perform the task
— = does not perform the task

(continued)

Appendix A.
Entry-Level Knowledge and Skills Assessment *(cont.)*

Occupational Therapists and Occupational Therapy Assistants Will Have Entry-Level Knowledge and Skills to Assess:

	Occupational Therapist	Occupational Therapy Assistant *(Based on the Establishment of Service Competency and Supervision by an Occupational Therapist)*
Pre-Oral Phase *(continued)*		
Ability to bring food to mouth as supported or prevented by factors such as figure ground, depth perception, spatial relations, and motor planning	✓	—
Neuromotor components that support or interfere with adequate positioning	✓	—
Upper-extremity function and hand manipulation adequate for self-feeding	✓	—
Influence of motor activity involved in bringing food to mouth	✓	—
Ability to orient mouth to receive food (timing, positioning of structures)	✓	—
Initiation of eating as supported/prevented by level of alertness/arousal, orientation to task, recognition, and memory	✓	—
Persistence with feeding that is supported/prevented by level of arousal, attention span, initiation of activity, memory, and sequencing	✓	—
Carryover of skill to future feeding tasks is supported/ prevented by level of memory, learning, and generalization	✓	—
Factors that influence the willingness or unwillingness to eat (self-image, self-esteem, caregiver, family, feeder interaction, eating history, dying)	✓	—
Oral Phase		
Behaviors or reports that indicate pain or discomfort in the oral area	✓	✓
Behaviors that interfere with the oral phase (spitting foods, pocketing foods, refusing to swallow)	✓	✓
Level of awareness/sensation in the oral–motor area	✓	—
Level of reception and perception of tactile (texture), temperature, proprioception, and gustatory qualities of food and utensils	✓	—
Factors supporting/interfering with secretion management	✓	—

Appendix A.
Entry-Level Knowledge and Skills Assessment *(cont.)*

Occupational Therapists and Occupational Therapy Assistants Will Have Entry-Level Knowledge and Skills to Assess:

	Occupational Therapist	Occupational Therapy Assistant *(Based on the Establishment of Service Competency and Supervision by an Occupational Therapist)*
Oral Phase *(continued)*		
Respiratory control factors that permit safe and efficient bolus manipulation (mouth breathers, Adult Respiratory Distress Syndrome, bronchopulmonary dysplasia), chronic obstructive pulmonary disease, cardiopulmonary compromise	✓	—
Structural or neuromotor factors (reflexes, range of motion, muscle tone, strength, endurance) that support or interfere with oral–motor function	✓	—
Level of coordinated movements (praxis) of oral structures (cheeks, lips, jaw, tongue, palate, teeth) with or without foods	✓	—
Oral structures' ability to work together to contain, form, and propel the bolus	✓	—
Bolus manipulation supported/compromised by memory, attention span, orientation, and problem solving	✓	—
Speed of the oral phase adequate to support sufficient oral intake	✓	—
Pharyngeal Phase		
Behaviors, reports, or symptoms that indicate pain or discomfort localized to the pharyngeal area	✓	—
Presence of signs and symptoms indicating possible pharyngeal dysfunction or clinical signs indicating possible aspiration (e.g., coughing, choking, tachypnea)	✓	—
Esophageal Phase		
Behaviors, reports, or symptoms that indicate pain or discomfort in the esophageal area	✓	—
Presence of refluxed material from the stomach into the esophagus, pharynx, or oral cavity	✓	—

Occupational Therapists and Occupational Therapy Assistants Will Have Entry-Level Knowledge and Skills to:

Instrumentation		
Understand formal instrumentation used by therapists or other professionals to evaluate the oral, pharyngeal, and esophageal phase of the swallow, including, but not limited to, videofluoroscopy, ultrasonography, fiberoptic endoscopy, scintigraphy, and manometry	✓	—

(continued)

Appendix A.
Entry-Level Knowledge and Skills Assessment *(cont.)*

Occupational Therapists and Occupational Therapy Assistants Will Have Entry-Level Knowledge and Skills to:

Discharge Planning *(Discharge Planning is Addressed Throughout the Intervention Process)*	**Occupational Therapist**	**Occupational Therapy Assistant** *(Based on the Establishment of Service Competency and Supervision by an Occupational Therapist)*
Collaborate with client, family, caregivers, and team members to formulate discharge needs	✓	—
Provide appropriate referrals, follow-up plans, and reevaluation related to discharge needs	✓	—
Develop and document discharge and follow-up programs and resources in accordance with discharge environment	✓	—
Provide for educational needs related to feeding, eating, and swallowing management and establishment of proficiency of recommendations with client and family	✓	—
Implement discharge and follow-up plan with client, family, caregivers, and team members to promote transition to discharge environment and integration of intervention management techniques	✓	—
Terminate intervention when client has achieved maximum benefit from services	✓	—

Entry-Level Knowledge and Skills Intervention

Occupational Therapists and Occupational Therapy Assistants Will Have Entry-Level Knowledge and Skills to:

Context	**Occupational Therapist**	**Occupational Therapy Assistant** *(Based on the Establishment of Service Competency and Supervision by an Occupational Therapist)*
Consider cultural practices in selecting foods, utensils, and mealtime setting	✓	✓
Provide environmental modifications to promote appetite and feeding/eating performance (e.g., location, timing, seating, lighting)	✓	✓
Use eating/feeding activities appropriate for developmental status/life phase	✓	✓
Facilitate social interactions that support feeding performance	✓	✓
Plan intervention within the context of person's medical condition, particularly considering specific restrictions and limitations, expected progression, and outcome	✓	—

Appendix A.
Entry-Level Knowledge and Skills Intervention *(cont.)*

Occupational Therapists and Occupational Therapy Assistants Will Have Entry-Level Knowledge and Skills to:

Pre-Oral Phase	Occupational Therapist	Occupational Therapy Assistant (Based on the Establishment of Service Competency and Supervision by an Occupational Therapist)
Facilitate olfactory stimulation	✓	✓
Provide verbal or physical cues	✓	✓
Use sensitization and desensitization techniques	✓	✓
Facilitate oral hygiene	✓	✓
Facilitate visual–perceptual activity and body schema awareness	✓	✓
Increase awareness on affected/neglected side	✓	✓
Facilitate strategies to minimize visual field deficits and enhance acuity	✓	✓
Modify environment to enhance attention	✓	✓
Help client/caregiver to develop problem-solving methods	✓	✓
Use communicative strategies to increase participation in feeding	✓	✓
Use techniques to attain and maintain optimal level of arousal	✓	✓
Provide appropriate positioning and seating equipment	✓	✓
Provide nonnutritive oral stimulation, techniques, and/or exercises	✓	✓
Facilitate upper-extremity control and hand function (dexterity, strength, coordination)	✓	✓
Facilitate oral–motor control through exercises, play, and games	✓	✓
Improve self-esteem to increase engagement in self-feeding	✓	✓
Structure mealtime habits	✓	✓
Implement nutritional recommendations	✓	✓
Manipulate feeding schedule to facilitate hunger	✓	—
Select, modify, and establish set-up of mealtime equipment	✓	—
Facilitate postural control	✓	—
Fabricate upper-extremity orthotics	✓	—
Use behavior modification	✓	—

(continued)

Appendix A.
Entry-Level Knowledge and Skills Intervention *(cont.)*

Occupational Therapists and Occupational Therapy Assistants Will Have Entry-Level Knowledge and Skills to:

	Occupational Therapist	Occupational Therapy Assistant (Based on the Establishment of Service Competency and Supervision by an Occupational Therapist)
Oral Phase		
Provide nonnutritive oral stimulation and exercises (jaw, lip, cheeks, tongue)	✓	✓
Use desensitization techniques	✓	✓
Maintain appropriate position during mealtime (facilitate stability or movement)	✓	✓
Time the introduction of food to facilitate coordinated respiration	✓	✓
Facilitate placement of food in mouth and use of utensils	✓	✓
Use verbal, written, tactile cues to initiate, maintain, and follow through (chew, swallow) with feeding/eating task	✓	✓
Provide an environmental modification program	✓	✓
Facilitate oral compensatory strategies for altered sensation, structure, or function	✓	—
Select and modify equipment for feeding	✓	—
Grade or alter qualities of bolus (e.g., texture, taste, temperature)	✓	—
Provide a behavior modification program	✓	—
Pharyngeal Phase		
Facilitate head and neck positioning for swallowing (e.g., chin tuck, head turns)	✓	—
Facilitate compensatory swallow techniques	✓	—
Esophageal Phase		
Modify position before, during, and after feeding task	✓	—
Refer to gastrointestinal service when appropriate	✓	—

Appendix B.
Advanced-Level Knowledge and Skills

Occupational Therapist	Occupational Therapy Assistant
I. *Eating function*—The occupational therapist with advanced-level knowledge and skills has built upon foundational knowledge of the eating process, thus enhancing the depth and specificity of evaluation and intervention. The occupational therapist has developed	I. *Eating function*—The occupational therapy assistant with advanced-level knowledge and skills has built upon foundational knowledge of the eating process for the purpose of providing more comprehensive intervention. The occupational therapy assistant has developed
A. Extensive knowledge of anatomy and physiology of the phases of eating for the purpose of assessing structural, neuromotor, and sensory factors that support or interfere with function and of determining intervention strategies	A. Advanced knowledge of anatomy and physiology of the phases of eating
1. Pre-oral phase	1. Pre-oral phase
2. Oral phase	2. Oral phase
3. Pharyngeal phase	3. Pharyngeal phase
4. Esophageal phase	4. Esophageal phase
B. Extensive knowledge of airway functions, including protective responses and respiratory control factors that affect swallowing and eating.	B. Advanced knowledge of airway functions, including protective responses and respiratory control factors that affect swallowing and eating.
II. *Specialized client populations and settings*—The occupational therapist with advanced-level knowledge and skills has gained extensive knowledge and experience in the feeding, eating, and swallowing needs of specific client populations or clients in specific settings. The increased depth of knowledge allows the occupational therapist to provide services to clients who are more medically fragile or whose problems/needs are more complex than those addressed by entry-level therapists. By developing expertise with specific client populations, occupational therapists with advanced-level knowledge and skills not only provide services that represent "best practice" but also contribute to the development of new and innovative approaches to evaluation and intervention for that population. Areas of expertise that may be developed include	II. *Specialized client populations and settings*—The occupational therapy assistant with advanced-level knowledge and skills has gained extensive knowledge and experience in the feeding, eating, and swallowing needs of specific client populations or clients in specific settings. The increased depth of knowledge allows the occupational therapy assistant with advanced-level knowledge and skills to provide services to clients who are more medically fragile or whose problems/needs are more complex than those addressed by the occupational therapy assistant with entry-level knowledge and skills. Areas of expertise that may be developed include
A. Specific medical diagnoses	A. Specific medical diagnoses
1. In-depth knowledge of diagnosis, including potential impact on feeding, eating, and swallowing	1. In-depth knowledge of diagnosis, including potential impact on feeding, eating, and swallowing
2. Common medications used and their interaction with the feeding, eating, and swallowing process; advising regarding oral administration of medications (e.g., crushing meds, through nasogastric tube, changing to liquid suspension)	2. Common medications used and their interaction with the feeding, eating, and swallowing process
3. Dietary needs or restrictions	3. Dietary needs or restrictions
4. Specialized equipment that may be used and can affect feeding, eating, and swallowing (e.g., tracheostomy tubes, ventilators, feeding tubes)	4. Specialized equipment that may be used and can affect feeding, eating, and swallowing (e.g., tracheostomy tubes, ventilators, feeding tubes)
B. Specialized settings such as general intensive care units and neonatal intensive care units (AOTA, 1993)	B. Specialized settings such as intensive care units (AOTA, 1993)

(continued)

Appendix B.
Advanced-Level Knowledge and Skills *(cont.)*

Occupational Therapist	Occupational Therapy Assistant
C. Specific developmental, social, or cultural factors	C. Specific developmental, social, or cultural factors
1. In-depth knowledge of age-related expectations, such as feeding processes in infants and children and the effects of aging on feeding	1. In-depth knowledge of age-related expectations, such as feeding processes in children and the effects of aging on feeding
2. Extensive knowledge of particular cultural groups and the influence of their custom on eating, particularly for persons with feeding, eating, and swallowing problems	2. Extensive knowledge of particular cultural groups and the influence of their custom on eating, particularly for persons with feeding, eating, and swallowing problems
3. Extensive knowledge of social or emotional factors that can influence feeding	3. Extensive knowledge of social or emotional factors that can influence feeding
III. *Instrumental evaluation*—The occupational therapists with advanced-level knowledge and skills may develop the following skills for instrumental evaluations relevant to their area of practice. These assessment techniques require specialized formal training and equipment. They may include, but are not limited to, videofluoroscopy, cervical auscultation, ultrasonography, fiberoptic endoscopy, scintigraphy, manometry, electromyography, and manofluorography.	III. *Instrumental evaluation*—The occupational therapy assistants with advanced-level knowledge and skills may develop the following skills for those instrumental evaluations relevant to their area of practice.
A. Knowledge and application of instrumental techniques, including purpose, indications for use, limitations, reliability, and validity	A. Knowledge of the instrumentation techniques, including purpose, indications for use, limitations, reliability, and validity
B. Ability to recommend appropriate instrumental evaluation	B. Ability to assist the occupational therapist in carrying out the assessment
C. Collaboration with other professionals in carrying out the instrumental evaluation and interpretation of data	
D. Ability to independently carry out the assessment, including interpretation of data and implementation of recommendations	
E. Ability to use results effectively in evaluation and intervention	
IV. *Specialized interventions*—Occupational therapists with advanced-level knowledge and skills have knowledge and skills of all existing intervention procedures in their specialty area and can provide the clinical judgment and rationale for selection of any procedure being used. They are aware of new interventions and potential applications from other fields. Skills may be developed in using specialized interventions that include, but are not limited to	IV. *Specialized interventions*—Occupational therapy assistants who have advanced-level knowledge and skills of specialized intervention procedures in their specialty area in order to implement intervention recommendations made by the occupational therapist. Skills may be developed in implementing specialized interventions that include, but are not limited to
A. Interventions to facilitate oral performance, improve pharyngeal swallow, and potentially reduce the risk of aspiration, if present. Use of these interventions is based on the results of instrumental evaluation of function, with safety to the client as a primary concern. Examples include	A. Interventions to improve pharyngeal swallow and esophageal function. Use of these interventions is based on results of instrumental evaluation of function by the occupational therapist. Examples Include
1. Compensatory swallowing techniques/strategies	1. Compensatory swallowing techniques
2. Thermal or tactile stimulation	2. Thermal or tactile stimulation
3. Grading or altering the bolus size/texture/changing consistency of liquids/route of administering medications orally	3. Grading or altering the bolus size/texture
4. Specialized positioning	4. Specialized positioning

Appendix B.
Advanced-Level Knowledge and Skills *(cont.)*

Occupational Therapist	Occupational Therapy Assistant

B. Enteral feeding
 	
   1. Knowledge of purpose, types, indications, limitations, and precautions
 	
   2. Ability to integrate enteral feeding systems into occupational therapy intervention plan
 	
   3. Ability to make recommendations regarding use of or need for enteral feeding systems
 	
C. Oral appliances (prosthodontics)
 	
   1. Knowledge of purpose, indications, limitations, and precautions
 	
   2. Ability to fabricate or collaborate on fabrication
 	
   3. Client training and education
 	
V. *Training and education*—Occupational therapists who have advanced-level knowledge and skills that should be disseminated to others. Through formal and informal methods, occupational therapists with advanced-level knowledge and skills should provide training and education to other occupational therapists, occupational therapy assistants, students, staff members, and professionals from related fields.
	B. Enteral feeding
	
	   1. Knowledge of purpose, types, indications, limitations, and precautions
	
	C. Oral appliances (prosthodontics)
	
	   1. Knowledge of purpose, indications, limitations, and precautions
	
	V. *Training and education*—Occupational therapy assistants with advanced-level knowledge and skills provide training and education to clients, family, and staff members, in collaboration with an occupational therapist.

Definitions—Common Terminology

Adaptive feeding equipment
Equipment used to support optimal feeding performance and to compensate for associated deficits related to coordination, strength, praxis, range of motion, or positioning.

Airway protection
Methods designed to prevent accidental loss of food, medications, or liquids into the airway while eating or drinking.

Aspiration
The entry of secretions, fluids, food, or any foreign substance below the vocal cords and into the lungs; may result in aspiration pneumonia, which may be fatal.

Bolus
The mass of food or liquid that is orally processed and swallowed.

Cervical auscultation
A method of assessing the pharyngeal swallow by listening to stereotypical sounds using the stethoscope.

Chin tuck
An intervention strategy where the head is flexed (chin tucked downward toward the chest) during the swallow allowing the anterior structures of the pharynx posteriorly resulting in a smaller entrance to the larynx; this strategy reduces the chance of food or liquid to fall into the airway.

Clearing techniques
Strategies used to clear the mouth or pharynx of food or liquid residue.

Clinical evaluation
The observation of feeding, eating, and swallowing, including client/caregiver interaction, positioning, food consistencies, method of intake, food preferences, oral structures, oral–motor patterns, tone, tactile responses, strength, fatigue, time required for mealtime activities, oral reflexes, sucking, coordination, labial, lingual, velar, facial, mandibular, dentition.

Clinical feeding, eating, and swallowing evaluation
A comprehensive evaluation, not including instrumentation, that examines the client's ability to feed, eat, and initiate the swallowing process; also referred to as "bedside dysphagia evaluation."

Cranial nerves
Nerves that provide motor and sensory innervation to the head and neck.

Diet liberalization
The relaxation of standards of accepted diets as ways to treat illness or decrease symptoms related to dsyphagia.

Double/multiple swallows
A swallow strategy whereby two or more attempts are used to swallow the food, medications, or liquid.

Dysphagia
Difficulty with any stage of swallowing (oral, pharyngeal, esophageal); dysfunction in any stage or process of eating; includes any difficulty in the passage of food, liquid, or medicine during any stage of swallowing that impairs the client's ability to swallow independently or safely.

Eating
"…the ability to keep and manipulate food or fluid in the mouth and swallow it; eating and swallowing are often used interchangeably" (AOTA, 2006a).

Eating disorders
Dysfunction in eating and nutrition related to complex biological, psychological, and sociocultural factors that may result in a life-threatening illness, such as anorexia and bulimia nervosa.

Effortful/hard swallows
A swallow strategy whereby the tongue muscles are volitionally contracted with increased effort while swallowing; results in the base of the tongue moving posteriorly during the pharyngeal swallow, which helps to clear food material from the valleculae during swallow.

Electromyography (EMG)
A procedure by which skeletal muscles are electrically stimulated and changes in electrical activity are recorded. Paralysis of the pharyngeal constrictors and vocal cords can be determined.

Enteral feeding
Feedings that use the intestinal tract for absorption of nutrients; often called gastrostomy tube feedings.

Esophageal phase
The phase of swallowing in which the bolus travels through the esophagus into the stomach.

Esophageal state function
Includes upper esophagus/cricopharyngeal function, esophageal motility.

Feeding
"…the process of setting up, arranging, and bringing food [or fluid] from the plate or cup to the mouth; sometimes called self-feeding" (AOTA, 2006a).

Feeding, eating, and swallowing history
Includes medical diagnoses, past medical history, food allergies, gastrointestinal disorders, current medications, developmental level (as appropriate), nutritional status, neurological status, respiratory status, pertinent

diagnostic studies, feeding history including progression of solids and liquids, alternate/supplemental feeding interventions, positioning, cognition, behavior, communication, eating habits/patterns, methods of feeding, dietary restrictions.

Fiberoptic endoscopic evaluation of swallowing (FEES)

Process of passing a flexible fiberoptic endoscope through the nose and positioning it to observe structures and function of the swallowing mechanism to include the nasopharynx, oropharynx, and hypopharynx. The procedure is also known as fiberoptic endoscopic examination of swallowing and videoendoscopic swallowing study.

Food and liquid consistencies

Includes thin liquids, nectar-thick liquids, honey-thick liquids, puree, chopped, soft, solid food consistencies.

Gastrostomy tube

A tube placed surgically or endoscopically into the stomach through which fluids and nutrition are provided.

Graded tactile pressure

Includes deep touch, light touch, sustained touch, pulsing touch, symmetrical touch, asymmetrical touch.

Grading/altering bolus

Manipulation of the food or liquid to change its properties related to temperature, size, or texture.

Instrumental assessment

An assessment of swallowing using radiological or imaging procedures; may include but is not limited to modified barium swallow, fiberoptic endoscopy, ultrasound, scintigraphy, electromyography, and manometry.

Jejunostomy tube

A tube placed into the jejunum of the small intestine during surgery through which enteral feedings are provided.

Manofluorography

Simultaneous videofluoroscopy and manometry by which oropharyngeal and esophageal pressure and bolus information are recorded. This procedure is also known as pharyngeal manofluorography and videomanometry.

Manometry

A procedure by which the strength, timing, and sequencing of pressure events in the esophagus are measured by a catheter with pressure transducers. Alone, it is an ineffective tool for the diagnosis of oropharyngeal dysphagia (Bastian, 1998).

Mendelsohn maneuver

A swallowing technique to facilitate prolonged laryngeal elevation during the swallow; results in keeping the upper esophageal sphincter open longer to allow passage of the bolus.

Nasogastric tube

A tube used to provide feedings directly into the stomach through a tube inserted in the nose into the stomach.

National Dysphagia Diet (NDD)

From the National Dysphagia Diet Task Force (2000) of the American Dietetic Association, these diet levels aim to establish standard terminology and practice applications of dietary texture modification in dysphagia management. Diet levels include the following:

NDD Level I: Dysphagia–Pureed (homogenous, very cohesive, pudding-like, requiring very little chewing ability)

NDD Level II: Dysphagia–Mechanical Altered (cohesive, moist, semisolid foods, requiring some chewing)

NDD Level III: Dysphagia–Advanced (soft foods that require more chewing ability)
- Regular: All foods allowed
- Proposed levels of liquid viscosity are:
  - –Thin
  - –Nectar-like
  - –Honey-like
  - –Spoon-thick

Oral phase
The phase of swallow in which the bolus of food or liquid is propelled to the pharynx by the tongue.

Oral preparatory phase
The phase of swallowing during which the bolus of food or liquid is masticated by the teeth and gums and manipulated by the lips, cheek, and tongue to create a bolus of appropriate texture for swallowing; this phase also allows for sensory appreciation of bolus qualities.

Oral reflexes
Abnormal and primitive reflexes include hyperactive gag, tonic bite, tongue thrust, jaw jerk, rooting, sucking.

Oral stage function
Includes bolus intake and containment, bolus formation, bolus transit and clearing time, velar function, behavioral components, base of tongue contact to pharyngeal wall, residue post swallow.

Orogastric tube
Used to lavage or decompress the stomach; it must be removed prior to assessment.

Penetration
The entry of secretions, fluids, food, medications, or any foreign substance into the laryngeal vestibule at or above the level of the true vocal cords.

Pharyngeal phase
The phase of swallow when the swallowing response is initiated.

Pharyngeal state function
Includes nasopharyngeal insufficiency and reflux, vallecular function, pyriform sinus function, epiglottal function, timing of swallow response, initiation of pharyngeal swallow, timing of clearance, pharyngeal competence, pharyngeal wall residue, laryngeal elevation, laryngeal penetration, or aspiration risk.

Pleasure/recreational feedings
Meals or snacks that provide enjoyment and stimulation but that are not depended on to provide nutrition.

Pocketing
Retention of food between the teeth and cheek.

Pre-oral phase
The process in which food, medication, or drink is brought to the mouth either by the person engaged in eating or by the feeder.

Presentation
Includes temperature, texture, size, placement, utensil choice, flavor, rate, method of delivery.

Prosthodontics

Prosthetic appliances used to facilitate oral and/or pharyngeal function either inside or outside of the oral cavity. May also be used for cosmesis.

Reflux

Reflux of food, medication, liquids, and gastric juice from the stomach into the esophagus; also called gastroesophageal reflux disease (GERD).

Scintigraphy

A procedure by which a radioactive bolus is monitored during and after ingestion to assess and measure bolus transit and aspiration (Bastian, 1998).

Secretion management

The ability to retain, manipulate, and swallow one's own saliva.

Self-feeding

The process of setting up, arranging, and bringing food from the plate or cup to the mouth; sometimes just referred to as feeding.

Silent aspiration

Aspiration that occurs without coughing or overt choking, indicating motor and/or sensory deficits (if present) that inhibit protective responses.

Supraglottic swallow

A swallowing technique used for airway protection where the client is told to take a breath and hold it while swallowing and then coughs after the swallow; results in the voluntary closure of the vocal folds before, during, and after the swallow.

Swallowing

A complicated act where food, fluid, medication, or saliva is moved from the mouth through the pharynx and esophagus into the stomach (AOTA, 2006a).

Therapeutic feedings

Controlled delivery of food, medication, or liquid used to facilitate therapeutic outcomes to improve feeding, eating, and swallowing ability; not used as a primary source of nutrition or hydration.

Thickening agent

Substances used to increase the viscosity of liquids.

Total parenteral nutrition

A formula providing nutrients through an intravenous tube.

Ultrasonography

The use of high frequency sound waves to provide ultrasonic images of the upper digestive tract structures and motilities, bolus transit, and vallecular stasis. It is not effective to detect penetration or aspiration (Bastian, 1998).

Upper aerodigestive tract

The combined organs and tissues of the respiratory tract and the upper part of the digestive tract (including the lips, nose, mouth, tongue, pharynx, larynx, upper trachea, and upper esophagus).

VitalStim

A Food and Drug Administration (FDA)–cleared method to promote swallowing through the application of neuromuscular electrical stimulation to the swallowing muscles to strengthen and re-educate muscles and to facilitate motor control/function of the swallowing mechanism.

References

Accreditation Council for Occupational Therapy Education. (2006). *ACOTE standards and interpretive guidelines*. Retrieved September 19, 2006, from http://www.aota.org/nonmembers/area13/docs/acotestandards806.pdf

American Occupational Therapy Association. (1993). Occupational therapy roles. *American Journal of Occupational Therapy, 47*, 1087–1099.

American Occupational Therapy Association. (2002). Occupational therapy practice framework: Domain and process. *American Journal of Occupational Therapy, 56*, 609–639.

American Occupational Therapy Association. (2004). Guidelines for supervision, roles, and responsibilities during the delivery of occupational therapy services. *American Journal of Occupational Therapy, 58*, 663–667.

American Occupational Therapy Association. (2005a). Occupational therapy code of ethics. *American Journal of Occupational Therapy, 59*, 639–642.

American Occupational Therapy Association. (2005b). Standards of practice for occupational therapy. *American Journal of Occupational Therapy, 59*, 663–665.

American Occupational Therapy Association. (2006a). *AOTA specialty certification in feeding, eating, and swallowing: 2007 candidate handbook—Occupational therapists* [PDF, available from http://www.aota.org/memservices/certappprogram/cr_login.aspx]. Bethesda, MD: Author.

American Occupational Therapy Association. (2006b). Policy 1.44: Categories of occupational therapy personnel. *American Journal of Occupational Therapy, 60*, 683–684.

Bastian, R. W. (1998). Contemporary diagnosis of the dysphagic patient. In R. L. Plant & G. L. Schectiter (Eds.), The otolaryngologic clinics of North America. *Dysphagia in Children, Adults, and Geriatrics, 31*, 489–506.

National Dysphagia Diet Task Force. (2000). *National dysphagia diet: Standardization for optimal care*. Washington, DC: American Dietetic Association.

World Health Organization. (2001). *International classification of functioning, disability, and health (ICF)*. Geneva, Switzerland: Author.

Selected Readings

Adult Eating and Dysphagia Treatment

Bastian, R. W. (1998). Contemporary diagnosis of the dysphagic patient. In R. L. Plant & G. L. Schectiter (Eds.), The otolaryngologic clinics of North America. *Dysphagia in Children, Adults, and Geriatrics, 31*, 489–506.

Groher, M. E. (1997). *Dysphagia: Diagnosis and management* (3rd ed.). Boston: Butterworth-Heinemann.

Healthy People 2010. Retrieved March 5, 2007, from http://www.cdc.gov/nchs/datawh/nchsdefs/healthypeople2010.htm

Joint Commission on Accreditation of Healthcare Organizations. (2007). Retrieved March 5, 2007, from www.jointcommission.org

---

Note: This list of selected readings is not meant to be exhaustive but to suggest current resources for library building pertinent to eating and dysphagia treatment. Key words that are helpful in accomplishing a literature review search of this topic may include *dysphagia, feeding, eating, swallowing disorders, deglutition disorders,* and *dysphagia rehabilitation*.

Langmore, S. E., & Miller, R. M. (1994). Behavioral treatment for adults with oropharyngeal dysphagia. *Archives of Physical Medicine and Rehabilitation, 75,* 1154–1159.

Logemann, J. A. (1998). *Evaluation and treatment of swallowing disorders* (2nd ed.). Austin, TX: Pro-Ed.

Logsdon, B. (2002). Cultivating competence. *Advance for Directors in Rehabilitation, 11*(10), 71–73.

Neumann, S. (1993). Swallowing therapy with neurologic clients: Results of direct and indirect therapy methods in 66 clients suffering from neurological disorders. *Dysphagia, 8,* 150–153.

Neumann, S., Bartolome, D., Buchholz, D., & Prosiegal, M. (1995). Swallowing therapy of neurologic patients: Correlation of outcome with pretreatment variables and therapeutic methods. *Dysphagia, 10,* 1–5.

Clinical Dysphagia Assessment

Avery-Smith, W., Dellarosa, D. M., & Rosen, A. B. (1992). Clinical assessment of dysphagia in adults. *Occupational Therapy Practice, 3*(2), 51–58.

Avery-Smith, W., Rosen, A. B., & Dellarosa, D. (1997). *Dysphagia evaluation protocol.* San Antonio, TX: Therapy Skill Builders.

Depippo, K. L., Holas, M. A., & Reding, M. J. (1994). The Burke Dysphagia Screening Test: Validation of its use in patients with stroke. *Archives of Physical Medicine and Rehabilitation, 75,* 1284–1286.

Fleming, S. M., & Weaver, A. W. (1986). Index of dysphagia: A tool for identifying deglutition problems. *Dysphagia, 1,* 206–208.

Hardy, E. (1995). *Bedside evaluation of dysphagia.* Bisbee, AZ: Imaginart.

Hopper, P., & Holme, S. (1999). The role of fiberoptic endoscopy in dysphagia rehabilitation. *Journal of Head Trauma Rehabilitation, 5,* 475–485.

Leopold, N. A., & Kagel, M. C. (1997). Dysphagia—Ingestion or deglutition: A proposed paradigm. *Dysphagia, 12,* 202–206.

Shanley, C., & O'Loughlin, G. (2000). Dysphagia among nursing home residents: An assessment and management protocol. *Journal of Gerontology in Nursing, 26*(8), 35–48.

Eating Disorders

Bouley, B., & Sadik, C. (1992). Inpatient treatment of eating disorders within a cognitive–behavioral framework. *Occupational Therapy Practice, 3*(2), 1–11.

Giles, G. M. (1985). Anorexia nervosa and bulimia: An activity-oriented approach. *American Journal of Occupational Therapy, 39,* 510–517.

Martin, J. E. (1998). *Eating disorders, food, and occupational therapy.* London: Whurr.

Instrumental Dysphagia Assessment

Bastian, R. (1993). The videoendoscopic swallowing study: An alternative and partner to the videofluoroscopic swallowing study. *Dysphagia, 8,* 359–367.

Broniatowski, M. (1998). Fiberoptic endoscopic evaluation of dysphagia and videofluoroscopy. *Dysphagia, 13,* 22–23.

Langmore, S. E., Schatz, K., & Olsen, N. (1988). Fiberoptic endoscopic examination of swallowing safety: A new procedure. *Dysphagia, 2,* 216–219.

Leder, S. B., Sasaki, C. T., & Burrell, M. I. (1998). Fiberoptic endoscopic evaluation of dysphagia to identify silent aspiration. *Dysphagia, 13,* 19–21.

Logemann, J. A. (1993). *Manual for the videofluoroscopic study of swallowing* (2nd ed.). Austin, TX: Pro-Ed.

Perlman, A. L. (1993). Electromyography and the study of oropharyngeal swallowing. *Dysphagia, 8,* 351–355.

Silverman, K. H. (1994). The use of scintigraphy in the management of patients with pulmonary aspiration. *Dysphagia, 9,* 107–115.

Pediatric Eating and Dysphagia Treatment

Arvedson, J. C., & Brodsky, L. (1993). *Pediatric swallowing and feeding: Assessment and management.* San Diego, CA: Singular.

Backes, L., Deitz, J., Price, R., Glass, R., & Hays, R. (1994). The effect of oral support on sucking efficiency in pre-term infants. *American Journal of Occupational Therapy, 48,* 490–498.

Carruth, B. R., & Skinner, J. D. (2002). Feeding behaviors and other motor development in healthy children (2–24 months). *Journal of the American College of Nutrition, 21*(2), 88–96.

Clark, G. (1993). Oral–motor and feeding issues. In C. Royeen (Ed.), *AOTA Self-Study Series: Classroom applications for school-based practice.* Bethesda, MD: American Occupational Therapy Association.

Glass, R. P., & Wolf, L. S. (1994). Global perspective on feeding assessment in the neonatal intensive care unit. *American Journal of Occupational Therapy, 48,* 487–489.

Mathisen, B., Worrall, L., Masel, J., Wall, C., & Shepherd, R.W. (1999). Feeding problems in infants with gastro-oesophageal reflux disease: A controlled study. *Journal of Paediatrics and Child Health, 35*(2), 163–169.

Morris, S., & Klein, M. (2000). *Pre-feeding skills* (2nd ed.). San Antonio, TX: Therapy Skill Builders.

Nelson, C. A., Meek, M. M., & Moore, J. C. (1994). *Head–neck treatment issues as a base for oral–motor function.* Albuquerque, NM: Clinician's View.

Rogers, B. (2004). Feeding method and health outcomes of children with cerebral palsy. *Journal of Pediatrics, 145*(Suppl.2).

Schwarz, S. M. (2003). Feeding disorders in children with developmental disabilities. *Infants and Young Children, 16,* 317–330.

Sullivan, P. B., & Rosenbloom, L. (1996). *Feeding the disabled child.* London: Mac Keith Press.

Tuchman, D. N., & Walter, R. S. (1994). *Disorders of feeding and swallowing in infants and children: Pathophysiology, diagnosis, and treatment.* San Diego, CA: Singular.

Waterman, E. T., Koltai, P. J., Downey, J. C., & Cacace, A. T. (1992). Swallowing disorders in a population of children with cerebral palsy. *International Journal of Pediatric Otorhinolaryngology, 24,* 63–71.

Wolf, L. S., & Glass, R. P. (1992). *Feeding and swallowing disorders in infancy: Assessment and management.* San Antonio, TX: Therapy Skill Builders.

Miscellaneous

Mody, M., & Nagai, J. (1990). A multidisciplinary approach to the development of competency standards and appropriate allocation for patients with dysphagia. *American Journal of Occupational Therapy, 44,* 369–372.

Authors

This paper was originally authored in 2000 by the Eating and Feeding Task Force: Gloria Frolek Clark, MS, OTR/L, FAOTA *(Chairperson)*; Wendy Avery-Smith, MS, OTR; Lynn S. Wold, MA, OTR; Paige Anthony, COTA; and Suzanne E. Holm, MA, OTR, BCN.

In 2005–2006, the paper was revised and updated by Gloria Frolek Clark, MS, OTR/L, FAOTA *(Coordinator)* and

The AOTASB Feeding & Swallowing Specialty Certification Panel:

Pam Roberts, MSHA, OTR/L, CPHQ, FAOTA, *Chairperson*
Marcia S. Cox, MHS, OTR/L
Suzanne E. Holm, MA, OTR, BCN
Sharon T. Kurfuerst, MEd, OTR/L
Amy K. Lynch, MS, OTR/L
Linda Miller Schuberth, MA, OTR/L

for

The Commission on Practice
Susanne Smith Roley, MS, OTR/L, FAOTA, *Chairperson*

Adopted by the Representative Assembly 2007C76

Note: This document replaces the 2000 document, *Specialized Knowledge and Skills for Eating and Feeding in Occupational Therapy Practice*. Previously published and copyrighted in 2000 by the American Occupational Therapy Association and reprinted in 2003 (*American Journal of Occupational Therapy, 57*, 660–678).

Copyright © 2007, by the American Occupational Therapy Association. Previously published in the *American Journal of Occupational Therapy, 61*, 686–700.

Specialized Knowledge and Skills of Occupational Therapy Educators of the Future

Introduction

In 2006, the American Occupational Therapy Association (AOTA) articulated a *Centennial Vision* statement for the profession as it nears its 100th anniversary. This statement affirms that

> We envision that occupational therapy is a powerful, widely recognized, science-driven, and evidence-based profession with a globally connected and diverse workforce meeting society's occupational needs. (AOTA, 2007).

This vision reflects the long-standing commitment of the profession to serve society in ways that are relevant and forward-thinking. As social concerns evolve, occupational therapy practitioners must understand the occupational implications of broad contextual issues that affect health and well-being directly and indirectly. Global effort to deal with climate change, for example, are causing downward economic pressures on middle-class living standards, thus altering daily routines, limiting occupational opportunities, increasing chronic health conditions, and reducing access to health care (Kawachi & Wamala, 2006). Occupational therapy practitioners need not only know how to respond to evolving social needs; they need to do so quickly, creatively, and proactively.

Occupational therapy education is critical to the achievement of this vision in 2017 and beyond. The constellation of skills and attitudes occupational therapy practitioners must possess are the result of their inherent abilities and motivations refined into long-standing dispositions through a deliberate educational process. Indeed, occupational therapy education embodies the aspirations for the kind of society we wish to see. To talk about the purpose of the profession is also to talk about the purpose of occupational therapy education, as it is here where these aspirations are nurtured and shaped.

Use of This Document

Occupational therapy is essentially an educative profession. Occupational therapy practitioners are skilled at analyzing limitations that may result in diminished occupational participation and designing therapeutic programs through which people learn new skills or re-learn skills lost to illness, injury, or contextual constraints. While to some degree all occupational therapy practitioners are educators, this document focuses on recognized roles related to education in the profession (Academic Program Director, Academic Faculty, Academic Fieldwork Coordinator, and Fieldwork Educator). The purpose is to articulate the attributes practitioners should possess in such roles in order to have an enduring legacy in the fulfillment of the *Centennial Vision* and beyond. These attributes are described in the language of possibility, including the characteristics of innovator/visionary, scholar/explorer, leader, integrator, and mentor. Because the embodiment of these attributes is developmental, they are described in a continuum of experience from novice, intermediate, and advanced practitioner.

The context surrounding the educator will determine which attributes are most needed and/or appropriate. While all professionals will demonstrate some aspects of the attributes, not everyone is expected to achieve the advanced level in all the attributes. Indeed, because of experience, available opportunities, and personal curiosities and strengths, an educator will likely demonstrate some attributes at the novice level while demonstrating others at the intermediate and advanced levels. Therefore, the purpose of this document is not to identify rigid standards of performance but rather to serve as a guide of desired attributes toward which an educator may aspire in order to contribute to the fulfillment of the *Centennial Vision* and beyond.

It is recommended that this document be used as an aid in the articulation of the professional development plans of faculty. Such plans are essential in their growth and are required by the Accreditation Council for Occupational Therapy Education (ACOTE) for all program directors and faculty who teach two or more courses (ACOTE, 2006, Standard A.5.2).

Desired attributes include the following:

- *Innovator/Visionary:* Someone who embraces new directions, is forward-thinking, projecting into the future. This person thinks outside of the traditional confines of the profession to predict and propose how to meet future societal needs. A visionary can see past traditional boundaries to new possibilities at all levels of personal and societal life.

- *Scholar/Explorer:* A scholar/explorer is someone who seeks, uses, and produces knowledge and effectively disseminates new findings to internal and external audiences. These individuals use a critical, theoretically grounded, and systematic approach in their scholarly endeavors to produce outcomes that inform and address societal needs.

- *Leader:* Someone who analyzes past, present, and future trends and develops solutions to problems or strategies for taking advantage of opportunities by collaborating, inspiring, and influencing people to create a desired future.

- *Integrator:* Someone who seeks and finds divergent information, perceives meaningful relationships, and makes connections through analysis to create a new, more coherent understanding.

- *Mentor:* A trusted role model who inspires, encourages, influences, challenges, and facilitates the growth and development of others' goals and aspirations. This involves a collaborative process that may be between peers, colleagues, experienced and inexperienced individuals, practitioners and academicians, and others. The mentor may function in various roles such as educator, tutor, coach, counselor, encourager, consultant, etc.

As stated earlier, the embodiment of these attributes is developmental, and not all tributes are likely to be developed at the same time nor needed equally. An educator can demonstrate an attribute at a novice level while demonstrating another at an advanced level. In this document, *novice* performance is understood as beginning expertise, as when a person has had limited experience in an area and therefore has limited familiarity with the associated knowledge or its application. *Intermediate* performance is understood as consistent demonstration of and attribute in specific situations as a result of prior experience in those situations. Finally, *advanced* performance is understood as the ability to demonstrate an attribute in multiple situations, including some in which a person has no prior experience. Advanced performance denotes a high level of expertise.

In Tables 1 & 5, each attribute is represented, summarizing how it might be demonstrated in each educator role. It is assumed that the incumbent in a role has met or exceeded occupational therapy practitioner competencies described in the *Standards for Continuing Competence* (AOTA, 2005). The attributes are general statements and specific characteristics may not apply to all situations.

References

Accreditation Council for Occupational Therapy Education. (2006). *Standards and interpretive guidelines.* Available at http://www.aota.org/Educate/Accredit/StandardsReview/guide/42369.aspx

American Occupational Therapy Association. (2005). Standards for continuing competence. *American Journal of Occupational Therapy, 59,* 661–662.

American Occupational Therapy Association. (2007). AOTA's *Centennial Vision* and executive summary. *American Journal of Occupational Therapy, 61,* 613–614.

Kawachi, I., & Wamala, S. (2006). *Globalization and health.* New York: Oxford University Press.

by

Commission on Education:

René Padilla, PhD, OTR/L, FAOTA, *Chairperson*
Andrea Bilics, PhD, OTR/L
Judith C. Blum, MS, OTR/L
Paula C. Bohr, PhD, OTR/L, FAOTA
Jennifer C. Coyne, COTA/L
Jyothi Gupta, PhD, OTR/L
Linda Musselman, PhD, OTR, FAOTA
Linda Orr, MPA, OTR/L
Abbey Sipp, *ASD Liaison*
Patricia Stutz-Tanenbaum, MS, OTR
Neil Harvison, PhD, OTR/L , *AOTA Staff Liaison*

Adopted by the Representative Assembly 2009FebCS112

Note: This document replaces the following documents: *Role Competencies for a Professional-Level Program Director in an Academic Setting, 2003M167; Role Competencies for a Program Director in an Occupational Therapy Assistant Academic Setting, 2005C239; Role Competencies for a Professional-Level Occupational Therapist Faculty Member in an Academic Setting, 2003M168; Role Competencies for a Faculty Member in an Occupational Therapy Assistant Academic Setting, 2005C240; Role Competencies for an Academic Fieldwork Coordinator, 2003M169;* and *Role Competencies for a Fieldwork Educator, 2005M284.*

Table 1.
Innovator/Visionary

Experience	Academic Program Director	OT/OTA Faculty Member	Academic Fieldwork Coordinator	Fieldwork Educator
Novice	1. Analyzes the current curriculum to reflect the future needs of the program, profession, and society. 2. Analyzes institutional needs in order to identify new ways that the program can fulfill the institution's mission. 3. Develops curriculum that challenges and prepares students to identify and fulfill innovative practice roles.	1. Demonstrates the ability to prepare ethical and competent practitioners for both traditional and emerging practice settings. 2. Develops plan to maintain self abreast of the breadth and depth of knowledge of the profession in order to incorporate such knowledge in student learning. 3. Assists with the development of new learning processes that can enhance learning opportunities for students in the program. 4. Develops a plan of continued proficiency in emerging pedagogy through investigation, and formal and informal education.	1. Embraces new approaches for fieldwork, including in non-OT practice settings, international fieldwork, diverse settings. 2. Projects an exemplary curricular model representing the OT/OTA academic program.	1. Embraces new approaches for fieldwork in traditional or emerging practice settings. 2. Implements a model fieldwork program that reflects the curricular design of the academic program. 3. Uses innovation within own fieldwork setting to enhance student learning experience during fieldwork.
Intermediate	1. Projects future trends and societal needs of the profession and appropriately adapts the curriculum, including both the academic and fieldwork components. 2. Establishes a management plan that guides student development in the OT program and facilitates faculty development within the OT unit and the college/university community.	1. Proposes and implements nontraditional learning environments that facilitate development of competent and ethical professionals. 2. Participates in college-/university-wide committees and assists in propelling the institution forward in the future in order to meet projected societal needs. 3. Embraces the use and development of course materials and experiences that are innovative and non-traditional.	1. Proposes strategies that facilitate linkages between academic program curriculum and fieldwork practice opportunities. 2. Proposes strategies to support client centered, meaningful, occupation-based, and evidence-based outcomes of the OT process during fieldwork experiences.	1. Proposes strategies that facilitate collaborative partnerships between academic program curricula and fieldwork practice opportunities. 2. Proposes strategies to support client-centered, meaningful, occupation-based, and evidence-based outcomes of the OT process during fieldwork experiences.

Table 1.

Innovator/Visionary *(cont.)*

Experience	Academic Program Director	OT/OTA Faculty Member	Academic Fieldwork Coordinator	Fieldwork Educator
Intermediate		4. Assesses and predicts the effectiveness of new learning processes to enhance learning opportunities for students in the program.		3. Promotes innovation among fieldwork educators in OT as well as other disciplines in own and other related settings to enhance student learning experiences and interdisciplinary collaboration.
Advanced	1. Anticipates future directions of the profession in meeting societal needs by exploring new possibilities for strategic planning and identifying factors related to funding, resources, etc. 2. Identifies opportunities to engage with the community to promote OT as a profession in order to serve society's evolving needs. 3. Identifies new ways of applying the use of occupation that will lead to societal growth, prosperity and social justice.	1. Proposes innovative solutions and designs innovative strategies to address predicted future trends in education, practice, and research. 2. Proposes, builds, and sustains novel integrative collaborations across disciplines.	1. Predicts future directions for fieldwork environments in emerging practice areas and propose fieldwork opportunities for students. 2. Innovates strategies for providing fieldwork in emerging practice areas 3. Anticipates and prepares for the direction of legal and health care policy that influences fieldwork and designs strategies for compliance.	1. Predicts future directions of practice and fieldwork in emerging environments and develops fieldwork opportunities for students. 2. Consults with other fieldwork educators and sites to develop creative learning experiences for students. 3. Innovates strategies for providing fieldwork in emerging practice areas. 4. Anticipates and prepares for the direction of legal and health care policy that influences fieldwork and designs strategies for compliance.

Table 2.
Scholar/Explorer

Experience	Academic Program Director	OT/OTA Faculty Member	Academic Fieldwork Coordinator	Fieldwork Educator
Novice	1. Possesses requisite knowledge and skills to design and conduct independent research relevant to OT practice and education and to disseminate results. 2. Recognizes the importance of scholarship within the academic community in general and within own educational institution in particular. 3. Designs a curriculum that meets accreditation standards relating to the scholarly role and skills of entry-level practitioners. 4. Actively engages in scholarly activities within area of expertise. 5. Creates a scholarly environment in which faculty and students have substantive resources and infrastructure necessary for productive scholarship.	1. Effectively critiques and uses new research literature and educational materials that will promote critical thinking, evidence-based practice, and lifelong learning in preparing future practitioners. 2. Critically integrates theory and research evidence into practice and facilitates that process in learners. 3. Models behaviors that demonstrate the importance of scholarship to learners and practitioners. 4. Initiates research inquiry within contextually determined expectations, either independently or with a mentor.* 5. Initiates the processes to develop a line of inquiry for research.* *May not always be possible for faculty in an OTA program.*	1. Effectively critiques and utilizes new research literature and educational materials that will promote critical thinking, evidence-based practice, and lifelong learning in preparing future practitioners. 2. Facilitates fieldwork educators' ability to effectively critique and use new research literature and educational materials that will promote critical thinking, evidence-based practice, and lifelong learning in preparing future practitioners. 3. Critically integrates theory and research evidence into practice and facilitates that process in fieldwork educators. 4. Facilitates integration and agreement of the academic philosophy and curriculum design within the fieldwork site. 5. Identifies questions about the fieldwork learning experiences for future research. 6. Facilitates best practices in using scholarship of teaching and learning in practice settings.	1. Critically evaluates current research to reflect best practice in teaching and practice. 2. Engages in systematic literature reviews to support and enhance practice. 3. Recognizes scholarly role in client service provision and program evaluation. 4. Models engagement in evidence-based practice specific to setting and populations served. 5. Seeks current evidence and information regarding effective fieldwork education and educational methodologies. 6. Translates practice knowledge into learning modes appropriate for fieldwork students. 7. Identifies questions about the fieldwork learning experiences for future research. 8. Monitors and interprets fieldwork student learning outcomes and effectiveness of student fieldwork program. 9. Coordinates with the Academic Fieldwork Coordinator to monitor and interpret student fieldwork learning outcomes.

Table 2.
Scholar/Explorer *(cont.)*

Experience	Academic Program Director	OT/OTA Faculty Member	Academic Fieldwork Coordinator	Fieldwork Educator
Intermediate	1. Coordinates active research agenda within the occupational therapy program. 2. Facilitates interdisciplinary collaboration and cooperation in research.	1. Contributes to the production of new findings and educational materials that add to the knowledge base of the profession. 2. Actively cultivates knowledge, skills, and interests in students by incorporating evidence from research into practice. 3. Conducts scholarship independently and begins to identify a coherent line(s) of inquiry.* 4. Successfully advises and guides students and practitioners in research.* 5. Disseminates findings in a public format such as presentations and publications. 6. Seeks opportunities to serve as a reviewer, editor, or publisher of scholarly work to internal and external audiences. *May not always be possible for faculty in an OTA program.*	1. Synthesizes new research literature and educational materials that will promote critical thinking, evidence-based practice, and lifelong learning in preparing future practitioners. 2. Conducts workshops and training programs to facilitate fieldwork educators' ability to use evidence in fieldwork education. 3. Plans and engages in the scholarship of teaching and learning regarding fieldwork education. 4. Collaborates with fieldwork educators and faculty to conduct research regarding fieldwork.	1. Designs evidence-based practice learning opportunities for fieldwork students to enhance understanding of the OT process. 2. Contributes to the breadth and body of knowledge through collaborative research projects. 3. Generates a clinical research agenda in collaboration with clinical and academic colleagues. 4. Collaborates with Academic Fieldwork Coordinator and faculty to conduct research regarding fieldwork.
Advanced	1. Provides national leadership in the development of and/or implementation of scholarship that further establishes foundational knowledge and efficacy of occupational therapy interventions.	1. Develops collaborative opportunities in research and scholarly work with other faculty. 2. Effectively produces and disseminates new findings within and outside of the profession.	1. Creates and disseminates new resources for fieldwork educators and Academic Fieldwork Coordinators to incorporate best practices in fieldwork education through student–fieldwork educator collaboration.	1. Models for students the importance of practitioner scholarship by engaging in independent and/or collaborative research projects and program evaluation.

(continued)

Table 2.
Scholar/Explorer *(cont.)*

Experience	Academic Program Director	OT/OTA Faculty Member	Academic Fieldwork Coordinator	Fieldwork Educator
Advanced	2. Contributes to and/or leads national dialogue concerning the advancement of OT theory and practice through research and scholarship.	3. Establishes a well-defined scholarly agenda or lines of inquiry. 4. Provides leadership in advancing the profession's knowledge base. 5. Uses innovative methodologies to identify, analyze, and effectively address the changing needs of society at the local, national, or global levels. 6. Establishes a national or international reputation or recognition as an expert in their area of inquiry.	2. Conducts research with other Academic Fieldwork Coordinator and fieldwork educators 3. Uses research evidence to inform professional educational policy.	2. Engages in multi-site research.

Table 3.
Leader

Experience	Academic Program Director	OT/OTA Faculty Member	Academic Fieldwork Coordinator	Fieldwork Educator
Novice	1. Uses management and leadership skills related to finance, planning, policy, marketing, public relations, and legal issues in order to meet accreditation standards and fulfill the program and institutional missions within an increasingly challenging educational environment. 2. Uses excellent interpersonal skills and demonstrates the ability to relate to diverse groups, constituencies, and organizations. 3. Takes responsibility for the assessment process for specific and overall program evaluation to enable the individual faculty to assess, diagnose, and apply interventions necessary to ensure quality.	1. Facilitates student development toward leadership roles. 2. Models ethical and professional behavior to facilitate the transition from student to clinician, advocate, and future fieldwork educator. 3. Assesses course materials, objectives, and educational experiences to promote optimal learning for students. 4. Develops plan of continued competency in leadership skills as related to role of teaching. 5. Participates with faculty in identifying trends that may influence future student learning and preparation.	1. Takes responsibility to develop systems to manage data for record keeping, fieldwork contract agreements, confidential student health records, and so on to ensure compliance with standards and legal requirements of local, state, and federal jurisdictions. 2. Develops a working relationship between the institution and fieldwork sites to facilitate ongoing collaborative partnerships to support education and practice. 3. Assists and monitors students in the development of their successful transition from the academic to the fieldwork portion of the educational program. 4. Evaluates the ongoing effectiveness of the fieldwork program, including student performance and fieldwork site integration of academic curricular design.	1. Critically reviews site-specific fieldwork program to ensure that quality learning experiences reflect best practice. 2. Advocates for department-wide participation in fieldwork education. 3. Facilitates student's transition into practice.
Intermediate	1. Forms strategic alliances with critical constituent groups within and outside the program's organization that can assist and promote the program's goals.	1. Seeks and obtains leadership role as representative from OTA/OT/OS department on institution-wide committees and organizations where collaboration occurs between various disciplines of study.	1. Analyzes current and future trends in OT practice to develop fieldwork settings to reflect emerging practice.	1. Modifies site-specific fieldwork objectives to ensure that high-quality learning experiences reflect best practice.

(continued)

Table 3.
Leader *(cont.)*

Experience	Academic Program Director	OT/OTA Faculty Member	Academic Fieldwork Coordinator	Fieldwork Educator
	2. Builds and maintains systems that ensure that the program operates in concert with the mission of the institution and the mission of the academic unit in which the program is housed. 3. Seeks and accepts institutional leadership roles.	2. Analyzes past, present, and future trends to integrate practice, theory, literature, and research for instruction in evidence-based practice. 3. Collaborates with other faculty members on scholarship/research activities related to the advancement of occupational therapy, occupational science, teaching, and outcomes assessment.	2. Develops or explores innovative strategies of supervision for students in emerging practice areas. 3. Collaborates with other clinical coordinators within the institution to streamline policies and procedures with regard to student placements in fieldwork.	2. Educates colleagues and develops networks and programs to ensure fieldwork excellence. 3. Participates in knowledge generation by contributing to local, regional, and/or national fieldwork discussion/dialogues. 4. Participates in national initiatives that are collaborative efforts between educational institutions and fieldwork sites (e.s. backpack awareness month).
Advanced	1. Applies the processes of advancement (philanthropy), including identifying, cultivating, and securing gifts through the matching of potential donors with well-articulated needs. 2. Seeks and accepts leadership roles within the community as well as within state, national, and international associations.	1. Proposes innovative solutions and designs innovative strategies to address predicted future trends in education, practice, and research. 2. Proposes, builds, and sustains novel integrative collaborations across disciplines.	1. Develops national and international fieldwork student exchanges, placements, and programs. 2. Provides national and global leadership in the development of fieldwork education. 3. Develops and evaluates the ongoing effectiveness and quality of national and international fieldwork education. 4. Seeks and fully embraces the leadership role in the education of regional fieldwork consortiums.	1. Develops national models for fieldwork education in collaboration with other Fieldwork Educators and Academic Feildwork Coordinators across disciplines. 2. Shares innovative models of fieldwork supervision on a state, national, and international levels. 3. Seeks leadership roles in regional, national, and international fieldwork education.

Table 4.
Integrator

Experience	Academic Program Director	OT/OTA Faculty Member	Academic Fieldwork Coordinator	Fieldwork Educator
Novice	1. Forms strategic alliances with critical constituent groups within and outside the program's organization that can assist and promote the program's goals.	1. Develops a plan to continue proficiency in teaching through investigation, continuing education, and self-investigation. 2. Meets diverse learning needs of students and faculty. 3. Creates learning environments that facilitate the development of culturally sensitive, competent, and ethical professionals. 4. Independently seeks, selectively chooses relevant resources from OT and other disciplines, and disseminates information to promote advanced understanding in a variety of areas. 5. Develops a strategic plan for professional development that combines teaching, scholarship, and service.	1. Seeks close collaboration with fieldwork educators to facilitate student fieldwork learning and align clinical fieldwork program with curriculum design/outcomes. 2. Facilitates partnerships between program faculty and fieldwork educators. 3. Supports communication, collaboration, and connections between students and fieldwork educators to support the selection, matching, and scheduling of appropriate fieldwork experiences. 4. Designs culturally sensitive fieldwork programs and fieldwork objectives. Advocates for interdisciplinary fieldwork learning opportunities. 5. Collaborates with fieldwork educators and faculty to facilitate congruence of curriculum design and best practice.	1. Seeks close collaboration with academic programs to facilitate student fieldwork learning and align clinical fieldwork program with curriculum design/outcome. 2. Develops and/or modifies clinical fieldwork manual/objectives to reflect national standards and academic fieldwork objectives. 3. Collaborates with Academic Fieldwork Coordinator to ensure integration of curriculum design into the practice setting. 4. Designs culturally sensitive fieldwork programs and fieldwork objectives. 5. Facilitates collaborative learning among fieldwork students within the profession and across disciplines.
Intermediate	1. Integrates increasingly diverse sources of information in order to define problems, explore solutions, and formulate appropriate decisions that result in effective management of the academic unit to meet its mission.	1. Develops a framework from which to practice using divergent resources. 2. Demonstrates progress of professional development plan that combines teaching, scholarship, and service.	1. Analyzes current trends to create new fieldwork opportunities. 2. Facilitates development of Academic Fieldwork Advisory Panels that integrate diverse perspectives from the community.	1. Serves on Academic Fieldwork Advisory Panels. 2. Actively facilitates interdisciplinary fieldwork learning opportunities.

(continued)

Table 4.
Integrator *(cont.)*

Experience	Academic Program Director	OT/OTA Faculty Member	Academic Fieldwork Coordinator	Fieldwork Educator
Intermediate		3. Forms strategic alliances across disciplines to advance the profession.		3. Develops and/or modifies fieldwork student manual/objectives to reflect national standards and academic fieldwork objectives. 4. Functions as a practice resource for Academic Fieldwork Coordinators to enhance fieldwork collaboration and academic outcomes. 5. Models cultural sensitivity when designing fieldwork programs and fieldwork objectives.
Advanced	1. Fosters ongoing relationships among educators, researchers, and practitioners that address the needs of both the profession and society. 2. Creatively collaborates with consumers, interdisciplinary educators, and researchers to meet the increasingly complex needs of national and global communities. 3. Effectively utilizes various venues, such as regulatory bodies, nongovernmental organizations, legislatures, and other bodies such as the World Health Organization or the Centers for Disease Control and Prevention in order to promote the health and well-being of people through occupation.	1. Collaborates with diverse disciplines for information synthesis and dissemination. 2. Articulates and represents the role of OT in emerging areas of practice at the local, national, and international levels. 3. Creatively collaborates with consumers, interdisciplinary educators, and researchers to meet the increasingly complex needs of national and global communities. 4. Effectively uses various venues, such as regulatory bodies, nongovernmental organizations, legislatures, and other internationally recognized agencies in order to promote the health and well-being through occupation.	1. Bridges the gap between OT/OTA practitioner needs (evidence-based practice) and resources available through OT/OTA academic program and student fieldwork experiences. 2. Enhances relationships with regional/national/international fieldwork committees. 3. Creatively contributes to a national/ international understanding of the importance of fieldwork education by facilitating meaningful relationships and networking among practitioners, students, and educators.	1. Contributes to a more coherent understanding of health care service provision and a national fieldwork student network. 2. Develops/contributes to interdisciplinary experimental learning modules. 3. Serves on regional/national/international fieldwork committees. 4. Creatively contributes to a national and international understanding of the importance of fieldwork education by facilitating meaningful relationships and networking among practitioners, students, and educators.

Table 5.
Mentor

Experience	Academic Program Director	OT/OTA Faculty Member	Academic Fieldwork Coordinator	Fieldwork Educator
Novice	1. Serves as a model to mentor diverse faculty, students, alumni, and occupational therapy practitioners in their area of expertise. 2. Facilitates mentoring relationships within the academic institution. 3. Models professional and ethical behavior within the academic setting. 4. Instills in students the professional responsibility of seeking and offering mentoring relationships. 5. Analyzes personal and professional goals and acquires resources necessary to attain professional growth.	1. Demonstrates a competent and positive attitude that results in the mentoring of students in professional development in scholarship, research, and/or service. 2. Develops and fosters trusting relationships with practitioners interested in transitioning from practice into academia. 3. Identifies a variety of tangible and intangible resources that can enhance the professional growth of self and others. 4. Analyzes personal and professional goals and acquires resources necessary to attain professional growth. 5. Encourages potential students to develop relationships with OT/OTA practitioners, alumni, students, and faculty prior to entering the profession. 6. Facilitates the inclusion of a diverse community of faculty and students through the mentoring process.	1. Coaches and guides students to engage in appropriate professional and fieldwork education activities. 2. Creates a collaborative process between academic faculty and fieldwork educators. 3. Serves as a model and consultant for fieldwork educators to facilitate development of quality fieldwork programs. 4. Facilitates the growth of practitioners and fieldwork educators for implementing best practice principles during fieldwork education. 5. Analyzes personal and professional goals and acquires resources necessary to attain professional growth. 6. Encourages potential students to develop relationships with occupational therapy practitioners, students, alumni, and faculty prior to entering the profession. 7. Facilitates the inclusion of a diverse community of faculty and students through the mentoring process. 8. Serves as a model representative of the academic program locally and regionally.	1. Mentors students prior to and during fieldwork by functioning as a model. 2. Serves as a model to mentor diverse individuals and occupational therapy practitioners in their area of expertise. 3. Encourages potential students to develop relationships with occupational therapy practitioners, students, and faculty prior to entering the profession. 4. Analyzes personal and professional goals and acquires resources necessary to attain professional growth.

(continued)

Table 5.
Mentor (cont.)

Experience	Academic Program Director	OT/OTA Faculty Member	Academic Fieldwork Coordinator	Fieldwork Educator
Intermediate	1. Develops innovative strategies for negotiating creative, constructive, and ethical solutions to address interpersonal and academic issues within a complex environment. 2. Develops resources, policies and procedures/guidelines for faculty that can be used to facilitate progressively higher levels of responsibility at the department, university, community, and professional levels. 3. Uses a variety of methods and technology to expand mentoring relationships beyond the academic institution and the community it serves.	1. Identifies individuals or groups in need of mentoring who would otherwise not seek mentorship and encourages them to develop mentoring relationships to maximize their potential. 2. Participates in mentoring or coaching of junior faculty through constructive feedback and role modeling of work with students, practitioners, and peers. 3. Effectively mentors and functions as faculty advisor for student organizations. 4. Inspires others to serve as mentor to students, alumni, practitioners, and faculty. 5. Actively contributes to the accomplishment of long-term expectations and outcomes of mentor relationships necessary for own personal and professional growth. 6. Uses a variety of methods and technology to expand mentoring relationships beyond the academic institution and the community it serves.	1. Collaborates with fieldwork educators to promote effective and innovative learning opportunities for students. 2. Tutors and coaches non-OT fieldwork educators in their development as supervisors and their implementation of fieldwork experiences reflecting OT practice. 3. Models and facilitates development of innovative strategies to obtain excellence within the constraints of the fieldwork practice environment. 4. Coaches students, fieldwork educators, and Academic Fieldwork Coordinators to negotiate and problem solve challenging fieldwork dilemmas. 5. Creates effective resources reflecting current trends and emerging practice areas to sustain excellence in fieldwork education. 6. Influences the development of innovative programs to bridge the gap between fieldwork and didactic content into a cohesive curriculum design. 7. Uses a variety of methods and technology to expand mentoring relationships beyond existing fieldwork education network.	1. Identifies a variety of tangible and intangible resources that can be used to enhance the professional growth of self and others. 2. Recruits and guides inexperienced OT/OTA staff to develop in the role as a fieldwork educator. 3. Models excellence as a fieldwork educator and fieldwork site coordinator. 4. Models excellence and commitment to the tenets of the profession using occupational-based and evidence-based practice during the OT process. 5. Develops mentorship programs within the facility that reflect and promote interdisciplinary and intradisciplinary fieldwork excellence. 6. Uses a variety of methods and technology to expand mentoring relationships beyond the fieldwork site. 7. Develops innovative strategies for negotiating creative, constructive, and ethical solutions to address interpersonal and practice issues within a complex environment. 8. Serves as role model for other fieldwork educators.

Table 5.
Mentor *(cont.)*

Experience	Academic Program Director	OT/OTA Faculty Member	Academic Fieldwork Coordinator	Fieldwork Educator
Advanced	1. Anticipates and facilitates the development of future mentoring relationships within and outside the educational program to meet the needs of the profession and society. 2. Facilitates intra- and interdisciplinary mentoring relationships for faculty, students, alumni, and practitioners. 3. Models advocacy and acts as a change agent to fulfill the occupational and social justice vision of the profession both nationally and globally. 4. Identifies and addresses professional and societal trends that may present new ethical challenges for the profession and society. 5. Inspires others to develop new strategies and paradigms in response to societal issues.	1. Creates and shares networks, resources, and opportunities for growth of mentees at the national and international levels. 2. Develops and sustains programs across disciplines and geographical regions to foster mentees' successful performance in scholarship, teaching, and practice. 3. Models advocacy and acts as a change agent to fulfill the occupational and social justice vision of the profession both nationally and globally. 4. Develops innovative strategies for facilitating connections among students, educators, alumni, practitioners, and other colleagues for unusual, challenging, and/ or complex mentee needs or situations. 5. Anticipates and develops mentoring opportunities and programs designed to address disparities in health care, social injustices, issues within the profession, and society. 6. Develops innovative strategies for negotiating creative, constructive, and ethical solutions to address interpersonal and academic issues within a complex environment.	1. Models the creation of innovative fieldwork training programs globally to anticipate and meet the needs of the profession in the future. 2. Facilitates national and international networks among academic fieldwork coordinators to collectively and systematically address fieldwork issues. 3. Develops innovative strategies for negotiating creative, constructive, and ethical solutions that address interpersonal and academic issues within a complex environment. 4. Develops and sustains programs across disciplines and geographical regions to foster mentees' successful performance in scholarship, teaching, and practice. 5. Anticipates and develops mentoring opportunities and programs designed to address disparities in health care, social injustices, issues within the profession, and society. 6. Models advocacy and acts as a change agent to fulfill the occupational and social justice vision of the profession both nationally and globally.	1. Consults on the development of new fieldwork programs, supporting at other fieldwork sites, settings, and practice areas. 2. Develops national and international programs of mentorship excellence that connect students, practitioners, fieldwork educators, and academic fieldwork coordinators. 3. Anticipates and develops mentoring opportunities and programs designed to address disparities in health care, social injustices, issues within the profession, and society. 4. Models advocacy and act as a change agent to fulfill the occupational and social justice vision of the profession both nationally and globally.

Specialized Knowledge and Skills for Occupational Therapy Practice in the Neonatal Intensive Care Unit

Purpose

The purpose of this paper is to provide a reference for occupational therapists on the advanced knowledge and skills necessary to practice in a neonatal intensive care unit (NICU). Occupational therapy practice with infants in the NICU and their families is high risk and specialized, only appropriate for occupational therapists with advanced knowledge and skills in neonatal care.

Introduction

Occupational therapy philosophy and education provide the foundation for this profession to make a valuable contribution to neonatal practice (American Occupational Therapy Association [AOTA], 2004b). Specialized knowledge of neonatal medical conditions and developmental variability and abnormality in infants cared for in the NICU is essential to safe, effective practice. The therapist must recognize the complex medical needs and vulnerabilities of acutely ill or premature infants. These infants frequently are physiologically fragile and easily compromised by environmental conditions. Interactions and therapeutic interventions that may appear innocuous can trigger physiologic instability in an infant and can be life threatening. In fact, protecting the fragile neonate from excessive or inappropriate sensory aspects of the environment is often a more urgent priority than direct interventions or interactions with the infant. Occupational therapy approaches, such as sensory integration and neurodevelopmental intervention, are applicable within the NICU setting. However, these approaches may need to be modified according to the infant's medical status, physiological homeostasis, and developmental and family needs.

The special needs of families whose infants are in the NICU also must be recognized. The infant's medical status and uncertain outcome, the highly technical environment of the NICU, separation from parents, and potential maternal complications after labor and delivery may contribute to family stress or crisis. These situations often alter the parent–infant attachment process, which is essential to optimal infant developmental outcomes. Families are best served by an occupational therapist who is not only knowledgeable about infant needs, but also sensitive to family circumstances, priorities, concerns, and cultural beliefs. The occupational therapist must seek ways to establish supportive, collaborative, and therapeutic relationships with family members in order to foster the infant's optimal development.

The social and physical aspects of the environment can be stressful to both the infant and the family. All persons who interact with the infant constitute the social environment. The physical environment is composed of inanimate elements and properties (e.g., lighting, sound, bedding, equipment). The occupational therapist must understand the interplay of the social and physical features of the NICU and the way in which this interplay influences the infant, family, and staff members. This knowledge is used as a basis for the occupational therapy evaluation and contributes to effective intervention strategies.

Working within the social and physical bounds of the NICU environment, an important role of the occupational therapist is to assist each family to foster optimal infant development, including the encouragement of developmentally appropriate occupations, sensorimotor processes, and neurobehavioral organization. This must occur while considering the often fragile medical and physiological status of the infant. Through direct observation, intervention, consultation, education, and research, the occupational therapist collaborates with others to provide the infant with the most effective and appropriate social and physical environment.

The occupational therapist working in the NICU must have a basic knowledge of occupational therapy, pediatric experience, and specialized knowledge and skills related to the complex needs of high-risk infants, their families, and the NICU environment. Basic occupational therapy education includes knowledge of biological sciences, disease processes, mental health, and typical and atypical child and adult family development. Occupational therapy's domain of concern, encompassing the interaction among the biological, developmental, and social–emotional aspects of human function as expressed in daily activities and occupations, makes it particularly suited to address the needs of the developing infant and family (AOTA, 2002). The occupational therapy method of activity analysis and adaptation to achieve a functional outcome is valuable in promoting "goodness of fit" (i.e., the match between the infant's capabilities and the physical and social environment), as there is often a mismatch between the NICU environment, parental expectations, and the infant's capabilities.

Experience in pediatric occupational therapy is essential for practice in the NICU. This experience provides a perspective on the continuum of typical and atypical child development and on the significance of the family in the child's life. Experience in pediatric occupational therapy affords the practitioner opportunities for development of the critical thinking skills necessary for evaluation and intervention to promote competent occupational performance and emotional well-being of children and their families. Therefore, the therapist interested in practicing in the NICU should have experience in the following areas: pediatric occupational therapy with infants and young children, longitudinal follow-up of infants treated in the NICU, and collaboration with families.

In addition to basic occupational therapy education and pediatric experience, the occupational therapist working in the NICU requires advanced knowledge and skills to provide complex interventions to critically ill neonates and their families. These interventions require continuous evaluation and a dynamic approach to intervention planning. They also require knowledge of grief reactions, social structures, attachment, medical procedures, and other issues relating to the health and well-being of the family unit. Intervention in the NICU context is not a recommended area of practice for occupational therapy assistants because such knowledge and skills are beyond the scope of their practice. Since practice in the NICU requires advanced-level expertise and clinical reasoning, this area of practice also is not recommended for entry-level occupational therapists or occupational therapists who do not have the pediatric experience described above. Extensive continuing education; mentoring by an occupational therapist experienced in neonatal care; and graded, closely supervised, mentored practice are recommended for any occupational therapist entering neonatal practice. Supervision often is required until the therapist demonstrates competency in working with infants and their families in the NICU environment (AOTA, 2004a).

The specialized knowledge required for practice in the NICU includes familiarity with relevant medical conditions, procedures, and equipment; an understanding of the individualized developmental abilities and vulnerabilities of infants; an understanding of theories of neonatal neurobehavioral organization; working knowledge of family systems, early social–emotional development, infant mental health, and NICU ecology; and an understanding of multidisciplinary team collaboration. Most importantly, the NICU therapist must have a clear understanding of the manner in which these factors interact to influence behavior. The occupational therapist develops the necessary skills through continuing education and supervised mentored clinical experience in evaluation and intervention specific to the NICU. Neonatal practice requires advanced clinical reasoning skills. These skills include the flexibility to recognize and respond to unfamiliar situations and nuances of behavior, the ability to anticipate future directions of intervention, and the ability to perceive the clinical condition as a whole. The occupational therapist in the NICU applies these competencies with regard to the infant; the infant's family and caregivers; and the NICU environment, including staff. Specifically, the occupational therapist in the NICU designs an individualized intervention plan in collaboration with the family and others that incorporates the family's priorities and NICU contexts along with the individualized needs of the infant. This requires understanding the occupations and activities valued by families and the NICU culture; defining what factors limit each infant's participation or engagement in those occupations and activities; identifying factors that would constitute readiness for engagement in occupations and activities; and finally, delineating what physical and/or social environmental supports will maximize participation for both the infant and the family in the short term and in the long term.

Maintenance of clinical competency and an evidence-based approach to practice are both vitally important in the rapidly changing field of neonatology. Clinical competence can be sustained through regular supervision or a mentoring relationship, participation in peer study groups, reflective process, and formal and informal continuing education. An evidence-based approach to practice necessitates ongoing critical review of the relevant research, literature, and clinical tools available in this rapidly changing field of practice. An occupational therapy practitioner is knowledgeable about evidence-based research and applies it ethically and appropriately to the occupational therapy process (AOTA, 2005b).

Knowledge and Skills: The Infant, Family, and NICU Environment

The following information identifies the knowledge and skills needed to function as an occupational therapist in the NICU. This information is organized under the three main areas of occupational therapy concern described previously: the infant, the family, and the NICU environment.

The Infant

To be competent, the occupational therapist has to have an in-depth understanding of approaches to evaluation and intervention, including use of a developmentally supportive consultative model of service delivery. These approaches are presented in the literature specific to occupational therapy, neonatology, psychology, and infant and family studies. In addition, the therapist has to have a thorough understanding of medical factors and the potential risks they pose to normal fetal and infant growth and development. The therapist must understand and critically analyze this information within the context of occupational therapy practice and the specific philosophy of the NICU in which the occupational therapist works. The therapist develops an evaluation plan that includes use of appropriate standardized tools, parent or caregiver interviews, and observations of infant adaptation to the social and physical environments. The occupational therapist, in conjunction with the family and medical caregivers, then develops appropriate intervention strategies, individually suited to each infant and family.

For clarity in this paper, infant behavior is discussed separately from family and environmental concerns. However, in program implementation, the infant is assessed and treated within the context of the family and the NICU environment.

The following is a comprehensive outline of the essential knowledge base that an occupational therapist must possess for working with NICU infants.

I. Medical knowledge base as the foundation for understanding infant behavior

    A. General information

        1. Medical terminology and abbreviations used in the NICU

        2. Basic principles, uses, and potential complications of the medical equipment and procedures, including precautions and implications for the therapist and infant

        3. Medical complications frequently encountered, including pathophysiology, risks, precautions, and prognoses associated with specific conditions.

B. Specific knowledge

   1. NICU equipment

   2. Diagnostic procedures

   3. Medical procedures

   4. Nursing procedures and routines

   5. Respiratory support

   6. Thermoregulatory support

   7. Nutritional support

   8. Medication effects

   9. Infection control

   10. Institution-specific policies and procedures.

II. Factors that may influence infant and child development

A. Prenatal

   1. Maternal and fetal complications during pregnancy

   2. Genetic disorders, congenital anomalies, syndromes, isolated defects

   3. Teratogens (e.g., licit and illicit drug exposure, radiation, environmental contaminates)

   4. Infectious diseases (e.g., rubella, cytomegalovirus, herpes, toxoplasmosis, HIV)

   5. Social risk factors (e.g., poverty, inadequate support, stress, environmental toxins).

B. Perinatal

   1. Maternal complications during delivery

   2. Neonatal complications during delivery

   3. Gestational age and birth weight.

C. Postnatal conditions and complications

   1. Respiratory

   2. Cardiovascular

   3. Neurologic

   4. Sensory

   5. Orthopedic

   6. Gastrointestinal

   7. Metabolic

   8. Hemolytic

   9. Dermatologic

   10. Infectious disease

   11. Iatrogenic complications.

III. Knowledge of the developmental course, abilities, and vulnerabilities of infants in the NICU

    A. Differences in body structure and body functions, developmental progression, variations, deviations, and abnormalities in infants in relation to preterm, term, or postterm birth and/or prenatal, perinatal, or postnatal factors

        1. Infant neurobehavioral organization

            a. Physiologic (e.g., cardiorespiratory)

            b. States of arousal

            c. Regulatory abilities
               Sleep and waking states
               Circadian rhythms
               Typical and atypical patterns
               Self-regulation
               External regulation
               Medication effects/side effects

            d. Neurosocial (e.g., attention, interaction).

        2. Sensory development and processing of sensory information

            a. Sequential developmental progression in utero and adaptations to the extra-uterine environment

            b. Thresholds for stimulation within the sensory systems: tactile, vestibular, proprioceptive, visual, auditory, olfactory, gustatory

            c. Responses: arousal, attention, modulation, transition, range, decompensation

            d. Sensory acuity.

        3. Motor function

            a. Neuromotor development, including, but not limited to, muscle tone, posture, quality of movement, reflexes and reactions, and motor control

            b. Biomechanical factors, including, but not limited to, active and passive range of motion, strength, and orthopedic status.

        4. Social–emotional development

            a. Early communicative cues

            b. Self-regulation of interaction

            c. Initial formation of attachment relationships

            d. Temperament.

    B. Emerging competencies in infant occupation

        1. General factors that influence participation in daily life activities

            a. Postconceptional age and weight

            b. Physical and developmental maturation

            c. Physiological status and medical conditions

            d. Neurobehavioral organization

    e. Sensory processing

    f. Biomechanical and neuromotor function

    g. Social interaction

    h. Physical environment

    i. Social environment.

2. Specific activities

    a. Ability to cope with and participate in caregiving

       (1) Feeding process

          (a) Modes (e.g., breast, bottle, tube)

          (b) Function (e.g., ability to meet nutritional needs, physiologic cost, endurance)

          (c) Oral–motor mechanism (e.g., structure, function, quality)

          (d) Maturation of mechanical and neural control of sucking, swallowing, and breathing

          (e) Relationship among nutritive and non-nutritive sucking, respiration, and oxygenation

          (f) Positioning and handling

          (g) Feeding readiness cues

          (h) Physiologic issues, such as metabolic and neurologic

          (i) Competency of the infant as a partner

          (j) Relationship with primary caregivers

          (k) Tolerance of oral–facial and intraoral sensations.

       (2) Bathing

       (3) Dressing and diapering

       (4) Medical routines and procedures.

    b. Engaging in nurturing interactions

       (1) Skin-to-skin holding (kangaroo care)

       (2) Physical and social dialogue

       (3) Feeding.

    c. Interrelationship between medical and developmental domains

       (1) Present conditions

       (2) Future implications.

IV. Knowledge of evolving developmental approaches in the NICU

  A. Historical and current perspectives

    1. Supplemental stimulation

    2. Reduced stimulation

    3. Environmental neonatology

4. Individualized developmental care

5. Family-centered care

6. Relationship-based approach.

B. Modification and integration of current pediatric occupational therapy frames of reference (e.g., sensory integration, neurodevelopmental therapy, coping, dynamic systems).

V. Specific skills related to occupational therapy with infants in the NICU, including the ability to

A. Instruct, consult, and communicate with caregivers

B. Use NICU equipment appropriately and safely, including understanding of the purpose, basic operation, settings, and precautions of all relevant equipment

C. Conduct appropriate assessments

1. Determine appropriate timing of infant assessments on the basis of the infant's medical and physiological status, postconceptional age, and NICU and family routines

2. Select and administer formal and informal assessment procedures that are appropriate for postconceptional age and medical condition and that identify developmental abilities, vulnerabilities, and limitations in daily life activities and occupations as they are influenced by medical status and

   a. Neurobehavioral organization

   b. Sensory development and processing

   c. Motor function

   d. Pain

   e. Daily activity (e.g., feeding)

   f. Social–emotional development.

3. Assess the effects of physical environment, caregiving practices, positioning, and nurturance on the infant's neurobehavioral organization, sensory, motor, and medical status.

D. Formulate an individualized therapeutic intervention plan that supports the infant's current level of function and facilitates optimal social–emotional, physical, cognitive, and sensory development of the infant within the context of the family and the NICU

1. Determine appropriate timing of infant interventions on the basis of the infant's medical and physiological status, postconceptional age, and NICU and family bedside routines

2. Modify sensory aspects of physical environment according to infant sensory threshold

3. Participate with the infant and caregivers in occupational therapy interventions that reinforce the role of the family as the constant in the life of the infant and support the individual infant's medical and physiological status in order to

   a. Enhance infant neurobehavioral organization

   b. Facilitate social participation

   c. Promote optimal infant neuromotor functioning and engagement in daily life activities

   d. Promote developmentally appropriate motor function and engagement in daily life activities through the use of biomechanical techniques, when appropriate

   e. Facilitate well-organized infant behavior through adaptation of infant daily life activities.

E. Continuously observe and critically analyze subtle infant responses to the intervention program and modify as needed

F. Collaborate with family, NICU staff, and other persons who potentially may have an impact on infant well-being to

1. Create and maintain individualized developmental care plans

2. Incorporate the occupational therapy program into NICU routines

3. Modify intervention and discharge plans considering anticipated infant outcome.

G. Provide documentation that is objective, interpretive, thorough, and concise

H. Formulate discharge and follow-up plans in coordination with the interdisciplinary team and community resources to meet the developmental needs of the infant and family.

The Family

Parents and other family members are acknowledged to be the most important and consistent influence in the infant's life. Their occupational roles as primary caregivers and nurturers constantly need to be recognized and reaffirmed. Typically, parents are mediators of the infant's affective, sensory, and motor experiences. When an infant is hospitalized in the NICU immediately after birth, parents are not always able to play this mediation role. The bi-directional attachment process, which begins at delivery and in which both infant and parent play a part, can be disrupted. Since attachment provides a foundation for the infant's future development and independent function, its promotion is an important consideration for the occupational therapist. Therefore, the occupational therapist collaborates with family members, on-site and off-site, to facilitate the infant's optimal development, promote the parents' occupational roles, support parent–infant attachment, and ensure a successful transition from hospital to home and community.

The following outline summarizes the knowledge base that would enable an occupational therapist to provide services in the NICU from a family-centered perspective.

I. Knowledge of the family as a basis for collaboration

A. Family systems

1. Family structure, occupational roles, cultural identification, beliefs, values, and practices

2. Family resources: Sources and allocation (e.g., time, money, energy, social–emotional support)

3. Family adaptation: Adjustment to adding a new family member, adjustment to stressful situations

4. Needs, culture, and roles of family members, including siblings.

B. Adult learning styles

1. Individual differences in learning

2. Relationship between emotional state and learning capacities

3. Changes in parental focus during NICU course.

C. Parent–infant interactions: progression and individual differences

1. Parents' role in the infant's early social–emotional development

2. Attachment as an ongoing two-way process between parents and infant, including the importance of attachment to later developmental function and the influence of hospitalization on parents and infants on the attachment process

3. Development of synchronous interactions

4. Importance of parents' learning to accurately observe, interpret, and respond to their infant's unique cues.

D. The transition of the infant from hospital to home and community

1. Possible stresses and difficulties inherent in the transition process for the infant and each family member

2. Knowledge of community resources and local, state, and federal guidelines and services.

II. Specific skills related to occupational therapy with families of infants in the NICU. The occupational therapist

A. Identifies family hopes, dreams, expectations, attitudes, knowledge, strengths, priorities, preferred communication styles, and skills regarding daily care, play, and other interactions with the infant

B. Identifies family members' learning styles

C. Assists parents in feeling comfortable with their infant and as parents to a new family member

D. Guides family members in observing and interpreting their infant's behavior and in adapting their own behaviors in response to the infant's cues to elicit appropriate sensory, motor, and social responses

1. During daily life activities

2. During interactions involving exploration, attention, and orientation

3. While engaged in nurturing interactions.

E. Recognizes and acknowledges the infant's contribution and strengths in others' lives

F. Fosters successful parent–infant interactions via mutual problem solving, anticipatory guidance, modeling of behaviors, didactic and experiential education, and modification of the infant's environment

G. Integrates family observations and priorities in formulating occupational therapy intervention recommendations

H. Interprets and discusses occupational therapy evaluation findings in collaboration with the family

I. Adapts intervention approaches according to family culture, changing emotions, needs, and resources that may be influenced by the infant's changing medical status or other circumstances

J. Formulates and implements a discharge and follow-up plan with the family and other team members to ensure a smooth transition to the community, integrating occupational therapy goals into the overall goals and priorities of the family.

The NICU Environment

The neonate who is born prematurely or acutely ill is not well-adapted to the stressful and technologically complex environment of the NICU. This mismatch between the infant and the environment may have a deleterious effect on the infant's medical and developmental outcomes. Therefore, a primary intervention goal in the NICU is to provide the best match or fit between the infant and the NICU environment. Adapting or structuring the environment to enhance function is a well-accepted occupational therapy approach. However, this first requires knowledge of the various components of the environment as well as their interplay. The occupational therapist assesses the environment and collaborates with others to shape the infant's physical and social environment to provide a milieu of developmentally supportive care. The following competencies are essential:

I. Knowledge of the unique sensory properties of the NICU and their relationship to each infant's neurobehavioral organization

   A. *Tactile:* Timing, intensity, texture, handling for medical and nursing procedures, parent interaction

   B. *Proprioceptive–vestibular:* Timing, intensity, handling for medical and nursing procedures, parent interaction

   C. *Olfactory and gustatory experiences specific to the NICU* (timing, quality, intensity)

   D. *Auditory:* Intensity, duration, timing, animate versus inanimate

   E. *Visual:* Timing, ambient and focal light intensity, contents of visual field.

II. Knowledge of the social environment and its relationship to each infant's neurobehavioral organization, including interactions and relationships among

   A. Parents and infant

   B. Extended family members and infant

   C. Staff members and infant

   D. Parents and staff members

   E. Occupational therapist, parents, staff, and infant.

III. Knowledge of the physical environment and its relationship to each infant's maturation and behavioral organization

   A. Medical equipment and procedures as described under the medical knowledge base section

   B. Frequency, timing, duration, quality, and intensity of sensory input from medical equipment and procedures

   C. Sensory input from equipment, procedures, and staff activities that is disruptive to the infant's neurobehavioral organization.

IV. Knowledge of the NICU culture

   A. The NICU's specific philosophy of care, including its particular orientation toward acute and chronic care of infants

   B. The team members' roles, functions, attitudes, and positions in the organizational structure of the individual NICU

   C. The influence of NICU stressors (e.g., census changes and subsequent staffing patterns)

   D. Communication patterns and structure, both formal and informal, among staff members and between family and staff members

   E. Spoken and unspoken rules of behavior

   F. The effect of the physical and social environments on staff performance and morale

   G. Hospital administrative policies (e.g., confidentiality).

V. Specific skills related to occupational therapy in assessing and adapting the environment. The occupational therapist

   A. Assesses the sensory aspects of the NICU physical and social environments and its effect on infant well-being

B. Develops intervention strategies in collaboration with the family, NICU staff, and other team members to adapt the environment in order to foster optimal infant development and family interactions

   1. Communicates with all levels of staff to establish rapport and develop team commitment to developmental and family goals

   2. Integrates occupational therapy goals into the infant's medical priorities and the NICU setting.

C. Develops and implements strategies to influence philosophy and practice of developmental and family-centered care within the NICU

D. Assesses the effect of intervention strategies and revises the plan accordingly.

VI. Knowledge of structures that support occupational therapy practice in the NICU

The occupational therapist position exists within the NICU structure. The following knowledge and skills are needed to ensure integration of occupational therapy services into the NICU setting for optimal infant-family outcomes:

A. Ability to articulate the role and function of occupational therapists in the NICU to demonstrate their value and effectiveness

B. Ability to use relevant research literature to support occupational therapy practice in the NICU

C. Knowledge of the hospital's structure, mission, strategic plan, and fiscal priorities as they relate to both NICU and occupational therapy programs

D. Ability to identify and access sources of administrative and fiscal support to maintain occupational therapy services in the NICU

E. Knowledge of the larger local, state, and national health and social service systems as they influence policy and fiscal support for occupational therapy services in the NICU and early intervention services

F. Ability to identify sources of administrative and fiscal support for the practice of occupational therapy within the NICU from the community and the health care system at large

G. Knowledge of confidentiality guidelines (e.g., HIPAA).

Professional and Personal Characteristics Necessary for Occupational Therapists Practicing in the NICU

The NICU, as a critical care area, necessitates certain professional and personal characteristics. These characteristics include the following:

1. Ability to synthesize information from multiple sources, including research findings, and judiciously apply it to the NICU

2. Ability to observe the infant and environment for prolonged periods, without intervening, and to identify and understand subtle nuances of behavior and physiology

3. Interest in and ability to bring about changes in the infant's social and physical environments through direct intervention with the infant and family, consultation and collaboration with other team members, and implementation of policies and procedures at the organizational level

4. Understanding of one's interpersonal communication skills and style and the ability to modify them in response to family and staff behavior, learning styles, and needs

5. Commitment to seek ongoing knowledge, education, and peer consultation in this field

6. Ability to provide formal and informal educational programs for the hospital and the community

7. Insight into one's professional knowledge and skills

8. Ability to value, communicate, and collaborate with other NICU team members, community-based early intervention programs, and other resources

9. Understanding of and ability to articulate one's values and attitudes about

   a. The rights and responsibilities of families

   b. Relationships between cultural or religious beliefs and medical management decisions

   c. Working with infants who ultimately may not survive

   d. Working with infants who may have severe and permanent disabilities

   e. Working with families whose values, attitudes, behaviors, and life circumstances differ from one's own

   f. Allocating limited fiscal, personnel, and technological resources to sustain life.

10. Understanding of the *AOTA Code of Ethics* (2005a) as it applies to the NICU.

Definitions

Activity
"[T]he performance of a task or action by an individual" (World Health Organization [WHO], 2001, p. 10).

Activity Limitations
"[D]ifficulties an individual may have in executing activities" (WHO, 2001, p. 10).

Attachment
"A bond between an infant and a caregiver, usually its mother. Attachment is generally formed within the context of a family, providing the child with the necessary feelings of safety and nurturing at a time when the infant is growing and developing. This relationship between the infant and his caregiver serves as a model for all future relationships" (Gale, 2005).

Body Functions
"[T]he physiological or psychological functions of body systems" (including psychological functions; WHO, 2001, p. 10).

Body Structures
"[A]natomical parts of the body, such as organs, limbs, and their components" (WHO, 2001, p. 10).

Bonding
See *Attachment*.

Clinical Reasoning Skills in Occupational Therapy
The process by which occupational therapists individualize and modify treatment. It includes not only the application of theory to practice, but also the treatment of the meaning of illness as experienced by the individual and family (Mattingly, 1991).

Environmental Factors
"[T]he physical, social, and attitudinal environment in which people live and conduct their lives" (WHO, 2001, p. 10).

Environmental Neonatology

The study of environment of newborn special care facilities and its impact on the medical and developmental status of at-risk infants (Gottfried & Gaiter, 1985).

Family

A unit composed of individuals who are linked by shared kinship, function, and/or responsibilities and who identify themselves in a common relationship (Crockenberg, Lyons-Ruth, & Dickson, 1993).

Family-Centered Care

A constellation of philosophies, attitudes, and approaches to the care of children with special health and developmental needs that recognizes that the family is the constant in the child's life and that parent–professional partnerships are essential to effective and high-quality service delivery (Dunst, Trivette, & Deal, 1988; Institute for Family-Centered Care, 1990).

Goodness-of-Fit

"When the properties of the environment and its expectations and demands are in accord with the organism's own capacities, characteristics, and style of behaving" (Chess & Thomas, 1999, p. 3).

Impairments

"[P]roblems in body function or structure such as a significant deviation or loss" (WHO, 2001, p. 10).

Infant Mental Health

"Infant" refers to children under 3 years of age. "Mental" includes social–emotional and cognitive domains. "Health" refers to the well-being of young children and families (Fraiberg, 1980). A multidisciplinary intervention approach for the "early identification of risk and treatment to reduce the likelihood of serious developmental failure and relationship disturbance" (Weatherston, 2002, p. 1).

Medical Caregivers

House staff involved in the care of infants in the NICU. Although personnel may vary between institutions, medical caregivers typically include nurses, physicians (e.g., neonatologists, attending physicians, residents, interns), therapists, pharmacists, nutritionists, and other personnel (adapted from U. S. National Library of Medicine, 2005).

Neurobehavioral Organization

An interrelationship among infant central nervous system integrity and maturation, behaviors, and the caregiving environment. The interrelationship is expressed in terms of self-regulation and mutual regulation of autonomic, motoric, state, and interactional functions (Als, 1982).

Neurosocial

The ability to interact as the nervous system matures in preterm infants. There are three developmental stages of neurosocial development: turning in, coming out, and reciprocity (Gorski, Davidson, & Brazelton, 1979).

NICU

Neonatal intensive care unit. Newborn Nurseries are designated as Basic (Level I), Specialty (Level II), or Subspecialty (Level III) on the basis of their responsibilities and the availability of special service. Basic Neonatal Care Nurseries (*Level I*) provide postnatal care to healthy newborn infants and are equipped to provide resuscitation and to stabilize ill newborn infants until they can be transferred to a neonatal intensive care facility. Specialty Care Nurseries (*Level II*) "provide care to infants who are moderately ill with problems that are expected to resolve rapidly or who are recovering from serious illness" after receiving subspecialty care. Subspecialty Nurseries (*Level III*) provide care to infants who are extremely premature, are critically ill, or require surgical management (American Academy of Pediatrics & American College of Obstetricians and Gynecologists, 2004, p. 134).

Participation

"[I]nvolvement in a life situation" (WHO, 2001, p. 10).

Participation Restrictions

"[P]roblems an individual may experience in involvement in life situations" (WHO, 2001, p. 10).

Physiologic Instability

Refers to a lack of balance or equilibrium within the autonomic nervous system. Signs of physiologic instability may include changes in cardiorespiratory status (heart rate, respiratory rate, decreased oxygen saturation), color changes (pale, dusky, mottled, flushed), or visceral cues (yawning, sneezing, gagging, spitting up, hiccupping, having bowel movement). Conversely, an infant with physiologic stability will be calm with stable color and vital signs (Als, 1986).

Regulatory Abilities

The infant's capacity to modulate or modify his or her own state of arousal and neurobehavioral organization (Als, 1982).

Relationship-Based Approach

An approach that is "guided by a neurodevelopmental framework for understanding preterm infants and depends on the capacities of professionals to collaborate with one another and with families in support of the infants medical, developmental, and emotional well being" (Als & Gilkerson, 1997, p. 178).

References

Als, H. (1982). Toward a synactive theory of development: Promise for the assessment of infant individuality. *Infant Mental Health Journal, 3,* 229–243.

Als, H. (1986). A synactive model of neonatal behavioral organization: Framework for the assessment of neurobehavioral development in the premature infant and for the support of infants and parents in the neonatal intensive care environment. *Physical and Occupational Therapy in Pediatrics, 6*(3/4), 3–53.

Als, H., & Gilkerson, L. (1997). The role of relationship-based developmentally supportive newborn intensive care in strengthening outcome of preterm infants. *Seminars in Perinatology, 21,* 178–189.

American Academy of Pediatrics, & American College of Obstetricians and Gynecologists. (2004). *Guidelines for perinatal care* (5th ed.). Elk Grove Village, IL: Author

American Occupational Therapy Association. (2002). Occupational therapy practice framework: Domain and process. *American Journal of Occupational Therapy, 56,* 609–639.

American Occupational Therapy Association. (2004a). Guidelines for supervision, roles, and responsibilities during the delivery of occupational therapy services. *American Journal of Occupational Therapy, 58,* 663–677.

American Occupational Therapy Association. (2004b). Scope of practice. *American Journal of Occupational Therapy, 58,* 673–677.

American Occupational Therapy Association. (2005a). Occupational therapy code of ethics (2005). *American Journal of Occupational Therapy, 59,* 639–642.

American Occupational Therapy Association. (2005b). Standards of practice for occupational therapy. *American Journal of Occupational Therapy, 59,* 663–665.

Chess, F., & Thomas, A. (1999). *Goodness of fit: Clinical applications from infancy through adult life.* Philadelphia: Brunner/Mazel.

Crockenberg, S., Lyons-Ruth, K., & Dickson, S. (1993). The family context of infant mental health: II. Infant development in multiple family relationships. In C. H. Zeanah (Ed.), *Handbook of infant mental health* (pp. 38–55). New York: Guilford.

Dunst, C. J., Trivette, C. M., & Deal, A. G. (1988). *Enabling and empowering families: Principles and guidelines for practice.* Cambridge, MA: Brookline Books.

Fraiberg, S. (1980). *Clinical studies in infant mental health.* New York: Basic Books.

Gale, T. (2005). *The Gale encyclopedia of children's health: Infancy through adolescence.* Farmington Hills, MI: Thomson Gale.

Gorski, P., Davidson, M. E., & Brazelton, T. B. (1979). Stages of behavioral organization in the high-risk neonate: Theoretical–clinical considerations. *Seminars in Perinatology, 3,* 61–73.

Gottfried, A. W., & Gaiter, J. L. (1985). *Infant stress under intensive care.* Baltimore: University Park Press.

Institute for Family-Centered Care. (1990). *Association for the care of children's health.* Washington, DC: Author.

Mattingly, C. (1991). What is clinical reasoning? *American Journal of Occupational Therapy, 45,* 979–996.

U.S. National Library of Medicine. (2005, December 13). *MedlinePlus medical encyclopedia.* Retrieved January 11, 2006, from http://www.nlm.nih.gov/medlineplus/ency/article/007241.htm

Weatherston, D. J. (2002). Introduction to the infant mental health program. In J. J. Shirilla & D. J. Weatherston (Eds.), *Case studies in infant mental health: Risk, resiliency, and relationships* (pp. 1–13). Washington, DC: ZERO to THREE.

World Health Organization. (2001). *International classification of functioning, disability, and health (ICF).* Geneva, Switzerland: Author.

Related Readings

Als, H., Duffy, F. H., McAnulty, G. B., Rivkin, M. J., Vajapeyam, S., Mulkern, R. V., et al. (2004). Early experience alters brain function and structure. *Pediatrics, 113,* 846–857.

Als, H., Gilkerson, L., Duffy, F. H., McAnulty, G. B., Buehler, D. M., VanderBerg, K., et al. (2003). A three-center randomized controlled trial of individualized developmental care for very low birth weight infants: Medical, neurodevelomental, parenting, and caregiving effects. *Journal of Developmental and Behavioral Pediatrics, 24,* 399–408.

Anzalone, M. E. (1994). Occupational therapy in neonatology: What is our ethical responsibility? *American Journal of Occupational Therapy, 48,* 563–566.

Browne, J. V. (2003). New perspectives on premature infants and their parents. *ZERO to THREE, 24*(2), 4–12.

Buehler, D., Als, H., Duffy, F., McAnulty, G., & Liederman, J. (1995). Effectiveness of individualized developmental care for low-risk preterm infants: Behavioral and electrophysiologic evidence. *Pediatrics, 96,* 923–932.

Carter, B. S. (2003). Collaborative decision making in the NICU: When life is uncertain, satisfice. *ZERO to THREE, 24*(2), 21–25.

Holloway, E. (1998). Relationship-based occupational therapy in the neonatal intensive care unit. In J. Case-Smith (Ed.), *Pediatric occupational therapy and intervention* (pp. 111–126). Boston: Butterworth-Heinemann.

Holloway, E. (in press). Fostering early parent–infant playfulness in the neonatal intensive care unit. In L. D. Parham & L. S. Fazio (Eds.), *Play in occupational therapy for children* (2nd ed.). St. Louis, MO: Mosby.

Hunter, J. G. (2005). Neonatal intensive care unit. In J. Case-Smith, (Ed.), *Occupational therapy with children* (5th ed., pp. 688–770). St. Louis, MO: Elsevier/Mosby.

Johnson, B. H., Abraham, M. R., & Parrish, R. N. (2004). Designing the neonatal intensive care until for optimal family involvement. *Clinics in Perinatology, 31,* 353–383.

McGrath, J. M., & Conliffe-Torres, S. (1996). Integrating family-centered developmental assessment and intervention into routine care in the neonatal intensive care unit. *Nursing Clinics of North America, 31,* 367–368.

Meyer, E. C., Lester, B. M., Boukydis, C. F. Z., & Bigsby, R. (1998). Family-based intervention with high-risk infants and their families. *Journal of Clinical Psychology in Medical Settings, 5,* 49–69.

Talmi, A., & Harmon, R. J. (2003). Relationships between preterm infants and their parents: Disruption and development. *ZERO to THREE, 24*(2), 13–20.

Vergara, E., & Bigsby, R. (2004). *Developmental and therapeutic interventions in the NICU.* Baltimore: Paul H. Brookes.

Authors

Revised by the 2005 Neonatal Intensive Care Unit Task Force
Elsie Vergara, ScD, OTR, FAOTA, *Chairperson*
Marie Anzalone, ScD, OTR, FAOTA
Rosemarie Bigsby, ScD, OTR, FAOTA
Delia Gorga, PhD, OTR, FAOTA
Elise Holloway, MPH, OTR
Jan Hunter, MA, OTR
Ginny Laadt, PhD, OTR/L
Susan Strzyzewski, MEd, OTR

for

The Commission on Practice
Susanne Smith Roley, MS, OTR/L, FAOTA, *Chairperson*

Adopted by the Representative Assembly 2006C404

This replaces the 2000 document "Specialized Knowledge and Skills for Occupational Therapy Practice in the Neonatal Intensive Care Unit" (*American Journal of Occupational Therapy, 54,* 641–648).

Specialized Knowledge and Skills in Technology and Environmental Interventions for Occupational Therapy Practice

Purpose

The purpose of this document is to describe the knowledge and skills that are necessary for occupational therapists and occupational therapy assistants[1] to provide ethical, competent occupational therapy services related to technology and environmental interventions. Intended for internal and external audiences, it provides information about occupational therapy practitioners' roles and collaborative partnerships with other professionals in technology and environmental interventions, outlines professional development and supervision guidelines, defines terms related to technology and environmental interventions, and describes entry- and advanced-level knowledge and skills. In this document, the phrase *technology and environmental interventions* represents the broad range and combination of technology, environmental interventions, and reasonable accommodation strategies. The emphasis is on technology and environmental interventions that support the ability of people with or without disabilities to fully participate in their daily lives in accessible environments and livable communities and through engagement in occupations.

Introduction

Occupational therapy practitioners have long-standing expertise in providing occupational therapy services to clients that incorporate technology and environmental modification, often in collaboration with other professionals. Clients include individuals, organizations, and populations (American Occupational Therapy Association [AOTA], 2008). When addressing technology and environmental interventions, occupational therapy practitioners consider the context in which people engage in daily life occupations that support their participation, health, and wellness. On the basis of their understanding of their clients' occupational engagement desires and needs, capacities, and contexts, occupational therapy practitioners collaborate with the client and with other professionals in the evaluation, design, fabrication, customization, modification, and application of new or existing technologies and environmental interventions. They also conduct outcome studies, support advocacy initiatives, offer guidance regarding funding resources and referrals, and provide training and consultation (Hammel & Angelo, 1996). Occupational therapy practitioners deliver technology and environmental-related services in a variety of settings, such as hospitals, rehabilitation centers, skilled nursing facilities, outpatient facilities, home health agencies, schools, work sites, industry, homes, and communities and in a variety of roles such as the primary service provider, team member, advocate, and expert consultant.

---

[1] *Occupational therapists* are responsible for all aspects of occupational therapy service delivery and are accountable for the safety and effectiveness of the occupational therapy service delivery process. *Occupational therapy assistants* deliver occupational therapy services under the supervision of and in partnership with an occupational therapist (AOTA, 2004a). When the term *occupational therapy practitioner* is used in this document, it refers to both occupational therapists and occupational therapy assistants (AOTA, 2006).

Occupational Therapy's Role in Technology and Environmental Modification

Technology and environmental interventions can support people's participation in occupations which, by definition, hold purpose and meaning for them. This is especially beneficial when the activities are otherwise too difficult or challenging. Occupational therapy practitioners collaborate with the client and other professionals to create a successful match among the client, the technology, and environmental interventions and the context for their use. As part of therapeutic services, occupational therapists are trained to conduct comprehensive evaluations to identify the skills and abilities of the client and to guide the recommendation for services. The evaluation includes the development of an occupational profile and selecting, administering, and interpreting assessments to analyze the occupational performance of individuals, organizations, and populations. This includes consideration of the client's performance skills, capacities, and performance patterns, the characteristics of the technology and the environmental interventions, the activity demands, and the contexts for the technology and environmental interventions. Occupational therapy assistants contribute to the evaluation process by gathering data and administering selected assessment tools or measures for which they have demonstrated competence (AOTA, 2004a).

During intervention, both occupational therapists and occupational therapy assistants select, administer, and adapt technologies and environments that support the intervention plan developed by the occupational therapist. The goal is to promote, improve, or maintain the ability of people to engage in basic and instrumental activities of daily living: work, education, leisure, play, social participation, and sleep occupations that are meaningful and necessary (AOTA, 2008). Examples include the selection and adaptation of computers and software to support education and work; the positioning and modification of speech and communication devices to facilitate social participation; the design and customization of seating devices, mobility equipment, and physical environments to promote play and leisure participation; the selection and training in the use of environmental controls and of vision and hearing technologies to support involvement in instrumental activities of daily living; and the fabrication and modification of assistive devices for self-care tasks. Interventions also may focus on advocacy initiatives, educational and training programs for organizations and populations, and policy development that promote accessible environments and livable communities.

When measuring the outcomes of interventions, occupational therapy practitioners focus on how the technology and environmental interventions support the client's health, participation (World Health Organization, 2001), and engagement in occupation (AOTA, 2008). The selected outcomes need to be measurable, reliable, and valid; sensitive to measuring change; reflective of clients' goals; and consistent with payer needs. Outcomes include subjective impressions such as improved competence, well-being, self-efficacy, hope, and quality of life (AOTA, 2008). Outcomes also include objective measurements such as improved efficiency, accessibility, task completion, independence or interdependence, and the ability of the client to assume or regain valued life roles and occupations.

Occupational therapy practitioners must adhere to state and agency regulatory laws when providing services across practice setting and the continua of care. Reimbursement for services may be available through various sources, including legislation (e.g., Individuals with Disabilities Education Improvement Act, Medicare), private insurance, Medicaid, and private pay.

Professional Development

For both occupational therapists and occupational therapy assistants, the progression from entry-level to advanced-level knowledge and skills related to technology and environmental interventions evolves through education and experience. At a level commensurate with their respective academic programs, occupational therapy and occupational therapy assistant students receive education in the structure and function of the human body, including the biological and physical sciences; human development throughout the life span and human behavior, including the behavioral and social sciences; and effects of mental and physical health, disease processes, genetic conditions, trauma, and context on occupational performance. They acquire foundational knowledge and skills regarding technology and environmental interventions, and they develop clinical-reasoning skills to consider the interplay of physical, cognitive, environmental, and sociocultural factors in providing effective services (AOTA, 2007a, 2007b, 2007c). Over time, as they advance in their education and arena of practice, occupational therapy practitioners may develop additional expertise in technology and environmental interventions. They ensure advanced knowledge and skills in technology and environmental interventions by maintaining and documenting competence in practice, education, and research and by participating in professional development, educational activities, and critical examination of available evidence (AOTA, 2004c). Examples include participating in local and national continuing education conferences such as those sponsored by AOTA, the Assistive Technology Industry Association (ATIA), Closing the Gap (CTG), the California State University National Conference (CSUN), and the Rehabilitation Engineering and Assistive Technology Society of North America (RESNA); completing postsecondary courses; and seeking advanced competency and specialty certification through AOTA or external organizations such as RESNA. In addition, they gain higher level knowledge, skills, and clinical reasoning through experience and mentoring opportunities.

The occupational therapy practitioner's acquisition of advanced-level knowledge and skills related to technology and environmental interventions is individualized; thus, a practitioner may possess differing levels of expertise in a wide variety of skill areas and populations served by occupational therapy. For example, an occupational therapy practitioner may have advanced-level skills in computer and information technologies for students in school systems but only entry-level knowledge in vehicle modification and transportation for older adult populations. It is the ethical responsibility of occupational therapy practitioners to ensure that they are competent in the services they provide and routinely seek out new knowledge and techniques that apply to their practice (AOTA, 2004c).

Supervision Considerations

The amount of supervision provided to occupational therapy practitioners in the area of technology and environmental interventions directly relates to their training and experience and state practice acts. Occupational therapy assistants and entry-level occupational therapists should seek supervision and mentoring from a more experienced occupational therapist or an occupational therapist with advanced knowledge and skills in technology and environmental interventions. The occupational therapist and occupational therapy assistant also may supervise other non-licensed personnel when providing technology and environmental modification to clients (AOTA, 2004a). Most state practice acts mandate the frequency and duration for supervision of entry-level occupational therapists, occupational therapy assistants, and non-licensed personnel. The occupational therapist has the primary role in evaluation and intervention planning; the occupational therapy assistant collaborates with the occupational therapist in the provision of specific interventions (AOTA, 2004a, 2004b, 2004c).

Terminology and Definitions

- *Assistive technology device (ATD):* "Any item, piece of equipment, or product system, whether acquired commercially, modified, or customized, that is used to increase, maintain, or improve functional capabilities of individuals with disabilities." *Assistive technology service* means "any service that directly assists an individual with a disability in the selection, acquisition, or use of an assistive technology device" (Assistive Technology Act of 2004, P.L. 108-364), including evaluation, fitting and customization, coordination of services, and training.

- *Basic technology:* Commonly used technologies or environmental interventions such as activities of daily living equipment and basic home modifications (Hammel & Angelo, 1996).

- ***Complex technology:*** Technology and environmental interventions that require advanced or specialized knowledge, training, and experience to evaluate, provide interventions, and measure outcomes such as custom seating and mobility and integrated systems (e.g., mobility + environmental control + computer access) (Hammel & Angelo, 1996).

- ***Electronic and information technology:*** Information technology, equipment, and interconnected systems or subsystems of equipment that are used in the creation, conversion, or duplication of data or information. It includes, but is not limited to, telecommunications products (e.g., telephones), information kiosks and transaction machines, Internet sites, multimedia, and office equipment such as copiers and fax machines (U.S. Access Board, 2000).

- ***Rehabilitative and educational technologies:*** Technology that is "used as a tool for remediation or rehabilitation," such as visual perception or cognitive training, improvement in motor control, or identification of letters and numbers. Depending on the client contexts, rehabilitation and educational technologies have the role of remediation, restoration, or acquisition of foundational skills (Cook & Polgar, 2008, p. 6).

- ***Technology:*** The combination of assistive, basic, complex, electronic and information, and rehabilitative and educational technologies.

- ***Technology and environmental competency (TEC):*** The combination of technology (e.g., assistive, electronic and information, rehabilitative), environmental interventions, and reasonable accommodation strategies used to increase, maintain, or improve functional capabilities of individuals with disabilities and/or create accessible environments (e.g., home, work, school, community, virtual).

- ***Universal design:*** The design of products and environments to be usable by all people, to the greatest extent possible, without the need for adaptation or specialized design (Center for Universal Design, 1997).

Entry- and Advanced-Level Knowledge and Skills

The appendix provides a matrix that outlines the entry- or advanced-level knowledge and skills that occupational therapists and occupational therapy assistants should demonstrate when providing occupational therapy services related to technology and environmental interventions. An *X* denotes the minimum knowledge and skills that the occupational therapist or occupational therapy assistant should demonstrate to practice competently at that level; an *A* denotes that the occupational therapist or the occupational therapy assistant may assist or contribute information but is not able to perform the task alone and requires supervision. Occupational therapy practitioners have a professional responsibility to work within their own level of competency, as well as within the scope of practice as defined and regulated by state licensure and *Occupational Therapy Code of Ethics*, including the duty to maintain high standards of competency within a practice area and to seek out supervision and continuing education in those areas of practice that are above their level of competency (AOTA, 2004b, 2005).

References

American Occupational Therapy Association. (2004a). Guidelines for supervision, roles, and responsibilities during the delivery of occupational therapy services. *American Journal of Occupational Therapy, 58,* 663–667.

American Occupational Therapy Association. (2004b). Scope of practice. *American Journal of Occupational Therapy, 58,* 673–677.

American Occupational Therapy Association. (2004c). Standards of practice for occupational therapy. *American Journal of Occupational Therapy, 52,* 866–869.

American Occupational Therapy Association. (2005). Occupational therapy code of ethics (2005). *American Journal of Occupational Therapy, 59,* 639–642.

American Occupational Therapy Association. (2006). Policy 1.44: Categories of occupational therapy personnel. In *Policy manual* (2007 ed., pp. 33–34). Bethesda, MD: Author.

American Occupational Therapy Association. (2007a). Accreditation standards for a doctoral-degree-level educational program for the occupational therapist. *American Journal of Occupational Therapy, 61,* 641–651.

American Occupational Therapy Association. (2007b). Accreditation standards for a master's-degree-level educational program for the occupational therapist. *American Journal of Occupational Therapy, 61,* 652–661.

American Occupational Therapy Association. (2007c). Accreditation standards for an educational program for the occupational therapy assistant. *American Journal of Occupational Therapy, 61,* 652–661.

American Occupational Therapy Association. (2008). Occupational therapy practice framework: Domain and process (2nd ed.). *American Journal of Occupational Therapy, 62,* 625–683.

Assistive Technology Act of 2004, P.L. 108-364, 108 Cong., 118 SAT. 1707(2004).

Center for Universal Design. (1997). *Principles of universal design.* Raleigh, NC: Author.

Cook, A. M., & Polgar, S. M. (2008). *Cook and Hussey's assistive technologies principles and practice.* St. Louis, MO: Mosby/Elsevier.

Hammel, J., & Angelo, J. (1996). Technology competencies for occupational therapy practitioners. *Assistive Technology, 8*(1), 34–42.

U. S. Access Board. (2000, December 21). Electronic and Information Technology Accessibility Standards (Section 508). *Federal Register.* Retrieved September 5, 2008, from http://www/access-board.gov/508

World Health Organization. (2001). *International classification of functioning, disability and health (ICF).* Geneva, Switzerland: Author.

Authors

This document is based on the work of Hammel and Angelo (1996) and on a motion from the April 2006 Representative Assembly. The knowledge and skills were revised by the Technology Special Interest Section Standing Committee with consultation from a panel of international experts from external organizations with occupational therapy and technology expertise and developed into a Knowledge and Skills Paper.

This 2008 paper was revised by
Joy Hammel, PhD, OTR/L, FAOTA, *Chairperson*
Daniel Knowland, OTR/L
Roger Smith, PhD, OT, FAOTA
Lynn Gitlow, PhD, OTR/L, ATP
Robin Jones, COTA, ROH
Susan Leech, EdD, OTR, ATP
Beth Goodrich, MEd, MS, OTR, ATP
Brent Braveman, PhD, OTR/L, FAOTA

With contributions from

Janet V. DeLany, DEd, OTR/L, FAOTA
Kim Hartmann, PhD, OTR/L, FAOTA

for

The Commission on Practice
Susanne Smith Roley, MS, OTR/L, FAOTA, *Chairperson*

Adopted by the Representative Assembly 2008CO107

Note: This document replaces the 2004 Statement *Assistive Technology Within Occupational Therapy Practice.*

Copyright © 2009, by the American Occupational Therapy Association. To be published in the *American Journal of Occupational Therapy, 63*(November/December).

Appendix.

Specialized Knowledge and Skills in Technology and Environmental Interventions

X = able to perform the task. A = assists with the task. ■ = does not perform the task.

		Entry-Level		Advanced	
	Knowledge and Skills	OTA	OT	OTA	OT
	All knowledge and skills assume active collaboration with the client, consumer, or user of the technology and environmental solutions, significant others relevant to the situation (e.g., family, caregivers), service delivery team members, and other relevant stakeholders (e.g., case managers, funders, advocates) throughout the process.				
A.	**Evaluation**				
A.1	*Upon referral for services, screen for occupational performance capacities and limitations, screen for environmental supports and barriers, and identify if the need for a comprehensive OT evaluation exists.*	A	X	A	X
A.2	*Determine technology and environmental needs as part of a comprehensive OT evaluation that includes occupational profile and an analysis of occupational performance.*				
A.2.a	Evaluate the client's occupational and participation needs in areas of occupation (e.g., basic and instrumental activities of daily living, education, work, play, leisure, social participation, sleep) and the potential need for technology and environment applications to support these needs.	A	X	A	X
A.2.b	Evaluate the client's contexts, including cultural, virtual, temporal (e.g., chronological, developmental, life cycle, disability status), and environments (physical, social) for their influence on technology and environmental access, application, and use.	A	X	A	X
A.2.c	Assess prior and current use of technology and environmental interventions across existing roles, occupations, activities, and contexts.	A	X	A	X
A.2.d	Evaluate and analyze the activity demands, the client's performance skills and performance patterns, and client factors across contexts of potential technology and environmental use, including transitions between contexts.	A	X	A	X
A.2.e	Screen and identify the level of technology and environmental intervention needed, ranging from none to basic to advanced/complex.	A	X	A	X
A.2.f	Communicate range of relevant and related interventions that could be considered (e.g., technology, environmental modification, training, pharmacology, surgery, therapy).	A	X	A	X

(continued)

Appendix.
Specialized Knowledge and Skills in Technology and Environmental Interventions *(cont.)*

X = able to perform the task. A = assists with the task. ■ = does not perform the task.

	Knowledge and Skills	Entry-Level		Advanced	
		OTA	OT	OTA	OT
A.2.g	Refer clients to appropriate professionals for technology and environmental resources when the services the client needs or seeks are beyond the scope of practice and competency level of the OT practitioner.	X	X	X	X
A.3	*Conduct a BASIC technology and environmental evaluation.*				
A.3.a	Evaluate basic technology and environmental needs within areas of occupation (e.g., basic and instrumental activities of daily living, work, education, play, leisure, social participation, sleep).	A	X	A	X
A.3.b	Compare and contrast different basic technology and environmental features and access methods in relation to the client, activity and environmental needs, supports, demands, and constraints.	A	X	X	X
A.3.c	Integrate basic theoretical information from OT, occupational science, and other disciplines into the plan (e.g., physical therapy, speech and language pathology, audiology, disability studies, engineering, rehabilitation engineering, education, ergonomics, psychology, public health, sociology, anthropology, architecture, urban planning).	A	X	A	X
A.3.d	Interpret and integrate basic technology and environmental evaluation results into intervention or service delivery plan and also outcome measures, reevaluating as needed.	A	X	A	X
A.3.e	Develop occupational goals, anticipated outcomes, and intervention plans, incorporating basic technology and environmental applications as appropriate.	A	X	A	X
A.3.f.	Coordinate evaluation of OT-related needs within interdisciplinary basic technology and environmental services.	A	X	A	X
A.4	*Conduct specialized or complex technology and environmental evaluations (assumes A.1–A.3 met).*				
A.4.a	Conduct advanced evaluation of complex or specialized technology and environmental applications (e.g., those related to computer access, seating and positioning needs, mobility and driving programs, sensory needs, environmental control, communication alternatives).	A	A	A	X
A.4.b	Utilize information resources on specialized or complex technology and environmental applications within decision making.	A	A	X	X

Appendix.
Specialized Knowledge and Skills in Technology and Environmental Interventions *(cont.)*

X = able to perform the task. A = assists with the task. ■ = does not perform the task.

		Entry-Level		Advanced	
	Knowledge and Skills	**OTA**	**OT**	**OTA**	**OT**
A.4.c	Compare and contrast different complex, specialized, or integrated technology and environmental features and access methods in relation to the client, contexts, activity, and environmental needs, supports, demands, and constraints.	A	A	X	X
A.4.d	Integrate advanced technology and environmental theoretical information from OT, occupational science, and other disciplines into the intervention or service delivery plan and also outcome measures.	A	A	A	X
A.4.e	Evaluate relationship of materials and different design choices, including advantages, trade-offs, and constraints within complex technology and environmental plans.	A	A	X	X
A.4.f	Interpret and integrate results of complex technology and environmental evaluation into intervention or service delivery plans and also outcome measures, reevaluating as needed.	A	A	A	X
A.4.g	Develop advanced technology and environmental goals, anticipated outcomes, and intervention plans, with incorporation in OT intervention plan and outcome measures, as relevant.	A	A	A	X
B.	**Intervention**				
B.1	*Provide technology and environmental interventions as part of a comprehensive OT plan.*				
B.1.a	Provide basic interventions that optimize the client's performance skills, performance patterns, and body functions. Examples include daily living skills training, cognitive rehabilitation, strengthening, ergonomic practice, visual/perceptual rehabilitation, and energy conservation.	X	X	X	X
B.1.b	Provide basic interventions that optimize the client's engagement in areas of occupation within the home, work, school, and community contexts. Examples include environmental interventions, ergonomic design, ADA training, and disability awareness training to promote participation and accessibility.	X	X	X	X
B.1.c	Design, alter, and/or adapt tasks to meet the occupational and activity demands of the context. Examples include rewriting job descriptions, rearranging class schedules, sharing job duties, and comparing level of assistance to do task (attendant vs. technology).	X	X	X	X

(continued)

Appendix.
Specialized Knowledge and Skills in Technology and Environmental Interventions *(cont.)*

X = able to perform the task. A = assists with the task. ■ = does not perform the task.

	Knowledge and Skills	Entry-Level OTA	Entry-Level OT	Advanced OTA	Advanced OT
B.2	*Provide access to, delivery of, and training in basic technology and environmental applications.*				
B.2.a	Utilize design and fabrication principles within basic technology and environment applications, including consideration of mechanics/strength of materials, mechanical components, systems, and electrical circuits and components.	A	X	X	X
B.2.b	Incorporate universal design principles within technology and environmental applications (e.g., simplicity, ease of use, equitable access).	A	X	X	X
B.2.c	Address issues of repair and maintenance in basic technology and environmental applications, including basic repair, preventative maintenance training and schedules, and limitations and violations of warranty for mechanical, electrical, and electronic equipment.	X	X	X	X
B.2.d	Address factors related to cost and benefit/impact of custom versus commercial technology and environment applications.	A	X	A	X
B.2.e	Perform product trials, recommend product specifications, order technologies and environmental solutions, and install and train individuals in use, maintenance, and repair.	A	X	X	X
B.2.f	Utilize fabrication tools, materials, and machines as needed to match basic technology and environmental applications to user's needs.	X	X	X	X
B.2.g	Participate in the design, fabrication, and customization of basic technology and environmental applications within a defensible level of competence as appropriate to the case and the level of expertise required, with referral to advanced expertise as indicated.	X	X	X	X
B.2.h	Periodically reevaluate basic technology and environmental use, needs, and integration into everyday life.	A	X	A	X
B.3	*Provide access to, delivery of, and training in complex or specialized technology and environmental applications (assumes B.1–B.2 met).*				
B.3.a	Utilize advanced design and fabrication principles (e.g., design to address issues of corrosion, temperature, pressure over time, compatibility or integration of multiple technologies).	A	A	A	X
B.3.b	Utilize advanced environmental and universal design principles to match client needs and specific environmental demands (e.g., school, work, community, home).	A	A	A	X

Appendix.
Specialized Knowledge and Skills in Technology and Environmental Interventions *(cont.)*

X = able to perform the task. A = assists with the task. ■ = does not perform the task.

		Entry-Level		Advanced	
	Knowledge and Skills	**OTA**	**OT**	**OTA**	**OT**
B.3.c	Address issues of compatibility and integration of technologies (e.g., hardware and software interface) across different environments and systems/equipment.	A	A	X	X
B.3.e	Utilize fabrication tools, materials, and machines as needed to match user's needs.	A	X	X	X
B.3.f	Perform product trials and feature analyses; coordinate delivery and installation of technology and environmental interventions; and train technology and environmental user and important others in the use, repair, and maintenance of complex, specialized, and integrated technology and environmental applications (e.g., wheelchair, environmental control, augmentative communication for education and work).	A	X	A	X
B.3.g	Collaborate in the design, fabrication, and customization of complex or specialized technology and environmental applications within a defensible level of competence as appropriate to the case and the level of expertise required, with referral to specialized expertise as needed.	A	A	A	X
B.3.h	Periodically reevaluate complex technology and environmental use, needs, and integration into everyday life.	A	X	A	X
C.	**Evidence-Based Practice and Outcomes**				
C.1	*Participate in and apply results from evidence-based practice within OT and basic technology and environmental service delivery.*				
C.1.a	Identify and document the outcomes of OT and basic technology and environmental interventions, including those related to occupational performance, participation in daily life, emotional and physical health and wellness, prevention, quality of life, and consumer use and satisfaction.	X	X	X	X
C.1.b	Participate in OT and basic technology and environmental program evaluations and continuous quality improvement initiatives to improve the effectiveness and efficiency of service delivery.	X	X	X	X
C.1.c	Participate in OT, occupational science, and basic technology and environmental research.	X	X	X	X
C.1.d	Critically analyze and apply evidence-based research within OT and basic technology and environmental practice.	A	X	A	X

Appendix.
Specialized Knowledge and Skills in Technology and Environmental Interventions *(cont.)*

X = able to perform the task. A = assists with the task. ■ = does not perform the task.

	Knowledge and Skills	Entry-Level		Advanced	
		OTA	OT	OTA	OT
C.2	*Participate in evidence-based practice within OT and complex or specialized technology and environmental delivery (assumes D.1 knowledge and skills met).*				
C.2.a	Identify and document the outcomes of OT and advanced technology and environmental interventions, including those related to occupational performance, participation in daily life, emotional and physical health and wellness, prevention, quality of life, and consumer use and satisfaction.	A	A	A	X
C.2.b	Participate in OT and advanced technology and environmental quality improvement and program evaluation activities.	A	A	A	X
C.2.c	Participate in OT, occupational science, and advanced technology and environmental research.	A	A	X	X
C.2.d	Critically analyze and apply evidence-based research within OT, occupational science, and advanced technology and environmental practice.	A	A	A	X
D.	**Resource Coordination and Advocacy**				
D.1	*Provide and coordinate OT and basic technology and environmental resources, services, and supports.*				
D.1.a	Understand and apply technology and environmental-related legislation and policies across the delivery process (e.g., ADA, IDEA, Technology Act).	X	X	X	X
D.1.b	Utilize and link clients and consumers to basic technology and environmental information resources (e.g., product databases, vendors, legislation and policies, funding/reimbursement sources, additional services, user groups, conferences, continuing education, advocacy organizations, legal).	X	X	X	X
D.1.c	Effectively communicate the role of OT practitioners in providing a global, occupation-based perspective encompassing technology and environmental use and delivery.	X	X	X	X
D.1.d	Describe the contributions of other disciplines and their roles within technology and environmental service delivery (e.g., rehabilitation engineering, physical therapy, speech and language pathology, audiology, engineering, education, vocational rehabilitation, case management).	X	X	X	X
D.1.e	Describe the role of distributors, vendors, suppliers, manufacturers, designers, and fabricators within technology	X	X	X	X

Appendix.
Specialized Knowledge and Skills in Technology and Environmental Interventions *(cont.)*

X = able to perform the task. A = assists with the task. ■ = does not perform the task.

	Knowledge and Skills	Entry-Level		Advanced	
		OTA	OT	OTA	OT
	and environmental delivery.				
D.1.f	Describe mechanisms, regulations, and policies regarding delivery and funding/ reimbursement of basic OT and technology and environmental applications.	X	X	X	X
D.1.g	Strategize different sources of funding (e.g., government funding, foundation grants, loan programs, private resources) within different settings (e.g., inpatient, community, schools, worksite) to improve access, including shared or matched funding strategies.	X	X	X	X
D.1.h	Justify and document the provision of OT and basic technology and environmental services and solutions for reimbursement.	X	X	X	X
D.1.i	Participate in advocacy activities related to technology and environment on an individual case level, and collaborate with consumer to become an informed self advocate for his or her own needs.	X	X	X	X
D.1.j	Participate in advocacy activities related to technology and environmental on a systems change level, and collaborate with the disability community in technology and environmental activism.	X	X	X	X
D.1.k	Maintain the *Occupational Therapy Code of Ethics* and *Standards of Practice* in primary discipline or field (e.g., therapy, engineering, education) and within technology and environmental service delivery.	X	X	X	X
D.2	*Provide and coordinate complex or specialized technology and environmental resources (assumes D.1 met).*				
D.2.a	Utilize and link clients and consumers to complex or specialized technology and environmental information resources (e.g., product databases, vendors, legislation and policies, funding/reimbursement sources, additional services, user groups, conferences, continuing education, advocacy organizations, legal assistance).	X	X	X	X
D.2.b	Describe mechanisms for obtaining reimbursement of OT and complex or specialized technology and environmental services.	A	A	A	X
D.2.c	Justify and document the provision of OT and complex or specialized technology and environmental services.	A	A	A	X
D.2.d	Maintain the *Occupational Therapy Code of Ethics* and *Standards of Practice* in specialized fields of technology and environmental service delivery (e.g., seating and mobility, computer access).	X	X	X	X

Position Papers

Complementary and Alternative Medicine (CAM)

Purpose of Paper

The American Occupational Therapy Association, Inc. (AOTA) asserts that complementary and alternative medicine (CAM) may be used by occupational therapists and occupational therapy assistants as part of a comprehensive approach to enhance engagement in occupation (Giese, Parker, Lech-Boura, Burkhardt, & Cook, 2003). Because the use of CAMs is expanding in various health care practices, the purpose of this paper is to define the appropriate use of complementary and alternative medicine within the scope of occupational therapy practice.

Explanation of CAMs

The National Center for Complementary and Alternative Medicine (NCCAM) of the National Institutes of Health has identified five domains of CAM practice and defines *complementary and alternative medicine* as "a group of diverse medical and health care systems, practices, and products that are not presently considered to be part of conventional medicine" (NCCAM, 2002). The five domains of CAM practice are (1) alternative medical systems, (2) mind–body interventions, (3) biologically based treatments, (4) manipulative and body-based methods, and (5) energy therapies. Though the terms *complementary* and *alternative* often are interchanged, the commonly accepted distinction between them is that alternative medicine is practiced *in place of* conventional medicine, while complementary practices are accessed *in conjunction with* allopathic medical practices. The newer terms *integrative medicine* and *blended medicine* also are used to reference complementary medicine. The definition of complementary and alternative medicine is, by its very nature, dynamic. Practices contained within the definition of CAMs change as some become adopted into conventional health, and new ones emerge (Giese et al., 2003).

CAM services, though often paid for privately, increasingly are covered by insurance companies and health maintenance organizations (Astin, Pelletier, Marie, & Haskell, 2000; Cleary-Guida, Okvat, Oz, & Ting, 2001; Wolsko, Eisenberg, Davis, Ettner, & Phillips, 2002). Factors that compel third-party payers to include selected CAMs in health care policies include cost-effectiveness, consumer demand, demonstrated clinical efficacy, and state mandate (Pelletier & Astin, 2002; Pelletier, Astin, & Haskell, 1999). Further support for the use of CAMs is provided by the funding for research and training of CAM practices by the NCCAM.

Research is important to determine the efficacy and effectiveness of CAM practices in health and wellness arenas. The current number of outcomes studies for any specific CAM method is small. Research that does exist generally has limited and nonrandomized sample sizes and inconsistently defined terms, thereby reducing the power of the evidence and the ability to generalize results. Results that do exist show mixed evidence on the efficacy of CAM practices. These findings suggest the need for more studies to validate the efficacy of specific CAM practices with scientific evidence using randomized, controlled trials.

Use of CAMs Within Occupational Therapy Practice

Occupational therapists and occupational therapy assistants have used various CAM techniques in the delivery of occupational therapy services. CAMs may be used within the scope of occupational therapy practice when they are used as preparatory methods or purposeful activities to facilitate the ability of clients to engage in their daily life occupations.

Occupational therapy values engagement in occupations and has as its core mission to support participation in context (AOTA, 2002). Occupations are "activities . . . of everyday life, named, organized, and given value and meaning by individuals and a culture" (Law, Polatajko, Baptiste, & Townsend, 1997). Occupations encompass activities of daily living, instrumental activities of daily living, education, leisure skills, play, social participation, and work (AOTA, 2002). The occupational therapist is responsible for all aspects of occupational therapy service delivery and is accountable for the safety and effectiveness of the occupational therapy service delivery process. The occupational therapy assistant is responsible for providing safe and effective occupational therapy services under the supervision of and in partnership with the occupational therapist (AOTA, 2004b).

To determine whether to use CAMs in the delivery of occupational therapy services, occupational therapists and occupational therapy assistants must evaluate the client, develop an intervention based on the client's needs and priorities, and conduct outcomes measurement. The evaluation enables the occupational therapist and the occupational therapy assistant to gain an understanding of the client's strengths, priorities, and current limitations in carrying out daily occupations. Evaluation and intervention address factors that influence the client's occupational performance, including how the client performs the daily life occupations, the demands of those occupations, and the environments where those occupations are performed. As part of the evaluation and the intervention, the occupational therapist and the occupational therapy assistant must determine whether the use of CAMs is consistent with the client's cultural practices, priorities, and needs; is safe to use; and is an appropriate approach to facilitate the ability of the client to participate in daily life occupations. Outcomes are measured to determine the effectiveness of occupational therapy services and future therapeutic interventions with the client. The occupational therapist and the occupational therapy assistant must measure whether the use of CAMs resulted in positive outcomes.

Some CAM techniques currently being utilized in occupational therapy include guided imagery, massage, myofascial release, meditation, yoga, and behavioral relaxation training (Lindsay, Fee, Michie, & Heap, 1994; Scott, 1999). Because individuals receiving occupational therapy services are embedded in their cultures and because some CAM practices are embedded within particular cultures, occupational therapists and occupational therapy assistants need to understand how those cultures influence where and when to use CAM techniques. Outcome studies continue to need to be conducted to determine the efficacy and effectiveness of using CAM techniques during occupational therapy intervention to enable individuals to engage in their daily life occupations.

The *Occupational Therapy Code of Ethics* (AOTA, 2000) mandates safe and competent practice, holding occupational therapy professionals responsible for the maintenance of high standards of competence. CAM techniques used within the scope of occupational therapy practice may require additional training, competency examinations, certification, and regulatory knowledge. The use of specific CAM techniques may be subject to federal, state, and often local municipal regulations that govern practice, advertising, ethics, professional terminology, and training. It is the responsibility of the occupational therapist and the occupational therapy assistant to know and comply with applicable laws and regulations associated with CAM techniques as well as those mandated for the occupational therapy profession. Occupational therapists and occupational therapy assistants must abide by state regulations when billing for occupational therapy services that incorporate the use of CAMs. They must distinguish between when they are using CAMs within the scope of occupational therapy practice and when they are using CAMs as a primary approach beyond the scope of occupational therapy practice (AOTA, 2002, 2004a).

Issues of client safety and health care worker safety are salient to all areas of occupational therapy practice. The use of CAMs requires attention to client safety in consumer decision making, client interventions, and professional education and training. The risks and benefits of CAMs used in occupational therapy should be communicated to clients as standard practice in a client-centered, evidence-based approach to care.

Summary

Occupational therapy professionals facilitate proficient and satisfying engagement in the significant tasks and meaningful activities of life. Complementary and alternative medical practices, systems, and products may be appropriately incorporated into occupational therapy practice as a way to encourage a client's engagement in meaningful occupations. Scientific studies are needed to validate the safety and efficacy of CAM methods within occupational therapy practice. Advanced-level training and continuing education are important to acquire the knowledge and skill to utilize CAM methods, to address the concerns for patient safety and informed consent, and to meet the rigors of regulatory requirements.

References

American Occupational Therapy Association. (2000). Occupational therapy code of ethics (2000). *American Journal of Occupational Therapy, 54,* 614–616.

American Occupational Therapy Association. (2002). Occupational therapy practice framework: Domain and process. *American Journal of Occupational Therapy, 56,* 609–639.

American Occupational Therapy Association. (2004a). *Definition of occupational therapy practice for the AOTA Model Practice Act.* (Available from the State Affairs Group, American Occupational Therapy Association, 4720 Montgomery Lane, Bethesda, MD 20814)

American Occupational Therapy Association. (2004b). Guidelines for supervision, roles, and responsibilities during the delivery of occupational therapy services. *American Journal of Occupational Therapy, 58,* 663–667.

Astin, J. A., Pelletier, K. R., Marie, A., & Haskell, W. L. (2000). Complementary and alternative medicine use among elderly persons: One-year analysis of a Blue Shield Medicare supplement. *Journals of Gerontology, Series A, Biological Sciences and Medical Sciences, 55*(1), M4–M9.

Cleary-Guida, M. B., Okvat, H. A., Oz, M. C., & Ting, W. (2001). A regional survey of health insurance coverage for complementary and alternative medicine: Current status and future ramifications. *Journal of Alternative and Complementary Medicine, 7,* 269–273.

Giese, T., Parker, J. A., Lech-Boura, J., Burkhardt, A., & Cook, A. (2003). *The role of occupational therapy in complementary and alternative medicine* [White Paper]. Adopted by the AOTA Board of Directors 6-22-03. (Available from American Occupational Therapy Association, 4720 Montgomery Lane, Bethesda, MD 20814)

Law, M., Polatajko, H., Baptiste, W., & Townsend, E. (1997). Core concepts of occupational therapy. In E. Townsend (Ed.), *Enabling occupation: An occupational therapy perspective* (pp. 29–56). Ottawa, ON: Canadian Association of Occupational Therapists.

Lindsay, W. R., Fee, M., Michie, A., & Heap, I. (1994). The effects of cue control relaxation on adults with severe mental retardation. *Research in Developmental Disabilities, 15,* 425–437.

National Center for Complementary and Alternative Medicine. (2002). *What is complementary and alternative medicine?* Retrieved July 14, 2002, from http://www.nccam.nih.gov/health/whatiscam/

Pelletier, K. R., & Astin, J. A. (2002). Integration and reimbursement of complementary and alternative medicine by managed care and insurance providers: 2000 update and cohort analysis. *Alternative Therapies in Health and Medicine, 8*(1), 38–39, 42, 44.

Pelletier, K. R., Astin, J. A., & Haskell, W. L. (1999). Current trends in the integration and reimbursement of complementary and alternative medicine by managed care organizations (MCOs) and insurance providers: 1998 update and cohort analysis. *American Journal of Health Promotion, 4,* 125–133.

Scott, A. H. (1999). Wellness works: Community service health promotion groups led by occupational therapy students. *American Journal of Occupational Therapy, 53,* 566–574.

Wolsko, P. M., Eisenberg, D. M., Davis, R. B., Ettner, S. L., & Phillips, R. S. (2002). Insurance coverage, medical conditions, and visits to alternative medicine providers: Results of a national survey. *Archives of Internal Medicine, 162,* 281–287.

Additional Reading

Bausell, R. B., Lee, W. L., & Berman, B. M. (2001). Demographic and health-related correlates to visits to complementary and alternative medical providers. *Medical Care, 9,* 190–196.

Burkhardt, A., & Parker, J. (1998, November 26). OT perspective: Complementary care survey results. *OT Week, 12*(48), 4.

Carlson, J. (2003). *Complementary therapies and wellness: Practice essentials for holistic healthcare.* Upper Saddle River, NJ: Prentice Hall.

Eisenberg, D. M., Davis, R. B., Ettner, S. L., Appel, S., Wilkey, S., Van Rompay, M., et al. (1998). Trends in alternative medicine use in the United States, 1990–1997: Results of a follow-up national survey. *Journal of the American Medical Association, 280,* 1569–1575.

Eisenberg, D. M., Kessler, R. C., Van Rompay, M. I., Kaptchuk, T. J., Wilkey, S. A., Appel, S., et al. (2001). Perceptions about complementary therapies relative to conventional therapies among adults who use both: Results from a national survey. *Annals of Internal Medicine, 135,* 344–351.

Kaboli, P. J., Doebbeling, B. N., Saag, K. G., & Rosenthal, G. E. (2001). Use of complementary and alternative medicine by older patients with arthritis: A population-based study. *Arthritis and Rheumatology, 45,* 398–403.

Ni, H., Simile, C., & Hardy, A. M. (2002). Utilization of complementary and alternative medicine by United States adults: Results from the 1999 national health interview survey. *Med Care, 40,* 353–358.

Author

Terry Giese, MBA, OT/L, FAOTA

for

The Commission on Practice
Sara Jane Brayman, PhD, OTR/L, FAOTA, *Chairperson*

Adopted by the Representative Assembly 2005C217

Note: This document replaces the 2003 AOTA White Paper "Complementary and Alternative Medicine."

The Importance of Occupational Therapy Assistant Education to the Profession

The American Occupational Therapy Association (AOTA) recognizes the value, necessity, and viability of occupational therapy assistant (OTA) education at the associate degree and certificate levels. Occupational therapy assistants are collaborative partners in the profession's pursuit to achieve its *Centennial Vision*. OTA education provides a sound foundation for practice for the development of competent skill sets to fulfill various professional roles. These roles include direct client care, collaboration with all levels of practice, and advocacy in both traditional and non-traditional care settings.

Meeting the *Centennial Vision* relies on the profession to help enable people "to improve their physical and mental health, secure well-being, and enjoy higher quality of life" (AOTA, 2007, p. 613). OTA education provides the knowledge base for occupational therapy assistant practitioners to successfully provide occupation-based intervention across the life span and the skills to promote healthy occupational choices in the communities they serve. The collaboration of occupational therapists and occupational therapy assistants in service delivery ensures greater affordability and accessibility of occupational therapy services for all populations so that more of society's occupational needs can be met effectively.

In addition, meeting the *Centennial Vision* relies on the profession's ability to "ensure a diverse workforce for multiple roles" (AOTA, 2007, p. 613). OTA programs are designed to meet the needs of a diverse student body, which often are representative of the surrounding community in which the graduates ultimately become employed and serve. OTA graduates are poised to practice within the challenges of traditional and emerging areas of practice with an entrepreneurial spirit that further augments the *Centennial Vision* statement.

OTA education cultivates leadership and mentorship skills in students, preparing them to assume leadership roles within the profession and their communities. OTA education includes the dissemination of knowledge and development of skills needed for occupational therapy assistant practitioners to participate in research and scientific inquiry. Collaboration in research aids the profession in its efforts to be science-driven and promotes the wider use of evidence-based practice in traditional and emerging areas of practice.

The Commission on Education recognizes that OTA education adds an important and valued dimension to the provision of occupational therapy services. The Commission on Education is committed to the support of OTA education by seeking role clarification and promoting collaboration between associate degree/certificate and professional levels of education in occupational therapy to ensure the profession meets the *Centennial Vision* and society's occupational needs.

Reference

American Occupational Therapy Association. (2007). AOTA's *Centennial Vision* and executive summary. *American Journal of Occupational Therapy, 61,* 613–614.

Prepared by

Judith C. Blum, MS, OTR/L

Jennifer C. Coyne, COTA/L

Linda Orr, MPA, OTR/L

for

The Commission on Education
René Padilla, PhD, OTR/L, FAOTA, *Chairperson*

Adopted by the Representative Assembly 2008CC40

Note: This paper replaces the 2002 position paper *The Viability of Occupational Therapy Assistant Education.*

Copyright © 2008, by the American Occupational Therapy Association. Previously published in the *American Journal of Occupational Therapy, 62,* 705–706.

Obesity and Occupational Therapy

Obesity is a significant and wide-ranging health and social problem in the United States. Occupational therapy is a health care profession that is qualified to provide interventions with individuals, groups, and society to effect change to promote optimum health. Occupational therapy services are often used directly and indirectly to influence weight management and related health concerns through attention to lifestyle and engagement in fulfilling activities. The purpose of this paper is to explain to persons within and outside of the profession the role of occupational therapists and occupational therapy assistants[1] in addressing the impact of obesity on people's ability to engage in daily activities.

Overview of Domain and Process of Occupational Therapy

Since its founding, occupational therapy has been a healing profession whose practitioners "focus on assisting people to engage in daily life activities that they find meaningful and purposeful" (American Occupational Therapy Association [AOTA], 2002, p. 610). Occupational therapy practitioners[2] apply their knowledge about engagement in occupation—that is, "everyday life activity" (AOTA, 2002)—to help clients who may be experiencing disease, impairment, disability, dissatisfaction, or adverse circumstances to participate in their daily life in a manner that supports their health and well-being. By working with clients from this perspective, occupational therapy practitioners use everyday life activities therapeutically to improve the health and quality of life of consumers and to prevent future disease or illness. AOTA and its members are committed to improving individual quality of life; promoting community health; and supporting primary, secondary, and tertiary prevention for the management of obesity (AOTA, 2006a). This paper illustrates the growing dangers of the obesity epidemic on health and describes the specific and effective services provided by occupational therapy practitioners in a variety of practice settings for clients at risk for or experiencing the negative health effects of obesity throughout the life span. It also explains how the occupational therapy profession provides expertise and leadership in working with the problem of obesity in our society as it affects individuals, families, groups, and populations across the life span.

Background on the Issue of Obesity

Being *overweight* (defined as having a body mass index [BMI] of 25 to 30) or obese reduces the likelihood of a person's participation in physical activity, including leisure time activity (Trost, Owen, Bauman, Sallis, & Brown, 2002). Although only 9% of Americans believe that they have a weight problem (Lee & Oliver, 2002), an all-time high 30.9% of Americans today are considered clinically *obese*, defined by having a BMI of over 30 (Centers for Disease Control and Prevention [CDC], 2004). The prevalence of *severe obesity* (defined as being 100 pounds overweight or more) is rising substantially faster than obesity (Sturm, 2003). Risk for obesity is elevated for individuals who have disabilities, fewer years of education, or poorer

---

[1]*Occupational therapists* are responsible for all aspects of occupational therapy service delivery and are accountable for the safety and effectiveness of the occupational therapy service delivery process. *Occupational therapy assistants* deliver occupational therapy services under the supervision of and in partnership with an occupational therapist (AOTA, 2004).

[2]When the term *occupational therapy practitioner* is used in this document, it refers to both occupational therapists and occupational therapy assistants (AOTA, 2006b).

economic or job status, as well as for Latino and African American women (CDC, 2006; Cousins et al., 1992; Friedman & Brownell, 1996; Wardle, Waller, & Jarvis, 2002). A number of studies have demonstrated that obesity appears correlated with increased risk of both acute and chronic diseases, including type II diabetes, sleep apnea, chronic low back pain, hypertension, breast cancer, prostate cancer, colon cancer, cardiovascular disease, stroke, gall bladder disease, joint problems, activity limitations, reduced generalized health ratings, psychological issues, discrimination, and an increased mortality rate (Expert Panel on the Identification, Evaluation, and Treatment of Overweight in Adults, 1998). The related medical costs are estimated at $99.2 billion annually (Bungum, Satterwhite, Jackson, & Morrow, 2003). Equally troubling is that nearly one-third of children 6 to 19 years of age are considered at risk for overweight or are overweight (as defined in children as being at or above the 85th percentile of the sex-specific BMI-for-age growth chart), putting them at risk for a variety of these health-related concerns (Center for Health and Health Care in Schools, 2005). Societal issues—such as overexposure to junk food marketing; lack of safety in outdoor activities in lower income areas; steadily increasing food portion sizes; and the growing popularity of sedentary activities, including viewing television, playing seated video games, and using the computer— have contributed to the astonishing rise of overweight and obesity in childhood (Miller, Rosenbloom, & Silverstein, 2004). The prevalence of obesity in adults and overweight in children suggests no decline and remains a major public health concern (Hedley et al., 2004).

Job absenteeism, due directly or indirectly to obesity-related illness, results in costs as high as $25 billion per year (Bungum et al., 2003). In addition, obesity has been called the "last acceptable form of prejudice" (Chambliss, Finley, & Blair, 2004), often resulting in reduced education, housing, and employment opportunities (Puhl & Brownell, 2001); decreased access and use of health care and wellness services (Wallis, 2004); and restricted social participation due to negative portrayal in popular media (Greenberg, Eastin, Hofschire, Lachlan, & Brownell, 2003; Moloney, 2000). Such negative consequences can have a devastating impact on individuals throughout their life span, limiting their opportunities for or access to participation in their desired occupations.

Weight loss of as little as 5%–10% of initial body weight can result in significant improvements in measures of blood pressure, cholesterol levels, and glycemic control, as well as other improved health outcomes (Expert Panel, 1998; Fabricatore & Wadden, 2003; Manson, Skerrett, Greenland, & VanItallie, 2004). However, although long-term and appropriate weight loss has been shown to improve health conditions, short-term loss and rebounding with increased weight gain, inappropriate dieting methods, or extreme weight loss may have damaging effects. In the *Archives of Internal Medicine*, Manson et al. (2004) affirmed that the typical methods used by consumers who wish to lose weight consist of adhering to a short-term calorie-restricted diet, engaging in a "regular, not intense" or "irregularly active" exercise program, and/or a "quick fix" of fad diets or weight-loss drugs, followed by a return to unhealthy eating habits and a sedentary lifestyle (Heshka et al., 2003; Lowe, Miller-Kovach, Frye, & Phelan, 1999; Manson et al., 2004; Mokdad et al., 2001; Moloney, 2000; Puhn, 1996; Smith & Fremouw, 1987; Willet, 2001). With millions of Americans of all ages struggling—and failing—to achieve and maintain a healthy lifestyle using current methods for weight management, it is clear that health care consumers need to implement successful approaches to attaining effective and sustainable changes in lifestyle that influence weight and, more importantly, produce related improvements in overall health.

Occupational Therapy Role

Through their knowledge of psychosocial, physical, environmental, and spiritual factors, as well as cultural traditions and perspectives that influence performance, occupational therapy practitioners help consumers develop and implement an individualized, structured approach for lifestyle change. A randomized trial published in the *Journal of the American Medical Association* (Heshka et al., 2003) indicated that weight loss is more effectively achieved when a health care consumer is assisted through a structured program than when the client relies on self-help methods. Using their analysis and understanding of performance patterns related to daily life activities (Clark, 2000; Quiroga, 1995; Wilcock, 1998; Yerxa, 2002), occupational therapy practitioners provide interventions that are meaningful and effective and motivate participation by the client to modify daily life habits, roles, and patterns that contribute to the chronic condition of obesity.

When assessing needs, setting goals, and developing and implementing interventions, the occupational therapy practitioner works closely with the client in designing specific plans or programs to meet individual goals and desires in whatever areas of occupation(s) are affected by obesity. Occupational therapy intervention may focus on prevention, remediation/restoration, adaptation/compensation, and maintenance programs in either long-term or short-term settings.

Occupational therapy programs incorporate the client's personal preferences, circumstances, context, and needs into a customized healthy living regimen that takes into account any pre-existing medical conditions. These structured programs provide clients with an alternative that contrasts with the shortcomings of involvement in short-term programs, time-limited visits to spas and health centers, the feelings of deprivation associated with dieting, resistance to engaging in physical activity that one does not enjoy, and the lack of effectiveness of programs that do not emphasize participation in a variety of health-promoting elements beyond diet and exercise. Through education, strategies, and intervention planning, occupational therapy practitioners can help their clients build habits, which include engagement in health-promoting activities that allow them to maintain targeted changes that influence their weight within the complex dynamic of their everyday lives.

Occupational therapy interventions in the area of obesity may include but are not limited to the following: community programs of health promotion through lifestyle change; education programs; facilitating the development of new habits and routines; Lifestyle Redesign® programs; recommendation of home modifications; adaptations/equipment; compensatory training in ADL and IADL; wellness programs for children, teens, and adults; play and physical education in the schools; safe patient-handling programs in hospitals and skilled-nursing facilities; and postsurgical acute-care interventions. Occupational therapy practitioners are trained in the areas of adaptive equipment evaluation, home modification planning, task modification solutions, durable medical equipment considerations, compensatory strategies, caregiver training, and client resource development and advocacy (Foti, 2004, 2005). Therefore, occupational therapy practitioners also make an important contribution to the interdisciplinary practice of *bariatrics* (the medical investigation, prevention, and interventions for individuals with obesity that include diet and nutrition, exercise, behavior modification, lifestyle changes, and appropriate medications).

These and other occupational therapy services addressing obesity and related conditions may be covered by major health care payers, including Medicare, Medicaid, and private health insurance.

Conclusion

Occupational therapy addresses the prevention and concerns of obesity through a holistic and client-centered approach to lifestyle via participation in activities that promote health. Occupational therapy interventions not only facilitate weight loss but also enable clients to make a number of changes to performance in multiple areas of life, including incorporating appropriate productive and social activity as well as physical activity, to address obesity, thus improving health outcomes and maintaining long-term wellness.

References

American Occupational Therapy Association. (2002). Occupational therapy practice framework: Domain and process. *American Journal of Occupational Therapy, 56,* 609–639.

American Occupational Therapy Association. (2004). Guidelines for supervision, roles, and responsibilities during the delivery of occupational therapy services. *American Journal of Occupational Therapy, 58,* 663–667.

American Occupational Therapy Association. (2006a). *AOTA's statement on obesity* [Representative Assembly Coordinating Council (RACC) (2006C359)]. Retrieved August 24, 2006, from http://www.aota.org/members/area6/2006-ra/racc_B1b.pdf

American Occupational Therapy Association. (2006b). Policy 1.44: Categories of occupational therapy personnel. *American Journal of Occupational Therapy, 60,* 683–684.

Bungum, T., Satterwhite, M., Jackson, A. W., & Morrow, J. R. (2003). The relationship of body mass index, medical costs, and job absenteeism. *American Journal of Health Behavior, 27,* 456–462.

Center for Health and Health Care in Schools. (2005). *Childhood overweight: What the research tells us* (revised March 2005). Retrieved August 4, 2006, from http://www.healthinschools.org/sh/obesityfacts.asp

Centers for Disease Control and Prevention. (2004). Trends in intake of energy and macronutrients—United States, 1971–2000. *Morbidity and Mortality Weekly Report, 53(4),* 80–82.

Centers for Disease Control and Prevention. (2006). *People with disabilities are less healthy than those without disabilities* [Disability and Health State Chartbook, 2006—Profiles of Health for Adults with Disabilities (2006, September 12)]. Retrieved October 19, 2006, from http://www.cdc.gov/od/oc/Media/pressrel/r060912.htm

Chambliss, H. O., Finley, C. E., & Blair, S. N. (2004). Attitudes towards obese individuals among exercise science students. *Medicine and Science in Sports and Exercise, 36,* 468–474.

Clark, F. A. (2000). The concepts of habit and routine: A preliminary theoretical synthesis. *Occupational Therapy Journal of Research, 20*(Supplement 2000), 123–137.

Cousins, J. H., Rubovits, D. S., Dunn, J. K., Reeves, R. S., Ramirez, A. G., & Foreyt, J. P. (1992). Family versus individually oriented intervention for weight loss in Mexican American women. *Public Health Reports, 107,* 549–555.

Expert Panel on the Identification, Evaluation, and Treatment of Overweight in Adults. (1998). Clinical guidelines on the identification, evaluation, and treatment of overweight and obesity in adults. *American Journal of Clinical Nutrition, 68,* 899–917.

Fabricatore, A. N., & Wadden, T. A. (2003). Treatment of obesity: An overview. *Clinical Diabetes, 21(2),* 67–72.

Foti, D. (2004). Bariatric care: Practical problem solving and interventions. *Physical Disabilities Special Interest Section Quarterly, 27(4),* 1–3.

Foti, D. (2005). Caring for the person of size. *OT Practice, 10(2),* 9–14.

Friedman, M. A., & Brownell, K. D. (1996). A comprehensive treatment manual for the management of obesity. In V. Van Hasselt & M. Hersen (Eds.), *Sourcebook of psychological treatment manuals for adult disorders* (pp. 375–422). New York: Plenum.

Greenberg, B. S., Eastin, M., Hofschire, L., Lachlan, K., & Brownell, K. D. (2003). Portrayals of overweight and obese individuals on commercial television. *American Journal of Public Health, 93,* 1342–1348.

Hedley, A. A., Ogden, C. L., Johnson, C. L., Carroll, M. D., Curtin, L. R., & Flegal, K. M. (2004). Prevalence of overweight and obesity among U.S. children, adolescents, and adults, 1999–2002. *Journal of the American Medical Association, 291,* 2847–2850.

Heshka, S., Anderson, J. W., Atkinson, R. L., Greenway, F. L., Hill, J. O., Phinney, S. D., et al. (2003). Weight loss with self-help compared with a structured commercial program: A randomized trial. *Journal of the American Medical Association, 289,* 1792–1798.

Lee, T., & Oliver, J. E. (2002). *Public opinion and the politics of America's obesity epidemic.* Boston: Harvard University, John F. Kennedy School of Government, Research Working Papers Series.

Lowe, M. R., Miller-Kovach, K., Frye, N., & Phelan, S. (1999). An initial evaluation of a commercial weight loss program: Short-term effects on weight, eating behavior, and mood. *Obesity Research, 7*(1), 51–59.

Manson, J. E., Skerrett, P. J., Greenland, P., & VanItallie, T. B. (2004). The escalating pandemics of obesity and sedentary lifestyle: A call to action for clinicians. *Archives of Internal Medicine, 164,* 249–258.

Miller, J., Rosenbloom, A., & Silverstein, J. (2004). Childhood obesity. *Journal of Clinical Endocrinology and Metabolism, 89,* 4211–4218.

Mokdad, A. H., Bowman, B. A., Ford, E. S., Vinicor, F., Marks, J. S., & Koplan, J. P. (2001). The continuing epidemics of obesity and diabetes in the United States. *Journal of the American Medical Association, 286,* 1195–1200.

Moloney, M. (2000). Symposium on Obesity—Genes, drugs, and dietary treatment: Dietary treatments of obesity. *Proceedings of the Nutrition Society, 59,* 601–608.

Puhl, R., & Brownell, K. D. (2001). Bias, discrimination, and obesity. *Obesity Research, 9,* 788–805.

Puhn, A. (1996). *The 5-day miracle diet.* New York: Ballantine Books.

Quiroga, V. (1995). *Occupational therapy: The first 30 years, 1900–1930.* Bethesda, MD: AOTA Press.

Smith, M. E., & Fremouw, W. J. (1987). A realistic approach to treating obesity. *Clinical Psychology Review, 7,* 449–465.

Sturm, R. (2003). Increases in clinically severe obesity in the United States, 1986–2000. *Archives of Internal Medicine, 163,* 2146–2148.

Trost, S. G., Owen, N., Bauman, A. E., Sallis, J. F., & Brown, W. (2002). Correlates of adults' participation in physical activity: Review and update. *Medicine and Science in Sports and Exercise, 34,* 1996–2001.

Wallis, L. (2004). Overweight patients face prejudice in health care. *Nursing Standard, 18*(38), 6.

Wardle, J., Waller, J., & Jarvis, M. (2002). Sex differences in the association of socioeconomic status with obesity. *American Journal of Public Health, 92,* 1299–1304.

Wilcock, A. A. (1998). *An occupational perspective on health.* Thorofare, NJ: Slack.

Willet, W. C. (2001). *Eat, drink, and be healthy.* New York: Free Press.

Yerxa, E. J. (2002). Habits in context: A synthesis, with implications for research in occupational science. *OTJR: Occupation, Participation, and Health, 22,* 104–110.

Authors

Florence Clark, PhD, OTR/L, FAOTA
Faryl Saliman Reingold, MA, OTR/L
Katie Salles-Jordan, OTD, OTR/L

for

The Commission on Practice
Susanne Smith Roley, MS, OTR/L, FAOTA, *Chairperson*

Adopted by the Representative Assembly 2007C12

Occupational Therapy's Commitment to Nondiscrimination and Inclusion

The occupational therapy profession affirms the right of every individual to access and fully participate in society. This paper states the profession's stance on nondiscrimination and inclusion.

Nondiscrimination exists when we accept and treat all people equally. In doing so, we avoid differentiating between people because of biases or prejudices. The principle of equality as defined and supported in the core values of occupational therapy requires that "all individuals be perceived as having the same fundamental human rights and opportunities" (American Occupational Therapy Association [AOTA], 1993, p. 1085). We value individuals and respect their culture, ethnicity, race, age, religion, gender, sexual orientation, and capacities, consistent with the principles defined and described in the *Occupational Therapy Code of Ethics* (AOTA, 2005). Nondiscrimination is a necessary prerequisite for inclusion. *Inclusion* requires that we ensure not only that everyone is treated fairly and equitably but also that all individuals have the same opportunities to participate in the naturally occurring activities of society, such as attending social events, having access to public transportation, and participating in professional organizations. We also believe that when we do not discriminate against others and when we include all members of society in our daily lives, we reap the benefits of being with individuals who have different perspectives, opinions, and talents from our own.

We support nondiscrimination and inclusion throughout our profession. Our concerns are twofold—for the persons who receive occupational therapy services and for our professional colleagues. In professional practice, our evaluations and interventions are designed to facilitate our clients' engagement in occupations to support their health and participation in the various contexts and environments of their lives. This includes, but is not limited to, the individuals' cultural, personal, temporal, virtual, physical, and social contexts as described in the *Occupational Therapy Practice Framework* (AOTA, 2008). As occupational therapists and occupational therapy assistants, we assume a collaborative partnership with clients and their significant others to support the individual's right to self-direction.

We believe that inclusion is achieved through the combined efforts of clients, their families, and significant others; health, education, and social services professionals; legislators; community members; and others. We support all individuals and their significant others' rights to fully participate in making decisions that concern their daily occupations: activities of daily living, instrumental activities of daily living, rest and sleep, work, education, play, leisure, and social participation.

AOTA and its members recognize the legal mandates concerning nondiscriminatory practices. However, the concept of nondiscrimination is not limited to that which is dictated by law. This professional association, through its members, boards, commissions, committees, officers, and staff, supports the belief that all members of the occupational therapy professional community are entitled to maximum opportunities to develop and use their abilities. These individuals also have the right to achieve productive and satisfying professional and personal lives.

We are committed to nondiscrimination and inclusion as an affirmation of our belief that the interests of all members of the profession are best served when the inherent worth of every individual is recognized and valued. We maintain that society has an obligation to provide the reasonable accommodations neces-

341

sary to allow individuals access to social, educational, recreational, and vocational opportunities. By embracing the concepts of nondiscrimination and inclusion, we will all benefit from the opportunities afforded in a diverse society.

References

American Occupational Therapy Association. (1993). Core values and attitudes of occupational therapy practice. *American Journal of Occupational Therapy, 47,* 1085–1086.

American Occupational Therapy Association. (2005). Occupational therapy code of ethics. *American Journal of Occupational Therapy, 59,* 639–642.

American Occupational Therapy Association. (2008). Occupational therapy practice framework: Domain and process (2nd ed.). *American Journal of Occupational Therapy, 62,* 625–688.

Authors
Ruth H. Hansen, PhD, FAOTA
Jim Hinojosa, PhD, OT, FAOTA

for

The Commission on Practice
Mary Jane Youngstrom, MS, OTR, *Chairperson*

Adopted by the Representative Assembly 1999M4

Edited by the Commission on Practice 2004

Received by the Representative Assembly 2004C28

Edited by the Commission on Practice 2009

Note: This document replaces the 1995 Position Paper *Occupational Therapy: A Profession in Support of Full Inclusion,* the accompanying 1996 White Paper *The Role of the Occupational Therapy Practitioner in the Implementation of Full Inclusion,* and the 1999 and 2004 Position Paper *Occupational Therapy's Commitment to Nondiscrimination and Inclusion.*

Physical Agent Modalities: A Position Paper

The American Occupational Therapy Association (AOTA) asserts that physical agent modalities (PAMs) may be used by occupational therapists and occupational therapy assistants in preparation for or concurrently with purposeful and occupation-based activities or interventions that ultimately enhance engagement in occupation (AOTA, 2002, 2003). AOTA further stipulates that PAMs may be applied only by occupational therapists and occupational therapy assistants who have documented evidence of possessing the theoretical background and technical skills for safe and competent integration of the modality into an occupational therapy intervention plan (AOTA, 2003). The purpose of this paper is to clarify the appropriate context for use of PAMs in occupational therapy.

Physical agent modalities are those procedures and interventions that are systematically applied to modify specific client factors when neurological, musculoskeletal, or skin conditions are present that may be limiting occupational performance. PAMs use various forms of energy to modulate pain, modify tissue healing, increase tissue extensibility, modify skin and scar tissue, and decrease edema/inflammation. PAMs are used in preparation for or concurrently with purposeful and occupation-based activities (Bracciano, 2008).

Specific categories of physical agents include superficial thermal agents, deep thermal agents, and electrotherapeutic agents and mechanical devices.

- *Superficial thermal agents* include but are not limited to hydrotherapy/whirlpool, cryotherapy (cold packs, ice), Fluidotherapy,™ hot packs, paraffin, water, infrared, and other commercially available superficial heating and cooling technologies.

- *Deep thermal agents* include but are not limited to therapeutic ultrasound, phonophoresis, short-wave diathermy, and other commercially available technologies.

- *Electrotherapeutic agents* use electricity and the electromagnetic spectrum to facilitate tissue healing, improve muscle strength and endurance, decrease edema, modulate pain, decrease the inflammatory process, and modify the healing process. Electrotherapeutic agents include but are not limited to biofeedback, neuromuscular electrical stimulation (NMES), functional electrical stimulation (FES), transcutaneous electrical nerve stimulation (TENS), high-voltage galvanic stimulation for tissue and wound repair (ESTR), high-voltage pulsed current (HVPC), direct current (DC), iontophoresis, and other commercially available technologies (Bracciano, 2008).

- *Mechanical devices* include but are not limited to vasopneumatic devices and continuous passive motion (CPM).

PAMs are categorized as preparatory methods (AOTA, 2002) that also can be used concurrently with purposeful activity or during occupational engagement. Preparatory methods support and promote the acquisition of the performance skills necessary to enable an individual to resume or assume habits, routines, and roles for engagement in occupation.

The exclusive use of PAMs as a therapeutic intervention without application to occupational performance is not considered occupational therapy. When used, *PAMs are always integrated into a broader occupational therapy program* as a preparatory method for the therapeutic use of occupations or purposeful activities (AOTA, 2002).

Occupational therapists and occupational therapy assistants must have demonstrated and verifiable competence in order to use PAMs in occupational therapy practice. The foundational knowledge necessary for proper use of these modalities requires appropriate, documented professional education. Examples of professional education include continuing education courses, institutes at annual conferences, and accredited higher education courses or programs. Integration of PAMs in occupational therapy practice must include foundational education and training in biological and physical sciences. Modality-specific education consists of biophysiological, neurophysiological, and electrophysiological changes that occur as a result of the application of the selected modality. Education in the application of PAMs also must include indications, contraindications, and precautions; safe and efficacious administration of the modalities; and patient preparation including the process and outcomes of treatment (i.e., risks and benefits). Education should include essential elements related to documentation, including parameters of intervention, subjective and objective criteria, efficacy, and the relationship between the physical agent and occupational performance. Supervised use of the PAM should continue until service competency and professional judgment in selection, modification, and integration into an occupational therapy intervention plan is demonstrated and documented (AOTA, 2002).

The occupational therapist makes decisions and assumes responsibility for use of PAMs as part of the intervention plan. The occupational therapy assistant delivers occupational therapy services under the supervision of the occupational therapist. Services delivered by the occupational therapy assistant are selected and delegated by the occupational therapist (AOTA, 2004). When an occupational therapist delegates the use of a PAM to an occupational therapy assistant, both must comply with appropriate supervision and regulatory requirements and ensure that preparation, application, and documentation are based on service competency. That is, *only occupational therapists with service competency in this area may supervise the use of PAMs by occupational therapy assistants.*

The *Occupational Therapy Code of Ethics* (AOTA, 2005) mandates a safe and competent practice in the profession and provides guiding principles that must be applied to PAM use. Principle 4 states that "occupational therapy personnel shall achieve and continually maintain high standards of competence." Principle 4E states that "occupational therapy practitioners shall critically examine available evidence so they may perform their duties on the basis of accurate information," which obliges practitioners to maintain competency by involvement in lifelong learning. In addition, Principle 5 states that "occupational therapy personnel shall comply with laws and Association policies guiding the profession of occupational therapy" and requires practitioners to remain abreast of any revisions to rules, regulations, and laws as they relate to PAMs. All state laws and regulations related to PAM use have precedence over AOTA policies and positions.

References

American Occupational Therapy Association. (2002). Occupational therapy practice framework: Domain and process. *American Journal of Occupational Therapy, 56,* 609–639.

American Occupational Therapy Association. (2003). Physical agent modalities: A position paper. *American Journal of Occupational Therapy, 57,* 650–651.

American Occupational Therapy Association. (2004). Roles and responsibilities of the occupational therapist and the occupational therapy assistant during the delivery of occupational therapy services. *American Journal of Occupational Therapy, 58,* 663–667.

American Occupational Therapy Association. (2005). Occupational therapy code of ethics (2005). *American Journal of Occupational Therapy, 59,* 639–642.

Bracciano, A. G. (2008). *Physical agent modalities: Theory and application for the occupational therapist* (2nd ed.). Thorofare, NJ: Slack.

Authors
Scott D. McPhee, DrPH, OT, FAOTA
Alfred G. Bracciano, EdD, OTR, FAOTA
Barbara Winthrop Rose, OTR, CVE, CHT, FAOTA

for

The Commission on Practice
Sara Jane Brayman, PhD, OTR/L, FAOTA, *Chairperson*

Adopted by the Representative Assembly 2003M37

Edited by the Commission on Practice 2007

Psychosocial Aspects of Occupational Therapy

Introduction

Psychosocial dimensions of human performance are fundamental to all aspects of occupation and occupational therapy, with every client, and across all practice settings. *Occupation* is defined as "activities of everyday life, named, organized, and given meaning by individuals and a culture" (Law, Polatajko, Baptiste, & Townsend, 1979, p. 34). A key tenet of occupational therapy is that the loss of valued occupations may adversely affect an individual's sense of self and agency in the world. An individual's sense of self is influenced by the social, cultural, personal, psychological, and spiritual contexts in which these occupations occur (Kannenberg & Greene, 2003).

This position paper is intended for occupational therapists and occupational therapy assistants in practice, academic, research, advocacy, and administrative positions. Other audiences for this paper include regulatory boards, provider groups, policymaking bodies, accreditation agencies, professionals who may be seeking clarification about occupational therapy's scope of practice and domain of concern, and the general public.

Definition of *Psychosocial*

For the purposes of this paper, *psychosocial* is defined as pertaining to intrapersonal, interpersonal, and social experiences and interactions that influence occupational behavior and development (Mosey, 1996). While there is no one uniformly accepted definition of the term *psychosocial*, it is often used in a manner that includes psychological, cognitive, social, cultural, and spiritual aspects of occupation. Some key concepts in the psychosocial area of occupation include meaning, purpose, motivation, symbolic aspects of occupation, relationships, roles, and unconscious dynamics that may influence occupational behavior. Aspects of personality, temperament, energy, and drive also affect how people perform their meaningful daily life activities (AOTA, 2002).

The *International Classification of Function* and the *Occupational Therapy Practice Framework*

The *International Classification of Functioning, Disability, and Health (ICF)* was developed by the World Health Organization (WHO) to provide a taxonomic standard language and perspective within which to view functioning, disability, and health. The *ICF* defines health and health-related domains and defines functioning and disability as a dynamic interaction between health conditions and contexts, including personal and environmental factors (WHO, 2001). The *ICF* identifies interpersonal interactions, relationships, and social attitudes as factors that may have an impact on the outcome of various interventions and influence function (WHO, 2001). The *ICF* integrates medical and social models of health into a unified *biopsychosocial* model, which views health, disability, and function from a holistic perspective.

Similarly, the *Occupational Therapy Practice Framework: Domain and Process* was developed by the American Occupational Therapy Association (AOTA) to provide a unified framework within which to view occupational therapy (AOTA, 2002). The *Framework* defines the domain and process of occupational therapy. The domain of occupational therapy includes the personal, cultural, social, and spiritual contexts of a client's life that influence the meaning and the importance of the client's daily activities.

The process of occupational therapy is collaborative and client centered. An occupational therapist initiates the process by gathering information to develop an understanding of the client's history, experiences, values, interests, and capacities. Psychosocial factors influence how the therapist approaches the client, the nature of the therapeutic relationship, and the direction and the eventual outcomes of intervention.

Historical Perspectives

Psychosocial aspects of occupational therapy are grounded in the historical roots of the profession. Occupational therapy was founded by a diverse group of professionals concerned with the deleterious effects of inactivity on individuals. These founders envisioned occupational therapy as a holistic profession, focusing on the mind–body interrelationship and the importance of activities (or "doing") in helping those with both physical and psychological limitations in maintaining a positive life orientation (Mosey, 1996). They believed that humans brought to their occupations a complex mix of personal, physical, and psychological aspects and also were influenced by cultural, social, environmental, and political variables (Kielhofner, 1997). Today, occupational therapy remains a holistic profession, committed to assisting individuals and groups to engage in occupation to achieve and maintain full participation in society.

Education, Training, and Competencies

Occupational therapists and occupational therapy assistants are educationally prepared to address the psychosocial concerns of all their clients. The Accreditation Council for Occupational Therapy Education (ACOTE) standards for educational programs require content related to the psychosocial domain, including human development, knowledge, and understanding of normal and abnormal human behavior, as well as knowledge of how sociocultural diversity factors and lifestyle choices influence occupations (AOTA, 1999). Academic occupational therapy education programs typically provide education in the following areas:

- Therapeutic relationships

- Interviewing skills

- Administration of functional assessments

- Interpersonal and group dynamics

- Therapeutic group design and facilitation

- Program interventions in collaboration with clients, caregivers, and families

- Health promotion and wellness through engagement in meaningful occupations.

Occupational therapists and occupational therapy assistants who work in mental health practice settings may have additional knowledge and skills in areas such as psychiatric rehabilitation, supported employment, vocational rehabilitation, expressive therapy, substance abuse, and dual diagnosis treatment and prevention.

Service Provision

Individuals are referred to occupational therapy when they have experienced a disruption in their ability to take part in necessary and valued occupations. This disruption often elicits emotional and psychological responses, including denial, anger, fear, hopelessness, resistance to treatment, loneliness, sadness, grief, anxiety, and other responses. These issues transcend a specific diagnosis or practice setting and may not be the primary reason for the referral but must be understood and addressed if client-centered, meaning-ful, occupation-based outcomes are to be developed and met. Whether the individual is a teen with bi-polar disorder, a child with cerebral palsy, an adult with a spinal cord injury, or an elder with arthritis, psychosocial factors must be considered.

Occupational therapy services also may be offered to individuals and populations to support their engage-ment in meaningful occupation using wellness and health promotion models. When providing such serv-ices, occupational therapists and occupational therapy assistants must consider the psychosocial factors influencing engagement in the occupations. Examples of these services include a parenting group for adolescent mothers, a community living skills group for individuals residing in a homeless shelter, and a job-seeking skills program for teenagers.

Many occupational therapists and occupational therapy assistants work with individuals who have primary or significant diagnoses that negatively affect their ability to engage in occupations, including mental illness, substance abuse, traumatic brain injury, developmental disabilities, developmental delay, Alzheimer's disease, or dementia. Occupational therapists and occupational therapy assistants working with these individuals use psychiatric rehabilitation principles and techniques to help them set and achieve personally meaningful occupational goals. Examples include

- Teaching community mobility skills to an individual with a schizophrenic disorder,

- Training an individual with a major depressive disorder in effective strategies to manage stress,

- Collaborating with an individual diagnosed with substance abuse to establish alternative routines and habits that support a substance-free lifestyle,

- Training an individual with cognitive impairments to use simplified strategies to prepare meals, and

- Facilitating interaction skills so that a child with attention-deficit disorder may socialize appropriately with peers.

Occupational therapists and occupational therapy assistants work in hospitals, skilled nursing facilities, home health agencies, clinics, day treatment and partial hospitalization programs, schools, prisons, home-less shelters, vocational rehabilitation programs, independent living programs, and the community. In these and other settings, occupational therapy involves the process of evaluation, planning, intervention, and reevaluation to the remediation of occupational dysfunction (Crepeau, Cohn, & Schell, 2003). Occupational therapists and occupational therapy assistants function as program developers, program directors, independent living specialists, case managers, vocational specialists, consultants, and educa-tors, depending on the licensing and regulatory requirements of the state. Referrals to other mental health care professionals are made as needed for issues such as group and individual psychotherapy, medications, family therapy, and vocational training.

Case Vignettes

- A child with a feeding problem is evaluated by an occupational therapist. The teenage mother is insecure about her ability to feed the child and wants a feeding tube inserted. An intervention plan is developed that includes helping the mother to develop confidence in her abilities, identify learning needs, and master the necessary skills to feed her child.

- A child with a developmental disorder has difficulty following school routines, adapting to the chang-ing class schedule, and interacting with peers. The occupational therapist assesses the environment, adapts the child's routines, and consults with the teacher to help the child be more successful. She also meets with the teacher and the aide and identifies strategies for the child to be included in peer group activities. The child attends a weekly therapeutic play group led by an occupational therapy assistant.

- A teenage girl in high school is on probation for minor criminal offenses, has low academic achievement levels, and lacks any work experience or career goals. Additionally, she has a defiant attitude toward authority. The occupational therapist, in collaboration with other service providers, develops an intervention plan with the girl that includes completing high school; attending a life skills training program; seeking a part-time job; and developing community living skills, such as budgeting and money management. The occupational therapy assistant meets regularly with the girl to address the community living skills.

- An adult male with a spinal cord injury is angry and resentful about his disability status, fearful that he will not be able to function sexually, and unsure how he will support himself as a person with a disability. The occupational therapist and client collaborate to identify goals, which include addressing sexuality concerns related to function and initiating a vocational exploration. The occupational therapist also recommends that he seek counseling to help him adjust to his new situation.

- An adult female with a diagnosis of schizophrenia and substance abuse who attends a partial hospitalization program wants to complete her GED and live independently of her family. The occupational therapist completes the occupational profile, collaborates with the client to develop a recovery plan, and facilitates the client's enrollment for degree completion courses at a local adult school. The occupational therapy assistant teaches the client independent living skills, such as cooking and money management, under the supervision of the occupational therapist. The client also is referred to Alcoholics Anonymous and counseling to help her transition to independent living.

- An elderly male with arthritis, depression, and substance abuse is moved from independent living to a skilled nursing facility. In completing the occupational profile, the client identifies loss of valued roles and activities as problems. The occupational therapist collaborates with the client to identify activities of interest that are offered within the facility. The occupational therapist also introduces assistive devices that allow the client to resume a favorite hobby by compensating for his arthritic impairments and organizes a schedule of events that he can attend at the facility. The occupational therapist refers him to a community wellness program led by the occupational therapy assistant and also refers him to the on-site Alcoholics Anonymous meetings.

- An elderly woman with Alzheimer's disease becomes increasingly difficult to care for in her daughter's home. The occupational therapist consults with the daughter to identify adaptive strategies, including making the home safer for the client, developing a structured daily routine, and organizing shared responsibility for caregiving with other siblings. The occupational therapy assistant administers cognitive and functional assessments under the direction of the occupational therapist.

- Residents of a senior assisted-living facility from many different countries experience a sense of social isolation related to cultural and language differences. They also complain of too much unstructured leisure time. The occupational therapist evaluates the occupational needs of the residents in an initial focus group. Based on this needs assessment, the occupational therapist establishes a walking and light exercise group led by an occupational therapy assistant, organizes a monthly ethnic food potluck event, and develops a program that pairs residents with local high school students to present social events about their native cultures.

References

American Occupational Therapy Association. (1997). The psychosocial core of occupational therapy. *American Journal of Occupational Therapy, 51*, 868–869.

American Occupational Therapy Association. (1999). Standards for an accredited educational program for the occupational therapist. *American Journal of Occupational Therapy, 53*, 575–582.

American Occupational Therapy Association. (2002). Occupational therapy practice framework: Domain and process. *American Journal of Occupational Therapy, 56*, 609–639.

Crepeau, E., Cohn, E., & Schell, B. (2003). *Willard and Spackman's occupational therapy* (10th ed.). Philadelphia: Lippincott Williams & Wilkins.

Kannenberg, K., & Greene, S. (2003, June). Infusing occupation into practice: Valuing and supporting the psychosocial foundation of occupation (AOTA Continuing Education Article). *OT Practice, 8*(10), CE-1–CE-8.

Keilhofner, G. (Ed.). (1997). *Conceptual foundations of occupational therapy* (2nd ed.). Philadelphia: F. A. Davis.

Law, M., Polatajko, H., Baptiste, W., & Townsend, E. (1997). Core concepts of occupational therapy. In E. Townsend (Ed.), *Enabling occupation: An occupational therapy perspective* (pp. 29–56). Ottawa, ON: Canadian Association of Occupational Therapists.

Mosey, A. (1996). *Psychosocial components of occupational therapy.* Philadelphia: Lippincott-Raven.

World Health Organization. (2001). *International classification of functioning, disability, and health.* New York: Author.

Further Reading

Bruce, M., & Borg, B. (2002). *Psychosocial frames of reference for occupation-based practice* (3rd ed.). Thorofare, NJ: Slack.

Cara, E., & MacRae, A. (2004). *Psychosocial occupational therapy: A clinical practice* (2nd ed.). Albany, NY: Delmar.

Cole, M. (1998). *Group dynamics in occupational therapy* (2nd ed.). Thorofare, NJ: Slack.

Cottrell, R. (2000). *Proactive approaches in psychosocial occupational therapy.* Thorofare, NJ: Slack.

Creek, J. (Ed.). (1997). *Occupational therapy and mental health* (2nd ed.). New York: Churchill-Livingstone.

Fidler, G., & Velde, B. (1999). *Activities: Reality and symbol.* Thorofare, NJ: Slack.

Hellen, C. (1998). *Alzheimer's disease: Activity-focused care.* Boston: Butterworth-Heineman.

Hemphill-Pearson, B. (1999). *Assessments in occupational therapy mental health: An integrated approach.* Thorofare, NJ: Slack.

Ross, M., & Bachner, S. (1998). *Adults with developmental disabilities: Current approaches in occupational therapy.* Bethesda, MD: American Occupational Therapy Association.

Scott, A. (Ed.). (1998). *New frontiers in psychosocial occupational therapy.* New York: Haworth Press.

Author
Ruth Ramsey, MS, OTR/L

for

The Commission on Practice
Sara Jane Brayman, PhD, OTR/L, FAOTA, *Chairperson*

Adopted by the Representative Assembly 2004C25

Note: This replaces the 1997 document "The Psychosocial Core of Occupational Therapy" (previously published and copyrighted in 1997 by the *American Journal of Occupational Therapy, 51*, 868–869).

Scope of Practice

Statement of Purpose

The purpose of this document is to

A. Define the scope of practice in occupational therapy by

1. Delineating the domain of occupational therapy practice that directs the focus and actions of services provided by occupational therapists and occupational therapy assistants;

2. Delineating the dynamic process of occupational therapy evaluation and intervention services used to achieve outcomes that support the participation of clients in their everyday life activities (occupations);

3. Describing the education and certification requirements needed to practice as an occupational therapist and occupational therapy assistant;

B. Inform consumers, health care providers, educators, the community, funding agencies, payers, referral sources, and policymakers regarding the scope of occupational therapy.

Introduction

The occupational therapy scope of practice is based on the American Occupational Therapy Association (AOTA) document *Occupational Therapy Practice Framework: Domain and Process* (AOTA, 2008) and on the *Philosophical Base of Occupational Therapy*, which states that "the understanding and use of occupations shall be at the central core of occupational therapy practice, education, and research" (AOTA, 2006b, Policy 1.11). Occupational therapy is a dynamic and evolving profession that is responsive to consumer needs and to emerging knowledge and research.

This scope of practice document is designed to support and be used in conjunction with the *Definition of Occupational Therapy Practice for the Model Practice Act* (AOTA, 2004b). While this scope of practice document helps support state laws and regulations that govern the practice of occupational therapy, it does not supersede those existing laws and other regulatory requirements. Occupational therapists and occupational therapy assistants are required to abide by statutes and regulations when providing occupational therapy services. State laws and other regulatory requirements typically include statements about educational requirements to practice occupational therapy, procedures to practice occupational therapy legally within the defined area of jurisdiction, the definition and scope of occupational therapy practice, and supervision requirements.

It is the position of AOTA that a referral is not required for the provision of occupational therapy services and that "an occupational therapist accepts and responds to referrals in compliance with state laws or other regulatory requirements"(AOTA 2005a, Standard II.1, p. 664). State laws and other regulatory requirements should be viewed as minimum criteria to practice occupational therapy. Ethical guidelines that ensure safe and effective delivery of occupational therapy services to clients always influence occupational therapy practice (AOTA, 2005b). Policies of payers such as insurance companies also must be followed.

Occupational therapy services may be provided by two levels of practitioners—the occupational therapist and the occupational therapy assistant. Occupational therapists function as autonomous practitioners and are responsible for all aspects of occupational therapy service delivery and are accountable for the safety and effectiveness of the occupational therapy service delivery process.

The occupational therapy assistant delivers occupational therapy services under the supervision of and in partnership with the occupational therapist (AOTA, 2009). When the term *occupational therapy practitioner* is used in this document, it refers to both occupational therapists and occupational therapy assistants (AOTA, 2006a).

Definition of *Occupational Therapy*

AOTA's *Definition of Occupational Therapy for the Model Practice Act* defines *occupational therapy* as

> The therapeutic use of everyday life activities (occupations) with individuals or groups for the purpose of participation in roles and situations in home, school, workplace, community, and other settings. Occupational therapy services are provided for the purpose of promoting health and wellness and to those who have or are at risk for developing an illness, injury, disease, disorder, condition, impairment, disability, activity limitation, or participation restriction. Occupational therapy addresses the physical, cognitive, psychosocial, sensory, and other aspects of performance in a variety of contexts to support engagement in everyday life activities that affect health, well-being, and quality of life. (AOTA, 2004b)

Occupational Therapy Practice

Occupational therapists and occupational therapy assistants are experts at analyzing the performance skills and patterns necessary for people to engage in their everyday activities in the contexts and environments in which those activities and occupations occur. The practice of occupational therapy includes

A. Methods or strategies selected to direct the process of interventions, such as

1. Establishment, remediation, or restoration of a skill or ability that has not yet developed or is impaired.

2. Compensation, modification, or adaptation of activity or environment to enhance performance.

3. Maintenance and enhancement of capabilities without which performance in everyday life activities would decline.

4. Health promotion and wellness to enable or enhance performance in everyday life activities.

5. Prevention of barriers to performance, including disability prevention.

B. Evaluation of factors affecting activities of daily living (ADLs), instrumental activities of daily living (IADLs), education, work, play, leisure, and social participation, including

1. Client factors, including body functions (e.g., neuromuscular, sensory, visual, perceptual, cognitive) and body structures (e.g., cardiovascular, digestive, integumentary, genitourinary systems).

2. Habits, routines, roles, and behavior patterns.

3. Cultural, physical, environmental, social, and spiritual contexts and activity demands that affect performance.

4. Performance skills, including motor, process, and communication/interaction skills.

C. Interventions and procedures to promote or enhance safety and performance in activities of daily living (ADLs), instrumental activities of daily living (IADLs), education, work, play, leisure, and social participation, including

1. Therapeutic use of occupations, exercises, and activities.

2. Training in self-care, self-management, home management, and community / work reintegration.

3. Development, remediation, or compensation of physical, cognitive, neuromuscular, sensory functions, and behavioral skills.

4. Therapeutic use of self, including one's personality, insights, perceptions, and judgments, as part of the therapeutic process.

5. Education and training of individuals, including family members, caregivers, and others.

6. Care coordination, case management, and transition services.

7. Consultative services to groups, programs, organizations, or communities.

8. Modification of environments (e.g., home, work, school, community) and adaptation of processes, including the application of ergonomic principles.

9. Assessment, design, fabrication, application, fitting, and training in assistive technology, adaptive devices, and orthotic devices, and training in the use of prosthetic devices.

10. Assessment, recommendation, and training in techniques to enhance functional mobility, including wheelchair management.

11. Driver rehabilitation and community mobility.

12. Management of feeding, eating, and swallowing to enable eating and feeding performance.

13. Application of physical agent modalities and use of a range of specific therapeutic procedures (e.g., wound care management; techniques to enhance sensory, perceptual, and cognitive processing; manual therapy techniques) to enhance performance skills. (AOTA, 2004b)

Scope of Practice: Domain and Process

The scope of practice includes the domain (see Figure 1) and process (see Figure 2) of occupational therapy services. These two concepts are intertwined, with the *domain* defining the focus of occupational therapy and the *process* defining the delivery of occupational therapy (see Figure 3). The domain of occupational therapy is the everyday life activities (occupations) that people find meaningful and purposeful. Within this domain, occupational therapy services enable clients to engage (participate) in their everyday life activities in their desired roles, contexts and environments, and life situations. Clients may be individuals or persons, organizations or populations. The occupations in which clients engage occur throughout the life span and include

- ADLs (self-care activities);

- Education (activities to participate as a learner in a learning environment);

- IADLs (multistep activities to care for self and others, such as household management, financial management, and child care);

- Rest and sleep (activities relating to obtaining rest and sleep, including identifying need for rest and sleep, preparing for sleep, and participating in rest and sleep);

- Leisure (nonobligatory, discretionary, and intrinsically rewarding activities);

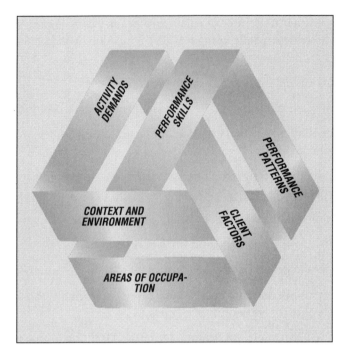

Figure 1. Occupational Therapy's Domain.
Supporting health and participation in life through engagement in
occupation (AOTA, 2008).

- Play (spontaneous and organized activities that promote pleasure, amusement, and diversion);

- Social participation (activities expected of individuals or individuals interacting with others); and

- Work (employment-related and volunteer activities).

Within their domain of practice, occupational therapists and occupational therapy assistants consider the repertoire of occupations in which the client engages the performance skills and patterns the client uses, the contexts and environments influencing engagement, the features and demands of the activity, and the client's body functions and structures. Occupational therapists and occupational therapy assistants use their knowledge and skills to help clients attain and resume daily life activities that support function and health throughout the lifespan. Participation in activities and occupations that are meaningful to the client involves emotional, psychosocial, cognitive, and physical aspects of performance. Participation in meaningful activities and occupations enhances health, well-being, and life satisfaction.

The domain of occupational therapy practice complements the World Health Organization's (WHO) conceptualization of participation and health articulated in the *International Classification of Functioning, Disability, and Health (ICF*; WHO, 2001). Occupational therapy incorporates the basic constructs of *ICF*, including environment, participation, activities, and body structures and functions, when addressing the complexity and richness of occupations and occupational engagement.

The process of occupational therapy refers to the delivery of services and includes evaluating, intervening, and targeting outcomes. Occupation remains central to the occupational therapy process. It is client-centered, involving collaboration with the client throughout each aspect of service delivery. During the evaluation, the therapist develops an occupational profile; analyzes the client's ability to carry out everyday life activities; and determines the client's occupational needs, problems, and priorities for intervention.

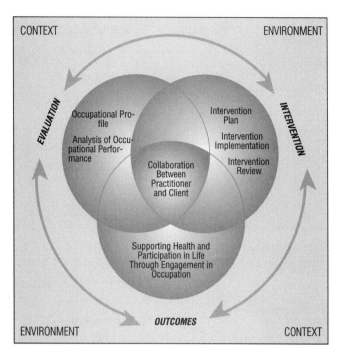

Figure 2. Occupational Therapy's Process.
Collaboration between the practitioner and the client is central to the
interactive nature of service delivery (AOTA, 2008).

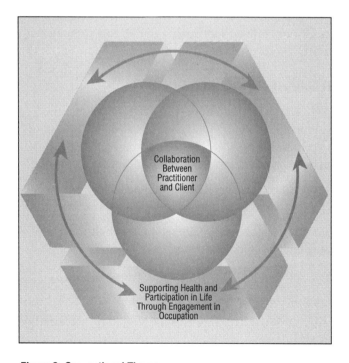

Figure 3. Occupational Therapy.
The domain and process are inextricably linked (AOTA, 2008).

Note: Mobius in figures 1 and 3 originally designed by Mark Dow. Used with permission.

AREAS OF OCCUPATION	CLIENT FACTORS	PERFORMANCE SKILLS	PERFORMANCE PATTERNS	CONTEXT AND ENVIRONMENT	ACTIVITY DEMANDS
Activities of Daily Living (ADL)* Instrumental Activities of Daily Living (IADL) Rest and Sleep Education Work Play Leisure Social Participation *Also referred to as *basic activities of daily living (BADL)* or *personal activities of daily living (PADL).*	Values, Beliefs, and Spirituality Body Functions Body Structures	Sensory Perceptual Skills Motor and Praxis Skills Emotional Regulation Skills Cognitive Skills Communication and Social Skills	Habits Routines Roles Rituals	Cultural Personal Physical Social Temporal Virtual	Objects Used and Their Properties Space Demands Social Demands Sequencing and Timing Required Actions Required Body Functions Required Body Structures

Figure 4. Aspects of Occupational Therapy's Domain.
All aspects of the domain transact to support engagement, participation, and health. This figure does not imply a hierarchy (AOTA, 2008).

Evaluation and intervention may address one or more aspects of the domain (see Figure 4) that influence occupational performance. Intervention includes planning and implementing occupational therapy services and involves therapeutic use of self, activities, and occupations, as well as consultation, education, and advocacy. The occupational therapist and occupational therapy assistant utilize occupation-based theories, frames of reference, evidence, and clinical reasoning to guide the intervention (AOTA, 2008).

The outcome of occupational therapy intervention is directed toward "supporting health and participation in life through engagement in occupations" (AOTA, 2008, p. 660). Outcomes of the intervention determine future actions with the client. Outcomes include the client's occupational performance, adaptation, health and wellness, participation, prevention, quality of life, role competence, self-advocacy, and occupational justice initiatives (AOTA, 2008, pp. 662–663).

Sites of Intervention and Areas of Focus

Occupational therapy services are provided to persons, organizations, and populations. People served come from all age groups. Practitioners work with individuals one to one, in organizations, or at the population level to address occupational needs and issues in mental health, work and industry, rehabilitation, disability and participation, productive aging, and health and wellness.

Along the continuum of service, occupational therapy services may be provided to clients throughout the life span in a variety of settings. The settings may include, but are not limited to, the following:

- Institutional settings (inpatient) (e.g., acute rehabilitation, psychiatric hospital, community and specialty-focused hospitals, nursing facilities, prisons)

- Outpatient settings (e.g., hospitals, clinics, medical and therapy offices)

- Home and community settings (e.g., home care, group homes, assisted living, schools, early intervention centers, day care centers, industry and business, hospice, sheltered workshops, transitional-living facilities, wellness and fitness centers, community mental health facilities)

- Research facilities.

Education and Certification Requirements

To practice as an occupational therapist, an individual

- Must have graduated from an occupational therapy program accredited by the Accreditation Council for Occupational Therapy Education (ACOTE®) or predecessor organizations,[1] and

- Must have successfully completed a period of supervised fieldwork experience required by the recognized educational institution where the applicant met the academic requirements of an educational program for occupational therapists that is accredited by ACOTE® or predecessor organization.

- Must have successfully passed the national certification examination for occupational therapists and/or met state requirements for licensure/registration.

To practice as an occupational therapy assistant, an individual

- Must have graduated from an occupational therapy assistant program accredited by ACOTE® or predecessor organizations, and

- Must have successfully completed a period of supervised fieldwork experience required by the recognized educational institution where the applicant met the academic requirements of an educational program for occupational therapy assistants that is accredited by ACOTE® or predecessor organizations.

- Must have successfully passed the national certification examination for occupational therapy assistants and/or met state requirements for licensure/registration.

AOTA supports licensure of qualified occupational therapists and occupational therapy assistants (AOTA, 2004a, Policy 5.3). State and other legislative or regulatory agencies may impose additional requirements to practice as occupational therapists and occupational therapy assistants in their area of jurisdiction.

References

Accreditation Council for Occupational Therapy Education. (2007a). Accreditation standards for a doctoral-degree-level educational program for the occupational therapist. *American Journal of Occupational Therapy, 61*, 641–651.

Accreditation Council for Occupational Therapy Education. (2007b). Accreditation standards for a master's-degree-level educational program for the occupational therapist. *American Journal of Occupational Therapy, 61*, 652–661.

Accreditation Council for Occupational Therapy Education. (2007c). Accreditation standards for an educational program for the occupational therapy assistant. *American Journal of Occupational Therapy, 61*, 662–671.

American Occupational Therapy Association. (2004a). Policy 5.3: Licensure. *Policy manual* (2008 ed., p. 64). Bethesda, MD: Author.

American Occupational Therapy Association. (2004b). Definition of occupational therapy practice for the AOTA Model Practice Act. (Available from the State Affairs Group, American Occupational Therapy Association, PO Box 31220, Bethesda, MD 20824-1220. E-mail: stpd@aota.org)

---

[1]Foreign-educated graduates of occupational therapy programs approved by the World Federation of Occupational therapy also may be eligible for certification/licensure as an occupational therapist provided that additional requirements are met.

[2]The majority of this information is taken from the *Accreditation Standards for a Doctoral-Degree-Level Educational Program for the Occupational Therapist* (ACOTE, 2007a), *Accreditation Standards for a Master's-Degree-Level Educational Program for the Occupational Therapist* (ACOTE, 2007b), and *Accreditation Standards for an Educational Program for the Occupational Therapy Assistant* (ACOTE, 2007c).

American Occupational Therapy Association. (2005a). Standards of practice for occupational therapy. *American Journal of Occupational Therapy, 59,* 663–665.

American Occupational Therapy Association. (2005b). Occupational therapy code of ethics (2005). *American Journal of Occupational Therapy, 54,* 614–616.

American Occupational Therapy Association. (2006a). Policy 1.44: Categories of occupational therapy personnel. In *Policy manual* (2008 ed., p. 10). Bethesda, MD: Author.

American Occupational Therapy Association. (2006b). Policy 1.11: The philosophical base of occupational therapy. In *Policy manual* (2008 ed., pp. 33–34). Bethesda, MD: Author.

American Occupational Therapy Association. (2008). Occupational therapy practice framework: Domain and process (2nd ed.). *American Journal of Occupational Therapy, 62,* 625–688.

American Occupational Therapy Association. (2009). Guidelines for supervision, roles, and responsibilities during the delivery of occupational therapy services. *American Journal of Occupational Therapy, 63.*

World Health Organization. (2001). *International classification of functioning, disability, and health (ICF).* Geneva, Switzerland: Author.

Additional Reading

Moyers, P., & Dale, L. (Eds.). (2007). *The guide to occupational therapy practice* (2nd ed.). Bethesda, MD: AOTA Press.

Authors

The Commission on Practice:
Sara Jane Brayman, PhD, OTR/L, FAOTA, *Chairperson, 2002–2005*
Gloria Frolek Clark, MS, OTR/L, FAOTA
Janet V. DeLany, DEd, OTR/L
Eileen R. Garza, PhD, OTR, ATP
Mary V. Radomski, MA, OTR/L, FAOTA
Ruth Ramsey, MS, OTR/L
Carol Siebert, MS, OTR/L
Kristi Voelkerding, BS, COTA/L
Patricia D. LaVesser, PhD, OTR/L, *SIS Liaison*
Lenna Aird, *ASD Liaison*
Deborah Lieberman, MHSA, OTR/L, FAOTA, *AOTA Headquarters Liaison*

for

The Commission on Practice
Sara Jane Brayman, PhD, OTR/L FAOTA, *Chairperson*

Adopted by the Representative Assembly 2004C23

Edited by the Commission on Practice 2005

Edited by the Commission on Practice 2009

This replaces the 2004 document Scope of Practice (previously published and copyrighted in 2004 by the *American Journal of Occupational Therapy 58,* 673–677).

Telerehabilitation

The purpose of this paper is to articulate the position of the American Occupational Therapy Association (AOTA) regarding the use of telerehabilitation technologies by occupational therapists and occupational therapy assistants.[1] Telerehabilitation is the clinical application of consultative, preventative, diagnostic, and therapeutic services via two-way interactive telecommunication technology.

The AOTA asserts that the same ethical and professional standards that apply to the traditional delivery of occupational therapy services also apply to the delivery of services received via telepractice. This document examines issues related to telerehabilitation and service provision, practitioner[2] qualifications, ethics, and reimbursement. Key terms related to telerehabilitation are defined in the Appendix. Occupational therapy practitioners are the intended audience for this document, although those who supervise or reimburse occupational therapy services also may find it helpful.

Service Provision

Over the past decade, computer and information technologies have become increasingly accessible and cost-effective as a means of providing educational and health care services. This has occurred simultaneously with an increased national emphasis on the quality of rural health care services, a focus on evidence-based outcomes, and a general increase in demand on practitioners' time and expertise. As a result, occupational therapy practitioners are initiating and participating in the use of telerehabilitation technology as a method of service delivery for (1) evaluation, (2) intervention, (3) consultation, (4) education, and (5) supervision of students and other personnel.

Telerehabilitation offers many new opportunities to provide occupational therapy services in alternative ways. Its effectiveness depends upon the specifics of the application, including the type and severity of disability, purpose of assessment, intervention goals, specifics of the technology, and infrastructure of both the local and remote sites. Current research and anecdotal reports regarding the use and efficacy of telepractice have yielded encouraging, but as yet inconclusive, preliminary findings. For the most part, research evidence cited in this document is specific to occupational therapy, though some studies related to the use of telecommunication and telerehabilitation technologies in allied health or medicine also are included, as appropriate.

---

[1] The *occupational therapist* is responsible for all aspects of occupational therapy service delivery and is accountable for the safety and effectiveness of the occupational therapy service delivery process. The *occupational therapy assistant* delivers occupational therapy services under the supervision of and in partnership with the occupational therapist (AOTA, 2004a).

[2] The term *practitioner* refers to an individual initially certified to practice as an occupational therapist or occupational therapy assistant or licensed or regulated by a state, district, commonwealth, or territory of the United States to practice as an occupational therapist or occupational therapy assistant and who has not had that certification, license, or regulation revoked due to disciplinary action (AOTA, 2004b).

Telerehabilitation for Evaluation

Cooper et al. (2002) and Shaw, Dreyer, Dreyer, and Wittman (2001) found that low-cost, "dial-up" methods of Internet connection may be effective for conducting interview assessments. Low-speed Internet connections also have been found to be adequate for observation of performance of daily living tasks (Shaw et al., 2001), overall assessment of sitting posture (Cooper et al., 2002), and collaboration regarding goal setting and intervention planning (Cooper et al., 2002). However, high-speed connections, specific assessment protocols, and clinicians experienced in the use of telerehabilitation technology are recommended for evaluations that require detailed observations of occupational performance or motor performance skills (Allegretti et al., 2004). Assessments conducted using telerehabilitation methods are often low cost for clients, particularly when they eliminate long-distance travel, but may be initially time-consuming for clinicians. Massman, Dodge, Fortman, Schwartz, and Solem (1999) suggest that as remote sites become more familiar with preparing clients for teleconsultations, telerehabilitation will become more efficient and cost-effective for clinicians and consumers.

Telerehabilitation in Intervention Planning, Implementation, and Follow-up Care

Research and documentation regarding the use of telerehabilitation methods for ongoing implementation of intervention is minimal at the time of this writing. Guilfoyle et al. (2003) investigated whether intervention plans developed following allied health (including occupational therapy) evaluation carried out via videoconferencing were comparable to those made following evaluations carried out face to face. Results indicated that despite the therapists' preference for working in person with their clients, intervention plans formulated via videoconferencing were reasonably similar to those formulated in face-to-face evaluation. Follow-up care conducted using telerehabilitation methods, including videophones and video-conferencing, has been managed successfully by medical personnel to address concerns such as pressure sores (Vesmarovich, Walker, Hauber, Temkin, & Burns, 1999), and by interdisciplinary teams to manage post-stroke care and rehabilitation for a client in a rural area (Clark, Dawson, Scheideman-Miller, & Post, 2002). No published studies or reports were found regarding the use of telerehabilitation methods for follow-up of specific occupational therapy services.

Telerehabilitation in Consultation

Wakeford (2002) documents the use of videoconferencing via a high-speed Internet connection to obtain consultation regarding specific areas of play performance for a young child with special needs. Cooper et al. (2002) describe the use of telerehabilitation methods to provide consultation regarding wheelchair mobility, and the Sister Kenny Institute in Minneapolis, Minnesota, routinely uses telerehabilitation technologies to provide consultation to a physical therapist in a remote clinic in American Samoa (White, 2003). As with evaluation, high-speed connections facilitate detailed observations, while low-speed connections or telecommunication methods other than computer based may be adequate for general observations, interviews, or other conversation-based collaboration.

Telerehabilitation in Education

Multi-point Internet videoconferencing has been used by the TelAbility Project (www.telability.org) in Chapel Hill, North Carolina, to provide evidence-based continuing education for physical and occupational therapy practitioners on topics such as constraint-induced movement therapy, music therapy interventions, and the use of specific standardized assessment tools in telerehabilitation. This was enhanced by the capability of the videoconferencing software to allow sharing of word-processing documents and videotaped case study information. Just as telerehabilitation methods may be used in consultative arenas that include practitioners and clients, those methods also may be used to support a continuing education model, particularly when interested parties are apart from one another and travel capabilities for clinicians are limited.

Telerehabilitation in Supervision of Students and Other Personnel

State licensure laws, institution-specific guidelines regarding supervision of occupational therapy students and personnel, the AOTA *Guidelines for Supervision, Roles, and Responsibilities During the Delivery of Occupational Therapy Services* (AOTA, 2004a), and the AOTA *Occupational Therapy Code of Ethics* (AOTA, 2000) must be followed, regardless of the method(s) of supervision chosen. However, the use of telecommunications technology may be used within those laws and guidelines as an adjunct to face-to-face methods, to support students and practitioners working in isolated or rural areas, and to allow students opportunities to pursue nontraditional fieldwork placements that cannot offer on-site supervision (Hubbard, 2000; Miller, Miller, Burton, Sprang, & Adams, 2003). At the time of this writing, there were no published studies regarding the use of telehealth technologies to provide supervision of occupational therapy assistants.

Practitioner Qualifications

Occupational therapy practitioners using telehealth technology as a method of service delivery should be competent in operating the system (hardware and software) or consistently have the support of technical assistance personnel. Practitioners also must have a working knowledge of the benefits and limitations of the technology, especially the interrelated issues of bandwidth and communication protocols across sites. Finally, practitioners should be competent in, and comfortable with, using on-camera skills that facilitate therapeutic and/or collaborative interactions. It is strongly recommended that occupational therapy practitioners using telerehabilitation as a method of service delivery develop their proficiency through various means, including, but not limited to, continuing education and on-site training by experts.

Ethical Issues

Client confidentiality can be a significant issue with the use of telerehabilitation interactions. Secure connections need to be established, and practitioners should seek the expertise of network professionals to ensure that firewalls are active or encryption techniques have been established with the connection. This is paramount with Internet-based connections, and assurances of compliance with the Health Insurance Portability and Accountability Act of 1996 (HIPAA) should be obtained. Consumers also should provide informed consent for the telerehabilitation service as well as be given the opportunity to refuse the service if they feel their safety or privacy will be compromised.

Billing and Reimbursement

Typically, occupational therapists and occupational therapy assistants using telehealth technologies to deliver services have relied on state and federal grants to support telerehabilitation projects. However, in some cases, practitioners have been able to negotiate fee-for-service with various third-party payers or, in some cases, private pay. A recent survey (Palsbo, 2004) conducted to assess current payment practices for telerehabilitation services by state Medicaid programs revealed that while most states reimburse *telemedicine* services (primarily provided by physicians and nurses), *telerehabilitation* (including occupational therapy, physical therapy, and speech–language therapy) is reimbursed in only four states (Hawaii, Louisiana, Minnesota, and Nebraska). The survey report did not indicate the frequency with which telerehabilitation services were billed or reimbursed in those states, nor the types of facilities or providers that were reimbursed. The report cited provider shortages in rural areas as the primary incentive for reimbursing telerehabilitation. Although Medicaid and other third-party payment are not yet widespread, they reflect a potential trend toward more routine reimbursement for telerehabilitation services.

Governmental Influences

State Regulations

Practitioners using telerehabilitation methods must comply with licensure laws and other state legislation regulating the practice of occupational therapy in the state or states in which those services are received. When telerehabilitation is used to provide individual client services (evaluation and intervention), the practitioner must be licensed in the state in which the client receives those services. The provision of consultation to another practitioner or continuing education content (e.g., workshop or seminar) using this technology may or may not be addressed by individual state regulations, and it is recommended that practitioners using the technology in these ways investigate those regulations to ensure compliance.

Federal Influence

In 1998, the National Institute on Disabilities and Rehabilitation Research established a Rehabilitation Engineering Research Center for Telerehabilitation, the purpose of which is to support research and development of rehabilitation consultation, assessment, monitoring, and intervention at a distance.

As of 2005, many of the Veterans Health Administration's (VHA) Veteran's Integrated Service Networks are using telerehabilitation technologies at VA Medical Centers and Health Care Systems, and the VHA's Rehabilitation Research and Development Service supports research to expand the use of telerehabilitation to address various rehabilitation health care issues (Veterans Health Administration, 2001, 2005).

Case Studies

Though there are a variety of methods and applications for telerehabilitation available within occupational therapy practice, the most common use currently occurs as consultation within the intervention process, with the intent of improving specific client outcomes. As noted in the literature cited in this document, the use of telehealth technology for the purposes of providing continuing education to practitioners and supervision to students and occupational therapy assistants shows promise, but is not yet well documented. The two cases presented here provide examples of the use of telerehabilitation for consultation to improve client outcomes.

Case 1: Margaret

Margaret lived in a rural area. She received occupational therapy services through a local hospital to address problems with occupational performance associated with right hemiparesis and painful, subluxed shoulder related to a recent stroke. The on-site (local) occupational therapist requested a tele-rehabilitation consult from a practitioner with specialized training in neurorehabilitation who practiced in a metropolitan hospital approximately 150 miles away. Margaret was evaluated via high-end video-conferencing equipment. During this 45-minute session, she and the local occupational therapist were asked to engage in several activities, which allowed the consulting occupational therapist to observe the effects of both limited range of motion and the presence of pain at the shoulder on occupational performance. The teleconsultation resulted in changes to the intervention plan (including the addition of a hemi-cuff sling and functional electrical stimulation to the shoulder) that advanced Margaret's progress toward her occupational performance goals.

Case 2: Rose

Rose is a charming, social 3½-year-old girl who was diagnosed with spastic quadriplegic cerebral palsy at birth. She received occupational therapy, physical therapy, speech–language therapy, and special education services at her preschool.

One of the concerns for which Rose's occupational therapist sought consultation was the potential for Rose to use powered mobility. The consulting site had professionals with expertise in this area but was located 150 miles away. Preliminary information, such as recent medical history and Rose's current levels of performance in play, self-care, communication, learning, and mobility, was sent in an organized format to the consulting site several days before the videoconference.

The consult question regarding the potential for using powered mobility led to a surprising outcome. One of the reasons the local therapists had asked the question was that Rose's family had minimal financial resources. Rose's family and therapists were concerned about using Rose's Medicaid or other financial resources to purchase a power wheelchair if she was not going to be able to use it. The therapists at the remote site agreed that Rose had good potential to use a power chair, then offered to loan a chair that was in their assistive technology inventory but not being used by anyone in their area. Arrangements were made to transport the chair to Rose's child care program, where she could work with her local therapists on learning to drive it. Although the chair required seating modifications and joystick adaptations and she needed practice, learning to use this chair gave Rose more options, specifically for joining friends in outdoor play, and in general for overall independence.

Summary

Though the use of telerehabilitation technologies is expanding quickly as a viable method of service delivery for many practitioners within the field of health care, there remain issues of efficacy, cost, reimbursement, legal and ethical ramifications, and practitioner competence. There is a significant need for occupational therapy practitioners to document, research, and publish on the efficacy of consultation, intervention, and follow-up services provided using telerehabilitation technologies. Further investigation of the use of telehealth technologies in professional development and supervision is needed to clarify effectiveness and efficiency, as demand for services, particularly in rural areas, threatens to exceed services available. Occupational therapy practitioners using telerehabilitation methods must adhere to the AOTA *Occupational Therapy Code of Ethics* (AOTA, 2000), maintain the AOTA *Standards of Practice* (AOTA, 2005), and comply with state regulations, ensuring both their proficiencies as practitioners and the well-being of their clients.

References

Allegretti, A., Fitzgerald, S., Schmeler, M., Cooper, R. A., Boninger, M. L., & Shapcott, N. (2004). Pelvic positioning evaluations for wheelchair selection: A comparison between in-person and video conferencing. In *Proceedings of the 20th International Seating Symposium* (pp. 215–216). Vancouver, Canada: RESNA.

American Occupational Therapy Association. (2000). Occupational therapy code of ethics. *American Journal of Occupational Therapy, 54,* 614–616.

American Occupational Therapy Association. (2002). Occupational therapy practice framework: Domain and process. *American Journal of Occupational Therapy, 56,* 609–639.

American Occupational Therapy Association. (2004a). Guidelines for supervision, roles, and responsibilities during the delivery of occupational therapy services. *American Journal of Occupational Therapy, 58,* 663–667.

American Occupational Therapy Association. (2004b). Policy 1.44: Categories of occupational therapy personnel. In *Policy manual* (2004 ed.). Bethesda, MD: Author.

American Occupational Therapy Association. (2005). *Standards of practice for occupational therapy* [draft]. (Available from the Practice Department, American Occupational Therapy Association, 4720 Montgomery Lane, Bethesda, MD 20814.)

Association of Telehealth Service Providers. (2004). *ATSP telemedicine glossary.* Retrieved January 23, 2004, from http://www.atsp.org/telemedicine/homepage.asp

Clark, P. G., Dawson, S. J., Scheideman-Miller, C., & Post, M. I. (2002). Telerehab: Stroke teletherapy and management using two-way interactive video. *Neurology Report, 26*, 87–93.

Cooper, R., Fitzgerald, S., Boninger, M. L., Cooper, R. A., Shapcott, N., Cohen, L., et al. (2002). Using telerehabilitation to aid in selecting a wheelchair. In R. Simpson (Ed.), *RESNA 2002 Annual Conference Proceedings* (pp. 245–247). Minneapolis, MN: RESNA Press.

Guilfoyle, C., Wootton, R., Hassall, S., Offer, J., Warren, M., & Smith, D. (2003). Preliminary experience of allied health assessments delivered face to face and by videoconference to a residential facility for elderly people. *Journal of Telemed Telecare, 9*, 230–233.

Hubbard, S. (2000, December 4 & 18). A case example of remote supervision. *OT Practice, 5*(24), 16–18.

Law, M., Polatajko, H., Baptiste, W., & Townsend, E. (1997). Core concepts of occupational therapy. In E. Townsend (Ed.), *Enabling occupation: An occupational therapy perspective* (pp. 29–56). Ottawa, ON: Canadian Association of Occupational Therapists.

Linkous, J. D. (2004). *Toward a rapidly evolving definition of telemedicine.* Retrieved January 22, 2004, from http://www.atmeda.org/news/definition.html

Massman, N. J., Dodge, J. D., Fortman, K. K., Schwartz, K. J., & Solem, L. D. (1999). Burns follow-up: An innovative application of telemedicine. *Journal of Telemedicine and Telecare, 5* (Suppl. 1), S52–S54.

Miller, T. W., Miller, J. M., Burton, D., Sprang, R., & Adams, J. (2003). Telehealth: A model for clinical supervision in allied health. *Internet Journal of Allied Health Sciences and Practice, 1*(2).

Palsbo, S. E. (2004). Medicaid payment for telerehabilitation. *Archives of Physical Medicine and Rehabilitation, 85*, 1188–1191.

Shaw, D. K., Dreyer, N. C., Dreyer, K. A., & Wittman, P. P. (2001). The efficacy of telemedicine in occupational therapy. *Journal of Allied Health, 30*(1), 39–42.

Vesmarovich, S., Walker, T., Hauber, R. P., Temkin, A., & Burns, R. (1999). Innovations in practice: Use of telerehabilitation to manage pressure ulcers in persons with spinal cord injuries. *Advances in Wound Care, 12*(5), 264–269.

Veterans Health Administration. (2001). *VA research: A foundation of veteran's health care. Annual report 2001.* Department of Veterans Affairs, Office of Research and Development. Retrieved March 23, 2005, from http://www1. va.gov/resdev/resources/pubs/docs/annrpt01.pdf

Veterans Health Administration. (2005). *VHA telerehabilitation overview.* Retrieved March 23, 2005, from http://www.va.gov/telehealth/Telerehabilitation/overview.asp

Wakeford, L. (2002, November 25). Using telehealth technology to provide services to children with special needs. *OT Practice, 7*(21), 12–16.

White, M. (2003, May). *Telerehabilitation: A primer for the OT practitioner.* Presented at the AOTA Annual Conference and Expo, Washington, DC.

Additional Resources

Canadian Occupational Therapy Association. http://www.caot.ca/

Journal of Telemedicine and Telecare. http://www.rsm.ac.uk/pub/jtt.htm

Rehabilitation Engineering Research Center (RERC) for Telerehabilitation. http://www.telerehab-nrh.org

Authors

Linn Wakeford, MS, OTR/L

Peggy P. Wittman, EdD, OTR/L, FAOTA

Matthew Wesley White, OTR/L

Mark R. Schmeler, MS, OTR/L, ATP

for

The Commission on Practice

Sara Jane Brayman, PhD, OTR/L, FAOTA, *Chairperson*

Adopted by the Representative Assembly 2005C241

Appendix: Definition of Terms

Bandwidth
The speed of a connection that determines the quality of the audio and visual connection.

Occupational Therapy
A profession that addresses engagement in occupations to support participation in context(s) (AOTA, 2002).

Occupations
"Activities of everyday life, named, organized, and given value and meaning by individuals and a culture" (Law, Polatajko, Baptiste, & Townsend, 1997, p. 34).

Plain Old Telephone System (POTS)
Standard analog home phone service, referred to as "dial-up" when Internet access is involved.

Protocol
In telepractice, a written document specifying standard operating policies and procedures for application of computer and information technologies to the delivery of services.

Telehealth
"The electronic provision of health care and information services for the direct benefit of individual patients and their families" (Association of Telehealth Service Providers, 2004).

Telehealth Technology
The hardware and software used in, as well as the overall process of, doing telemedicine and telerehabilitation.

Telemedicine
"The use of medical information exchanged from one site to another via electronic communications for the health and education of the patient or health care provider and for the purpose of improving patient care" (Linkous, 2004). *Note:* This is an older and more restrictive term than telehealth and implies delivery of physicians' services.

Telepractice
Service delivery characteristic of a particular profession, performed by means of telehealth technology rather than traditional face-to-face methods.

Telerehabilitation
The provision of rehabilitation services, such as occupational therapy, physical therapy, and speech–language therapy, using telehealth technology.

SECTION I.H.
Standards

Standards for Continuing Competence

AOTA's Standards for Continuing Competence

Continuing competence is a process involving the examination of current competence and the development of capacity for the future. It is a component of ongoing professional development and lifelong learning. Continuing competence is a dynamic, multidimensional process in which the occupational therapist and occupational therapy assistant develop and maintain the knowledge, performance skills, interpersonal abilities, critical reasoning, and ethical reasoning skills necessary to perform current and future roles and responsibilities within the profession.

Occupational therapists and occupational therapy assistants use these standards to assess, maintain, and document continuing competence. Basic to these standards is the belief that all occupational therapists and occupational therapy assistants share core values and knowledge guiding actions within their roles and responsibilities. The core of occupational therapy involves an understanding of occupation and purposeful activities and their influence on human performance. Occupational therapists and occupational therapy assistants have unique skills in activity analysis and activity synthesis and in critical and ethical reasoning. The profession is based on the values of client-centered holistic intervention and the right of an individual to be self-determining.

Standard 1. Knowledge

Occupational therapists and occupational therapy assistants shall demonstrate understanding and comprehension of the information required for the multiple roles and responsibilities they assume. The individual must demonstrate

- Mastery of the core of occupational therapy as it is applied in the multiple responsibilities assumed;

- Expertise associated with primary responsibilities;

- Integration of relevant evidence, literature, and epidemiological data related to primary responsibilities and to the consumer population(s) served; and

- Integration of current Association documents and legislative, legal, and regulatory issues into practice.

Standard 2. Critical Reasoning

Occupational therapists and occupational therapy assistants shall use reasoning processes to make sound judgments and decisions. The individual must demonstrate

- Deductive and inductive reasoning in making decisions specific to roles and responsibilities;

- Problem-solving skills necessary to carry out responsibilities;

- The ability to analyze occupational performance as influenced by environmental factors;

- The ability to reflect on one's own practice;

- Management and synthesis of information from a variety of sources in support of making decisions; and

- Application of evidence, research findings, and outcome data in making decisions.

Standard 3. Interpersonal Abilities

Occupational therapists and occupational therapy assistants shall develop and maintain their professional relationships with others within the context of their roles and responsibilities. The individual must demonstrate

- Use of effective communication methods that match the abilities, personal factors, learning styles, and therapeutic needs of consumers and others;

- Effective interaction with people from diverse backgrounds;

- Use of feedback from consumers, families, supervisors, and colleagues to modify one's professional behavior;

- Collaboration with consumers, families, and professionals to attain optimal consumer outcomes; and

- The ability to develop and sustain team relationships to meet identified outcomes.

Standard 4. Performance Skills

Occupational therapists and occupational therapy assistants shall demonstrate the expertise, aptitudes, proficiencies, and abilities to competently fulfill their roles and responsibilities. The individual must demonstrate expertise in

- Practice grounded in the core of occupational therapy;

- The therapeutic use of self, the therapeutic use of occupations and activities, the consultation process, and the education process to bring about change;

- Integrating current practice techniques and technologies;

- Updating performance based on current research and literature; and

- Quality improvement processes that prevent practice error and maximize client outcomes.

Standard 5. Ethical Reasoning

Occupational therapists and occupational therapy assistants shall identify, analyze, and clarify ethical issues or dilemmas to make responsible decisions within the changing context of their roles and responsibilities. The individual must demonstrate

- Understanding and adherence to the profession's *Code of Ethics,* other relevant codes of ethics, and applicable laws and regulations;

- The use of ethical principles and the profession's core values to understand complex situations; and

- The integrity to make and defend decisions based on ethical reasoning.

Authors

The Commission on Continuing Competence and Professional Development

Penelope Moyers, EdD, OTR/L, BCMH, FAOTA, *Chairperson*

Jane Case-Smith, EdD, OT/L, BCP, FAOTA

Mary Kay Currie, OT, BCPR

Coralie H. Glantz, OT/L, BCG, FAOTA

Jim Hinojosa, OT, PhD, BCP, FAOTA

Maria Elena E. Louch, OT/L, *AOTA Headquarters Liaison*

for

The Commission on Continuing Competence and Professional Development

Penelope Moyers, EdD, OTR/L, FAOTA, *Chairperson*

Adopted by the Representative Assembly 2005C243

Edited 2006

This document replaces the 1999 document *Standards for Continuing Competence* (*American Journal of Occupational Therapy, 53,* 559–560).

Standards of Practice for Occupational Therapy

Preface

This document defines minimum standards for the practice of occupational therapy. The *Standards of Practice for Occupational Therapy* are requirements for occupational therapists and occupational therapy assistants for the delivery of occupational therapy services. *The Reference Manual of Official Documents* contains documents that clarify and support occupational therapy practice (American Occupational Therapy Association [AOTA], 2004). These documents are reviewed and updated on an ongoing basis for their applicability.

Education, Examination, and Licensure Requirements

All occupational therapists and occupational therapy assistants must practice under federal and state law.

To practice as an occupational therapist, the individual trained in the United States

- Has graduated from an occupational therapy program accredited by the Accreditation Council for Occupational Therapy Education (ACOTE) or predecessor organizations;

- Has successfully completed a period of supervised fieldwork experience required by the recognized educational institution where the applicant met the academic requirements of an educational program for occupational therapists that is accredited by ACOTE or predecessor organizations;

- Has passed a nationally recognized entry-level examination for occupational therapists; and

- Fulfills state requirements for licensure, certification, or registration.

To practice as an occupational therapy assistant, the individual trained in the United States

- Has graduated from an associate- or certificate-level occupational therapy assistant program accredited by ACOTE or predecessor organizations;

- Has successfully completed a period of supervised fieldwork experience required by the recognized educational institution where the applicant met the academic requirements of an educational program for occupational therapy assistants that is accredited by ACOTE or predecessor organizations;

- Has passed a nationally recognized entry-level examination for occupational therapy assistants; and

- Fulfills state requirements for licensure, certification, or registration.

Definitions

Assessment
Specific tools or instruments that are used during the evaluation process.

Client
A person, group, program, organization, or community for whom the occupational therapy practitioner is providing services.

Evaluation
The process of obtaining and interpreting data necessary for intervention. This includes planning for and documenting the evaluation process and results.

Screening
Obtaining and reviewing data relevant to a potential client to determine the need for further evaluation and intervention.

Standard I: Professional Standing and Responsibility

1. An occupational therapy practitioner (occupational therapist or occupational therapy assistant) delivers occupational therapy services that reflect the philosophical base of occupational therapy and are consistent with the established principles and concepts of theory and practice.

2. An occupational therapy practitioner is knowledgeable about and delivers occupational therapy services in accordance with AOTA standards, policies, and guidelines and state and federal requirements relevant to practice and service delivery.

3. An occupational therapy practitioner maintains current licensure, registration, or certification as required by law or regulation.

4. An occupational therapy practitioner abides by the AOTA *Occupational Therapy Code of Ethics* (AOTA, 2000).

5. An occupational therapy practitioner abides by the AOTA *Standards for Continuing Competence* (AOTA, 1999) by establishing, maintaining, and updating professional performance, knowledge, and skills.

6. An occupational therapist is responsible for all aspects of occupational therapy service delivery and is accountable for the safety and effectiveness of the occupational therapy service delivery process.

7. An occupational therapy assistant is responsible for providing safe and effective occupational therapy services under the supervision of and in partnership with the occupational therapist and in accordance with laws or regulations and AOTA documents.

8. An occupational therapy practitioner maintains current knowledge of legislative, political, social, cultural, and reimbursement issues that affect clients and the practice of occupational therapy.

9. An occupational therapy practitioner is knowledgeable about evidence-based research and applies it ethically and appropriately to the occupational therapy process.

Standard II: Screening, Evaluation, and Re-evaluation

1. An occupational therapist accepts and responds to referrals in compliance with state laws or other regulatory requirements.

2. An occupational therapist, in collaboration with the client, evaluates the client's ability to participate in daily life activities by considering the client's capacities, the activities, and the environments in which these activities occur.

3. An occupational therapist initiates and directs the screening, evaluation, and re-evaluation process and analyzes and interprets the data in accordance with law, regulatory requirements, and AOTA documents.

4. An occupational therapy assistant contributes to the screening, evaluation, and re-evaluation process by implementing delegated assessments and by providing verbal and written reports of observations and client capacities to the occupational therapist in accordance with law, regulatory requirements, and AOTA documents.

5. An occupational therapy practitioner follows defined protocols when standardized assessments are used.

6. An occupational therapist completes and documents occupational therapy evaluation results. An occupational therapy assistant contributes to the documentation of evaluation results. An occupational therapy practitioner abides by the time frames, formats, and standards established by practice settings, government agencies, external accreditation programs, payers, and AOTA documents.

7. An occupational therapy practitioner communicates screening, evaluation, and re-evaluation results within the boundaries of client confidentiality to the appropriate person, group, or organization.

8. An occupational therapist recommends additional consultations or refers clients to appropriate resources when the needs of the client can best be served by the expertise of other professionals or services.

9. An occupational therapy practitioner educates current and potential referral sources about the scope of occupational therapy services and the process of initiating occupational therapy services.

Standard III: Intervention

1. An occupational therapist has overall responsibility for the development, documentation, and implementation of the occupational therapy intervention based on the evaluation, client goals, current best evidence, and clinical reasoning.

2. An occupational therapist ensures that the intervention plan is documented within the time frames, formats, and standards established by the practice settings, agencies, external accreditation programs, and payers.

3. An occupational therapy assistant selects, implements, and makes modifications to therapeutic activities and interventions that are consistent with the occupational therapy assistant's demonstrated competency and delegated responsibilities, the intervention plan, and requirements of the practice setting.

4. An occupational therapy practitioner reviews the intervention plan with the client and appropriate others regarding the rationale, safety issues, and relative benefits and risks of the planned interventions.

5. An occupational therapist modifies the intervention plan throughout the intervention process and documents changes in the client's needs, goals, and performance.

6. An occupational therapy assistant contributes to the modification of the intervention plan by exchanging information with and providing documentation to the occupational therapist about the client's responses to and communications throughout the intervention.

7. An occupational therapy practitioner documents the occupational therapy services provided within the time frames, formats, and standards established by the practice settings, agencies, external accreditation programs, payers, and AOTA documents.

Standard IV: Outcomes

1. An occupational therapist is responsible for selecting, measuring, documenting, and interpreting expected or achieved outcomes that are related to the client's ability to engage in occupations.

2. An occupational therapist is responsible for documenting changes in the client's performance and capacities and for discontinuing services when the client has achieved identified goals, reached maximum benefit, or does not desire to continue services.

3. An occupational therapist prepares and implements a discontinuation plan or transition plan based on the client's needs, goals, performance, and appropriate follow-up resources.

4. An occupational therapy assistant contributes to the discontinuation or transition plan by providing information and documentation to the supervising occupational therapist related to the client's needs, goals, performance, and appropriate follow-up resources.

5. An occupational therapy practitioner facilitates the transition process in collaboration with the client; family members; significant others; team; and community resources and individuals, when appropriate.

6. An occupational therapist is responsible for evaluating the safety and effectiveness of the occupational therapy processes and interventions within the practice setting.

7. An occupational therapy assistant contributes to evaluating the safety and effectiveness of the occupational therapy processes and interventions within the practice setting.

References

American Occupational Therapy Association. (1999). Standards for continuing competence. *American Journal of Occupational Therapy, 53,* 599–600.

American Occupational Therapy Association. (2000). Occupational therapy code of ethics (2000). *American Journal of Occupational Therapy, 54,* 614–616.

American Occupational Therapy Association. (2004). *The reference manual of the official documents of the American Occupational Therapy Association* (10th ed.). Bethesda, MD: Author.

Authors
The Commission on Practice
Sara Jane Brayman, PhD, OTR/L, FAOTA, *Chairperson*
Susanne Smith Roley, MS, OTR/L, FAOTA, *Chairperson-Elect*
Gloria Frolek Clark, MS, OTR/L, FAOTA
Janet V. DeLany, DEd, MSA, OTR/L, FAOTA
Eileen R. Garza, PhD, OTR, ATP
Mary V. Radomski, MA, OTR/L, FAOTA
Ruth Ramsey, MS, OTR/L
Carol Siebert, MS, OTR/L
Kristi Voelkerding, BS, COTA/L
Lenna Aird, COTA/L, *ASD Liaison*
Patricia D. LaVesser, PhD, OTR/L, *SIS Liaison*
Deborah Lieberman, MHSA, OTR/L, FAOTA, *AOTA Headquarters Liaison*

for

The Commission on Practice
Sara Jane Brayman, PhD, OTR/L, FAOTA, *Chairperson*

Adopted by the Representative Assembly 2005C218

Note: This document replaces the 1998 *Standards of Practice for Occupational Therapy*. These standards are intended as recommended guidelines to assist occupational therapy practitioners in the provision of occupational therapy services. These standards serve as a minimum standard for occupational therapy practice and are applicable to all individual populations and the programs in which these individuals are served.

SECTION I.I.
Statements

Academic Terminal Degree

Although there are doctoral-degree programs in occupational therapy and occupational science, currently it is customary for occupational therapy faculty to have a doctorate in related areas of science or social science, including but not limited to education, neuroscience, public health, psychology, policy, law, or sociology. Thus, a degree in any of these areas would be considered a terminal degree for occupational therapists in academia.

Prepared by

René Padilla, PhD, OTR/L, FAOTA

for

The Commission on Education
René Padilla, PhD, OTR/L, FAOTA, *Chairperson*

This replaces the 2003 document "Academic Terminal Degree" (*American Journal of Occupational Therapy, 58,* 648).

Adopted by the Representative Assembly 2008C4

Driving and Community Mobility

The purpose of this paper is to describe occupational therapy's contribution to driving and community mobility to practitioners within the profession and referral sources outside of the occupational therapy profession.

Community mobility, an instrumental activity of daily living (IADL), is defined as "moving self in the community and using public or private transportation, such as driving, or accessing buses, taxi cabs, or other public transportation systems" (American Occupational Therapy Association [AOTA], 2002, p. 620). Community mobility or transportation is essential for independence and access to engagement in other everyday life activities (occupations). Community mobility, specifically driving, contributes to quality of life (U.S. Department of Transportation, 2003b), autonomy (Hunt, 1993), fulfillment of life roles (Cox, Fox, & Irwin, 1988), access to leisure pursuits (Cobb & Coughlin, 1997), and engagement in other meaningful activities (Gillins, 1990). Loss of the fundamental role of driving and community mobility in adult life is exemplified by the feelings of loneliness, isolation, and depressive symptoms that often arise when one suddenly loses the ability to drive (Marottoli et al., 1997).

Driving and community mobility are included within the domain of occupational therapy (AOTA, 2002) and in the profession's *Scope of Practice* (AOTA, 2004b). Appendix A illustrates some of the aspects of driving and community mobility within the domain of occupational therapy practice and describes the complexity and influence of this critical IADL.

Service Provision

Populations Served

Occupational therapists and occupational therapy assistants address driving and other aspects of community mobility with clients of all ages. Intervention may address the following:

- Passenger safety by helping individuals access and ride safely in vehicles (e.g., designing mechanisms to assist children with disabilities get on and off the school bus, securing wheelchairs or car seats)

- Community mobility, including walking, biking, and riding as a passenger in a motor vehicle or on mass transit, to enhance independence and prevent injury

- Evaluation, education, and training of persons with learning disabilities, attention disorders, developmental disabilities, and acquired disabilities, such as brain injuries and amputations, in preparation of acquiring a first driver's license

- Evaluation and training of experienced drivers who have impairments or age-related changes that interfere with driving and community mobility

- Exploration of alternative transportation options with older adults and drivers of other ages who must temporarily abstain or retire from driving

- In addition to assisting individuals in engaging in driving and community mobility, occupational therapists and occupational therapy assistants work with communities, agencies, and groups to facilitate successful participation of all individuals. Efforts with community planners, school systems, governmental agencies, aging agencies, transit companies, community businesses, and health care organizations raise awareness of driving and community mobility issues and foster the implementation of alternatives to increase participation throughout the community by all community members.

Knowledge and Skill of Occupational Therapy Practitioners in Driving and Community Mobility

All occupational therapists and occupational therapy assistants possess the education and training necessary to address driving and community mobility as an IADL. Throughout the evaluation and intervention process, all practitioners recognize the impact of clients' aging, disability, or risk factors on driving and community mobility. Through the use of clinical reasoning skills, practitioners use information about client strengths and weaknesses in performance skills, performance patterns, contexts, and client factors to deduce potential difficulties with occupational performance in driving and community mobility.

Some occupational therapy practitioners specialize in driver rehabilitation and community mobility. These occupational therapists and occupational therapy assistants administer assessments specific to the requirements involved in driving and community mobility, including clinical assessments of vision, cognition, motor performance, reaction time, knowledge of traffic rules, and behind-the-wheel assessment of driving skills. They have additional training and expertise that enable them to recommend vehicle modifications and provide driver retraining. Many states require that occupational therapy driver rehabilitation specialists become licensed as professional driving instructors to be able to serve novice drivers or persons whose driver licenses have expired. AOTA asserts that occupational therapists and occupational therapy assistants require additional specialized training in driver rehabilitation prior to working directly in the area of driver assessment and intervention with clients who have health- or aging-related concerns.

Occupational therapists addressing community mobility assess clients as well as their communities to determine the client's ability to access transportation alternatives and utilize available resources and equipment. Individual assessments may include clinical testing similar to those in the area of driver rehabilitation. However, the focus of assessment is to determine the client's ability to access and utilize transportation resources. Assessment of the community context may involve analysis of the community resources available, location of supplemental agencies, accessibility of transportation alternatives, and policy review.

The nature of evaluation and intervention are different based on the role of the occupational therapist and the occupational therapy assistant. Consistent with the AOTA supervision guidelines (AOTA, 2004a), the occupational therapist carries the overall responsibility for the evaluation and intervention process. While the occupational therapist oversees the evaluation process, specific assessments may be delegated to the occupational therapy assistant if the occupational therapy assistant has demonstrated competency in administration of the individual assessment. The occupational therapist may delegate, on an individual client basis, any of the assessments in the driving evaluation, including clinic-based tests of vision, cognition, and motor performance or the behind-the-wheel assessment. The occupational therapist is responsible for interpreting the results of any assessments administered by the occupational therapy assistant and incorporating the results into the analysis of the entire evaluation. The occupational therapist also may delegate to the occupational therapy assistant the responsibility of implementing the intervention in accordance with the occupational therapist's plan and the client's treatment goals (AOTA, 2004a). The *Guidelines for Supervision, Roles, and Responsibilities During the Delivery of Occupational Therapy Services* (AOTA, 2004a) recommend that the occupational therapist and the occupational therapy assistant develop a collaborative plan for supervision which would be put into action during assessments and the intervention process. The supervision must follow state and federal regulations, as well as the policies of the workplace and the *Occupational Therapy Code of Ethics* (AOTA, 2000).

Both federal and state laws, as well as the activities of key professional organizations, influence delivery of and payment for occupational therapy services related to driving and community mobility. In the United States, the individual receiving services most often pays for driver evaluation and intervention. In general, specialized driver rehabilitation services are not currently considered covered services under Medicare benefits; however, there are a limited but growing number of states in which the Medicare carriers will reimburse for all or part of driver rehabilitation services. The Veterans Administration system provides driver rehabilitation services to veterans at select locations nationwide. State vocational agencies, Medicaid, workers' compensation, and private insurers may cover driver rehabilitation services and vehicle modification. See Appendix B for a summary of external influences on service delivery.

Case Studies

The following case studies illustrate the ways in which occupational therapists and occupational therapy assistants contribute to driving and community mobility in a variety of practice settings.

Rehabilitation Clinical Setting With Client-Centered Goal to Return to Driving

During the occupational therapy evaluation, a 78-year-old gentleman, Mr. Smith, expresses a desire to return to driving. Prior to a mild stroke that resulted in a fall and a right ankle fracture, Mr. Smith lived alone and needed his car for grocery shopping, access to medical appointments, transportation to his favorite fishing location, and visits with friends at the community clubhouse. The occupational therapist identifies residual impairments that are likely to be permanent in ankle mobility, affecting Mr. Smith's driving ability and safety. The occupational therapist communicates her concern about Mr. Smith's driving to the physician and recommends a driving evaluation. Throughout the therapeutic process, the therapist educates Mr. Smith regarding the impact of a right ankle fracture on driving performance safety and the need to participate in a thorough driving evaluation before driving again. Mr. Smith and the occupational therapist collaborate to identify options for alternative transportation until it is determined that Mr. Smith can safely resume driving.

Prior to discharge, the therapist makes a referral for a comprehensive driving evaluation. An occupational therapist who specializes in driver rehabilitation reviews Mr. Smith's discharge information. The occupational therapist performs a comprehensive driving evaluation, discusses various modifications for driving, and evaluates the client's ability to use these modifications in an equipped vehicle. An occupational therapy assistant trains Mr. Smith in the use of a left-foot gas pedal until he is competent, confident, and safe with the new equipment. The occupational therapist writes a prescription for the necessary equipment to be installed by a reputable equipment dealer. After installation, Mr. Smith returns so the occupational therapist can inspect the installation and ensure that Mr. Smith is able to use the equipment as it is installed in his own vehicle.

Specialized Occupational Therapy Driver Rehabilitation With the Novice Driver

An occupational therapist who specializes in driver rehabilitation has a contract with a local school system and receives referrals of young adults with disabilities as they approach driving age. Gary, a 16-year-old male with a diagnosis of attention deficit disorder, has expressed a desire to obtain a driver's license as he and his classmates reach this all-important milestone. An evaluation of his driving potential reveals the following strengths to performing this occupation: a strong determination to learn to drive, good upper and lower extremity coordination, and satisfactory visual and perceptual skills. Barriers include impulsivity, distractibility, and difficulty sustaining mental effort. During the behind-the-wheel evaluation, Gary demonstrates good beginning basic vehicle control skills but has a tendency to speed and has decreased visual scanning. His driving skills were observed to decrease sharply following approximately 30 minutes of driving. The occupational therapist prescribes a home program of exercises to improve visual scanning and sustained attention and discusses Gary's medication schedule with the physician. Additionally, the occupational therapist provides behind-the-wheel training to learn safe driving skills and improve communication with other road users and reinforces Gary's need to maintain a consistent medication regimen. Concurrently, Gary attends driver education classes at a local driving school as required by the state driver-licensing department. Upon the completion of all state requirements and the successful completion of the driving test, the client is issued his license without restrictions.

Community Mobility for the Adult Client

Mrs. Jones is a 33-year-old woman with a psychiatric disability who is concerned about driving after her medications have been changed. She reports to her physician that the anti-psychotic medications are making her very drowsy and that she got lost several times while driving. Mrs. Jones is referred to occupational therapy for community mobility training. The initial occupational therapy assessment reveals strengths in Mrs. Jones's motor performance, vision, and desire to be independent in moving around her community. Barriers to independence appear to be her impaired time management skills, fluctuating arousal and concentration levels, and periodic confusion. After the occupational therapist collaborates with Mrs. Jones to explore possible alternative modes of transportation, they determine that door-to-door service would be the safest transit for her in her community. The occupational therapist also collaborates with the transit agency regarding sensitivity training for schedulers and drivers. After successfully meeting the comprehensive community mobility goals, Mrs. Jones not only completes her therapy program but also is able to maintain her community involvement by using transportation systems to continue her employment, attend religious activities, and go shopping.

Summary

Attention to driving and community mobility is a growing area of concern due to the implications across the life span, association to occupational engagement, and relevance to other organizational entities (see Appendix B). The skills, knowledge base, and scope of practice of occupational therapy enhanced by additional training in driver rehabilitation place the profession of occupational therapy in the forefront of driving and community mobility services. The focus on injury prevention, engagement in occupation, and the intervention strategies used in driver rehabilitation and community mobility services are consistent with *The Philosophical Base of Occupational Therapy* (AOTA, 1995) and, therefore, warrant attention in all areas of occupational therapy practice.

References

American Medical Association Council on Ethical and Judicial Affairs. (1999). *Impaired drivers and their physicians* (No. 1-I-99). Chicago: Author.

American Occupational Therapy Association. (1995). The philosophical base of occupational therapy. *American Journal of Occupational Therapy, 49,* 1026.

American Occupational Therapy Association. (2000). Occupational therapy code of ethics. *American Journal of Occupational Therapy, 54,* 614–616.

American Occupational Therapy Association. (2002). Occupational therapy practice framework: Domain and process. *American Journal of Occupational Therapy, 56,* 609–639.

American Occupational Therapy Association. (2004a). Guidelines for supervision, roles, and responsibilities during the delivery of occupational therapy services. *American Journal of Occupational Therapy, 58,* 663–667.

American Occupational Therapy Association. (2004b). Scope of practice. *American Journal of Occupational Therapy, 58,* 673–677.

American Occupational Therapy Association. (2005). *About AOTA.* Retrieved March 25, 2005, from http://www.aota.org/general/about.asp

Association for Driver Rehabilitation Specialists (ADED). (2004). *Association for driver rehabilitation specialists.* Retrieved January 29, 2004, from http://www.aded.net

Cobb, R. W. & Coughlin, J. F. (1997). Regulating older drivers: How are the states coping? *Journal of Aging and Social Policy, 9,* 71–87.

Cox, J. L., Fox, M. D., & Irwin, L. (1988). Driving and the elderly: A review of the literature. *Physical and Occupational Therapy in Geriatrics, 7,* 7–12.

Gillins, L. (1990). Yielding to age: When the elderly can no longer drive. *Journal of Gerontological Nursing, 16,* 12–15, 39–41.

Hunt, L. (1993). Evaluation and retraining programs for older drivers. *Clinics in Geriatric Medicine, 9,* 439–449.

Marottoli, R. A., Mendes de Leon, C. F., Glass, T. A., Williams, C. S., Cooney, L. M., Jr., Berkman, L. F., et al. (1997). Driving cessation and increased depressive symptoms: Prospective evidence from the New Haven EPESE. Established populations for epidemiologic studies of the elderly. *Journal of the American Geriatrics Society, 5,* 202–206.

National Highway Traffic Safety Administration. (1999). *Safe mobility for older people notebook* (DOT HS 808 853). Springfield, VA: Author.

U.S. Department of Transportation. (2003a). *Model driver screening and evaluation program final technical report, Volume I: Project summary and model program recommendations* (DOT HS 809 582). Washington, DC: Author.

U.S. Department of Transportation. (2003b). *Safe mobility for a maturing society: Challenges and opportunities.* Washington, DC: Author.

Wang, C. C., Kosinski, C. J., Schwartzberg, J. G., & Shanklin, A. V. (2003). *Physician's guide to assessing and counseling older drivers.* Washington, DC: National Highway Traffic Safety Administration.

Authors
Wendy B. Stav, PhD, OTR/L, CDRS
Susan Pierce, OTR/L, CDRS
Carol J. Wheatley, OTR/L, CDRS
Elin Schold Davis, OTR/L, CDRS

for

The Commission on Practice
Sara Jane Brayman, PhD, OTR/L, FAOTA, *Chairperson*

Adopted by the Representative Assembly 2005C216

APPENDIXES

Appendix A. Domain of Occupational Therapy Specific to Driving and Community Mobility

Areas of Occupation	Community mobility is critical to performance of instrumental activities of daily living, education, work, leisure, and social participation.
Performance Skills (Motor, Process, Communication/Interaction Skills)	• Driving and community mobility require one to possess and execute adequate performance skills. Individuals must use motor skills, including posture, mobility, coordination strength and effort, and energy to maneuver the body through the environment, manipulate equipment, maintain a position, and sustain the activity through completion. • Driving and community mobility require sufficient process skills to draw from knowledge, temporal organization, organization of space and objects, adaptation, and energy while moving through the dynamic, unpredictable environment of the community. • Communication/interaction skills are used as individuals need to exchange information, relate, and physically communicate to move through a community in which other individuals are also mobile.
Performance Patterns (Habits, Routines, Roles)	Driving and community mobility involve performance patterns utilizing habits to operate equipment and routines to travel on an established route. Individuals fulfill the duties and responsibilities of life roles by engaging in community mobility.
Contexts (Cultural, Physical, Social, Personal, Spiritual, Temporal, Virtual)	The context in which driving and community mobility take place is critical in understanding who, what, where, when, how, and why individuals move through the community. The physical context relates to travel in urban or rural settings; on different types of roadways; over a street, sidewalk or path; or using underground, waterway, air, or land travel. The cultural context may dictate who operates an automobile while the social context influences independent versus group travel. An individual's personal context indicates whether travel will be performed as a passenger or operator based on age or socioeconomic status. Temporal context affects community mobility based on the stage of life, time of day, season of year, and duration driving. Recent technologies permit virtual engagement in community mobility through the use of computers and simulators.
Activity Demands	Driving and community mobility have many activity demands consisting of the objects and properties of tools used, space and social demands, sequence and timing, required actions, required body functions, and required body structures.
Client Factors	Individuals use their body functions—mental, sensory (including vision), neuromusculoskeletal, voice, and speech—as well as related body structures, to effectively and safely move about in the community.

Appendix B. External Influences on Occupational Therapy Practice Related to Driving and Community Mobility

Governmental Influences

Federal Government: National Highway Traffic Safety Administration (NHTSA)

NHTSA's mission is driver safety, with funding for programs and research on occupant protection specific to safety belt use, air bags, child passenger safety, graduated licensing, new drivers, vehicle modifications, and impaired driving due to alcohol or illegal drug use. A recent focus on older driver safety has generated programs including a Model Driver Screening and Evaluation Program (U. S. Department of Transportation, 2003a). Reports developed from NHTSA's initiative include *Safe Mobility for Older People* (NHTSA, 1999) and *Safe Mobility for a Maturing Society: Challenges and Opportunities* (U. S. Department of Transportation, 2003b). The latter report states the need to evaluate and improve driving skills, acknowledges the value of driver rehabilitation, and recognizes the contributions of the American Occupational Therapy Association to this field.

State Government: State Licensure Laws

Laws related to driving and community mobility vary by state and jurisdiction with regard to vision standards, medical reporting, legal immunity, and licensure laws. Therefore, occupational therapists and occupational therapy assistants must become knowledgeable of the statutes and guidelines specific to the state or jurisdiction of practice.

Professional Organizations

American Medical Association

- The American Medical Association (AMA) believes that older driver safety is a public health issue and that physicians play an important role in assuring the safety of older drivers (Wang, Kosinski, Schwartzberg, & Shanklin, 2003). The AMA has recently dedicated efforts to a safe driver initiative resulting in a physician training program and several publications.
- The AMA collaborated with aging, driver rehabilitation, and transportation experts nationwide to write guidelines for physician practice related to older drivers (Wang et al., 2003). The book advises a number of alternatives that physicians might pursue, such as referring older drivers to driver rehabilitation specialists.
- On December 7, 1999, the AMA's Council on Ethical and Judicial Affairs adopted a report outlining physicians' ethical obligation to address driving issues with their clients (AMA Council on Ethical and Judicial Affairs, 1999). The report included seven recommendations for physicians to recognize impairments and act on that knowledge when a patient's driving posed a strong threat to public safety.

Association for Driver Rehabilitation Specialists

The Association for Driver Rehabilitation Specialists (ADED) is a multidisciplinary group comprised of occupational therapy practitioners, driver educators, vehicle modification manufacturers and dealers, rehabilitation engineers, physical therapists and kinesiotherapists, and rehabilitation specialists (ADED, 2004). ADED provides certification for driver rehabilitation specialists (CDRS) by means of a portfolio review and standardized exam. ADED recently released *Best Practice Guidelines* for the CDRS.

American Occupational Therapy Association

The American Occupational Therapy Association (AOTA) provides standard-setting, advocacy, education, and research of the profession of occupational therapy to advance the quality, availability, use, and support of occupational therapy (AOTA, 2005). AOTA has created an Older Driver Initiative to coordinate multiple projects related to awareness and professional training. Projects include the following:

- An evidence-based literature review specific to driving and community mobility
- Practice guidelines for driver rehabilitation and community mobility for older adults
- Older Driver Microsite (www.aota.org/olderdriver)
- Specialty certification in driver rehabilitation and community mobility, targeted for availability in January 2006.

Occupational Therapy Fieldwork Education: Value and Purpose

The purpose of fieldwork education is to propel each generation of occupational therapy practitioners from the role of student to that of practitioner. Through the fieldwork experience, future practitioners achieve competence in applying the occupational therapy process and using evidence-based interventions to meet the occupational needs of a diverse client population. Fieldwork assignments may occur in a variety of practice settings, including medical, educational, and community-based programs. Moreover, fieldwork placements also present the opportunity to introduce occupational therapy services to new and emerging practice environments.

Fieldwork assignments constitute an integral part of the occupational therapy and occupational therapy assistant education curricula. Through fieldwork, students learn to apply theoretical and scientific principles learned from their academic programs to address actual client needs within the context of authentic practice environments. While on fieldwork, each student develops competency to ascertain client occupational performance needs to identify supports or barriers affecting health and participation and document interventions provided. Fieldwork also provides opportunities for the student to develop advocacy, leadership, and managerial skills in a variety of practice settings. Finally, the student develops a professional identity as an occupational therapy practitioner, aligning his or her professional judgments and decisions with the American Occupational Therapy Association (AOTA) *Standards of Practice* (AOTA, 2005b) and the *Occupational Therapy Code of Ethics* (AOTA, 2005a).

As students proceed through their fieldwork assignments, performance expectations become progressively more challenging. *Level I fieldwork* experiences occur concurrently with academic coursework and are "designed to enrich didactic coursework through directed observation and participation in selected aspects of the occupational therapy process" (Accreditation Council for Occupational Therapy Education [ACOTE], 2007a, 2007b, 2007c). *Level II fieldwork* experiences occur at or near the conclusion of the didactic phase of occupational therapy curricula and are designed to develop competent, entry-level, generalist practitioners (ACOTE, 2007a, 2007b, 2007c). Level II fieldwork assignments feature in-depth experience(s) in delivering occupational therapy services to clients, focusing on the application of purposeful and meaningful occupation and evidence-based practice through exposure to a "variety of clients across the life span and to a variety of settings" (ACOTE, 2007a, 2007b, 2007c).

The value of fieldwork transcends the obvious benefits directed toward the student. Supervising students enhances fieldwork educators' own professional development by providing exposure to current practice trends, evidence-based practice, and research. Moreover, the experience of fieldwork supervision is recognized by the National Board for Certification in Occupational Therapy (NBCOT) and many state regulatory boards as a legitimate venue for achieving continuing competency requirements for occupational therapy practitioners.

Another benefit to the fieldwork site for sponsoring a fieldwork education program is with the recruitment of qualified occupational therapy personnel. Through the responsibilities expected during Level II fieldwork, occupational therapy staff and administration are given opportunity for an in-depth view of a student's potential as a future employee. In turn, an active fieldwork program allows the student, as a potential employee, to view first-hand the agency's commitment to the professional growth of its occupational therapy personnel and to determine the "fit" of his or her professional goals with agency goals. The fieldwork program also creates a progressive, state-of-the-art image to the professional community, consumers, and other external audiences through its partnership with the academic programs.

In summary, fieldwork education is an essential bridge between academic education and authentic occupational therapy practice. Through the collaboration between academic faculty and fieldwork educators, students are given the opportunity to achieve the competencies necessary to meet the present and future occupational needs of individuals, groups, and indeed, society as a whole.

References

Accreditation Council for Occupational Therapy Education. (2007a). Accreditation standards for a doctoral-degree level educational program for the occupational therapist. *American Journal of Occupational Therapy, 61*, 641–651.

Accreditation Council for Occupational Therapy Education (2007b) Accreditation standards for a master's-degree level educational program for the occupational therapist. *American Journal of Occupational Therapy, 61*, 662–671.

Accreditation Council for Occupational Therapy Education. (2007c) Accreditation standards for an educational program for the occupational therapy assistant. *American Journal of Occupational Therapy, 61*, 652–661.

American Occupational Therapy Association. (2005a). Occupational therapy code of ethics (2005). *American Journal of Occupational Therapy, 59*, 639–642.

American Occupational Therapy Association. (2005b). Standards of practice for occupational therapy. *American Journal of Occupational Therapy, 59*, 663–665.

The Commission on Education
René Padilla, PhD, OTR/L, FAOTA, *Chairperson*
Andrea Bilics, PhD, OTR/L
Judith C. Blum, MS, OTR/L
Paula C. Bohr, PhD, OTR/L, FAOTA
Jennifer C. Coyne, COTA/L
Jyothi Gupta, PhD, OTR/L
Linda Musselman, PhD, OTR, FAOTA
Linda Orr, MPA, OTR/L
Abbey Sipp, *ASD Liaison*
Patricia Stutz-Tanenbaum, MS, OTR
Neil Harvison, PhD, OTR/L, *AOTA Staff Liaison*

Adopted by the Representative Assembly 2009FebCS115

This document replaces the document *The Purpose and Value of Occupational Therapy Fieldwork Education* 2003M41.

Occupational Therapy and Hospice

Within every person is a distinct and unique being that is unlike any life that has existed or will ever exist again (Moustakas, 1977, p. 1).

The purpose of this paper is to describe the contribution of occupational therapy to hospice care and to serve as a resource for occupational therapists and occupational therapy assistants, hospice agencies, policy makers, funding sources, and clients and caregivers who receive hospice services. *Hospice* refers to both a philosophy and a system of care that embody an individualized, humanistic approach to care for people who are dying. Hospice provides end-of-life care, with a focus on living and on dying.

Relationship of Occupational Therapy, Occupation, and Hospice

The basic philosophy of hospice is described in the *Standards of Practice for Hospice Programs:*

> Hospice provides support and care for persons in the last phases of incurable disease so that they may live as fully and as comfortably as possible. Hospice recognizes that the dying process is a part of the normal process of living and focuses on enhancing the quality of remaining life. Hospice affirms life and neither hastens nor postpones death. Hospice exists in the hope and belief that, through appropriate care and the promotion of a caring community sensitive to their needs, individuals and their families may be free to attain a degree of satisfaction in preparation for death. Hospice recognizes that human growth and development can be a lifelong process. Hospice seeks to preserve and promote the inherent potential for growth within individuals and families without regard to age, gender, nationality, race, creed, sexual orientation, disability, diagnosis, availability of a primary caregiver, or ability to pay. (National Hospice and Palliative Care Organization [NHPCO], 2002, p. ii)

Occupational therapists and occupational therapy assistants recognize that continued participation in daily activities (occupations) may serve dual purposes for hospice clients (Bye, 1998; Hasselkus, 1993; Hasselkus & Jacques, 1998). These occupations may provide a means of self-expression and engagement while also serving as a vehicle by which the client finds peace with the dying process and prepares for death.

Recent research explores the significance of occupations in the experience of hospice clients, their significant others,[1] and hospice team members. Four domains of occupation identified as elements in the dying process are (a) "'Doing the Things That Matter': Continuing Life," (b) "'Getting Everything in Order': Preparation for Death," (c) "'It Takes So Long to Die': Waiting," and (d) "'A Gentle Goodbye': Death and After-Death" (Jacques & Hasselkus, 2004, pp. 48–50). The investigators conclude "that occupation is the good death experience and that enabling occupation in an end-of-life care environment . . . can help bring about a good death experience for all involved in the dying process" (pp. 52–53).

To practice in hospice, an occupational therapy practitioner must be aware of his or her own values and beliefs about the dying process. In American society, there is a general discomfort with death and dying;

---

[1]In this document, the term *significant other* refers to others who are involved in the care and decisionmaking of a hospice client. It includes, but is not limited to, family, friends, partners, caregivers, and decision-making surrogates.

this discomfort also is evident in the culture of health care. In most health care settings, occupational therapy is provided to restore skills with the expectation of future occupations. In hospice, occupational therapy is provided to facilitate quality of life through engagement in occupations during the client's remaining days. Occupational therapists and occupational therapy assistants who work in hospice frame their practice on comfort and quality of life rather than on rehabilitation (Trump, 2001). The environment for hospice includes, but is not limited to, clients' homes, hospice care facilities, skilled nursing facilities, assisted living facilities, and independent senior homes. Occupational therapy may be provided to hospice clients in all of these settings.

Hospice teams are interdisciplinary. In addition to occupational therapy practitioners, teams may include counselors, clergypersons, and volunteers as well as physicians, nurses, social workers, dietitians, physical therapists, and speech–language pathologists. Occupational therapy assistants work in hospice with appropriate supervision. The supervising occupational therapist determines whether an occupational therapy assistant should be involved in a client's case based on the client's status, the intervention needs, and the service competencies of the occupational therapy assistant (AOTA, 2004). Client preferences and individual hospice policy and philosophy are considered when occupational therapists and occupational therapy assistants collaborate in hospice care.

Occupational Therapy Process

Evaluation

A hospice client may be referred for occupational therapy at any point during hospice care. Any member of the hospice team may identify the need for occupational therapy. The occupational therapist conducts an initial evaluation to identify the client's occupational needs and priorities. The occupational therapist seeks to understand the client's and caregivers' expectations of dying. *Caregivers* may include family or significant others who are offering care and assistance to the client. Emphasis is placed on cultural, spiritual, and social factors that influence those expectations. The evaluation includes interviewing the client and the family or significant others to determine their priorities and concerns.

Based on these priorities and concerns, the occupational therapist may specifically assess and analyze the client's or caregivers' skills. Although it is expected that a client receiving hospice services may have sustained declines in performance skills, the occupational therapist also assesses for the presence of intact or stable skills that can support continued performance of occupations. The occupational therapist analyzes the demands of activities important to the client and the supports and barriers of the environment as they affect these activities. The evaluation also may include assessment of caregivers' skills as they relate to providing assistance in specific activities to identify assistance strategies that are most compatible with these skills and capabilities. Identification of the client's needs and wishes, combined with analysis of performance, allows the occupational therapist to identify effective and client-centered occupational therapy interventions, which are then incorporated into the interdisciplinary hospice plan of care.

Intervention

The occupational therapist formulates an intervention plan in collaboration with the client, the client's significant others, and the hospice team. The intervention plan identifies the outcomes of intervention, the approaches to be used, and the mechanism for service delivery. Occupational therapy interventions are targeted toward creating a match or fit between the client's and caregivers' capabilities and the demands of the activities that are important to the client and caregivers.

In hospice, the approaches most commonly used by occupational therapy are modification (compensation, adaptation) and prevention. Occupational therapists and occupational therapy assistants focus on modifying the demands of activities or the habits and routines associated with the activity to match the abilities and tolerances of the client and caregivers. Practitioners also address interventions toward prevention. See Figure 1 for examples of interventions related to these approaches.

Intervention may be provided directly with the client, with the client and caregiver(s), or with caregivers only. Intervention directed toward caregivers is most often education and consultation to support their efficacy and satisfaction. Consultation with those providing care may include not only the client's family members or significant others but also other members of the hospice team, including volunteers. In this sense, occupational therapists and occupational therapy assistants may consult on hospice cases in which they provide direct services, as well as when they have no direct occupational therapy involvement.

Intervention review is the process of evaluating the effectiveness of the intervention and the progress toward targeted outcomes. Because hospice clients may experience sudden and sometimes unexpected declines in status, interventions may have to be modified significantly as their status changes. *Progress* is also defined by the nature of hospice care. Acceptance and improved quality of life is progress, even as a client's body systems and performance skills decline. The process of evaluating, intervening, and reevaluating is iterative rather than linear, as the client's needs and priorities evolve. Occupational therapy services may be appropriate at different points during the course of hospice care for a given client as the client's needs, priorities, and abilities change over time.

Outcomes

The ultimate outcome of hospice is a good death, with the focus on the client's and family's quality of life during the time that is left. The following case examples demonstrate how occupational therapy intervention may be provided to address different needs and priorities for hospice clients and their families.

- Gertrude was a grandmother with 11 grandchildren who lived near her and were very involved and supportive of her care. Gertrude moved into a hospice facility after a significant decline in her physical status. The hospice team was concerned about her refusal to follow her medication regime, even to control her severe pain. Occupational therapy was requested to address strategies for pain management. Upon evaluation and assessment of her priorities and needs, the occupational therapist determined that Gertrude was afraid of appearing confused or being lethargic when her grandchildren visited. She feared that she would frighten them or that they would not want to return to see her. She knew that she was lethargic and sometimes her speech was slurred when she took her pain medication, so she avoided taking it. Although she was alert when her grandchildren visited, her pain limited her ability to enjoy these visits or to participate in other activities that were important to her.

  The occupational therapist recommended changes in Gertrude's daily routines to accommodate her roles, her meaningful occupations, and her pain management needs. The hospice team collaborated with

Figure 1. Modification and Prevention Intervention Examples

Modification
• Reconfiguring the physical environment so that a client can continue to participate in social activities. • Introducing assistive devices or equipment to reduce the effort or time required for an activity of daily living (ADL) or leisure activity. • Adjusting daily routines to match the client's activity tolerance and needs for rest.

Prevention
• Preventing isolation by maintaining the client's ability to engage in his or her social context. • Preventing injury to the client or caregivers during caregiving tasks. • Preventing symptom exacerbation during activities. • Preventing risks associated with immobility as a client's physical mobility and physical tolerance decrease.

Gertrude and her family to develop a visitation schedule and a modified medication schedule so that family visits were not occurring at times when the medication's effects on Gertrude's alertness were most intense. With her anxiety about frightening her grandchildren lessened, Gertrude was more willing to take her medications regularly. The resulting effective management of her pain allowed her to increase her involvement in her valued occupations and maintain her role as a loving grandmother.

- Jacob resided in an assisted living facility (ALF) with his wife of 52 years. When Jacob's health condition was considered terminal, he elected into hospice care. Jacob, his wife, and the hospice team were concerned that as Jacob's abilities declined, his need for assistance might exceed the level permitted for him to remain in the ALF. Care provided by professionals or paraprofessionals was limited to a specific number of hours per week for Jacob to remain in the ALF, but care provided by Jacob's wife was not included in this limit. Because Jacob's wife was willing to provide care, a referral was made for occupational therapy to identify appropriate care strategies that Jacob's wife could manage safely.

  During the initial occupational therapy encounter, it became evident that Jacob's concern was not to burden his wife with his increasing needs for assistance. The hospice plan was modified to address this concern specifically through occupational therapy intervention. The occupational therapy assistant, under the supervision of the occupational therapist, implemented an intervention plan that involved both Jacob and his wife. The occupational therapy assistant instructed Jacob's wife in proper care techniques during the activities of daily living—bathing, dressing, and toileting—ensuring both her own and Jacob's safety. The occupational therapy assistant also prepared Jacob and his wife for further physical decline and planned for this decline with the family. This planning included introducing adaptive equipment and modifications to the home, which reduced the demands of important activities and made them manageable for Jacob and his wife. The occupational therapy assistant adapted Jacob's environment to allow him to continue to participate in his longstanding weekly poker party and to maintain his role as a vital and active member in the ALF. Jacob was able to stay in his home environment, his wife was able to care for him effectively, and he was able to maintain his roles as husband and community member during his last days as a result of these interventions.

- Maria wanted to maintain her role as a mother despite being diagnosed with terminal cancer. Because Maria had two small children, a referral was made to occupational therapy to identify strategies for her to participate in caring for her children and engaging in other occupations related to being a mother. The occupational therapist provided direct services to both Maria and her husband. The occupational therapist recommended positioning techniques to allow Maria to hold and to feed her toddler. Other interventions focused on strategies so that she could bathe her daughters, assist her older daughter with picking out clothes for school, and participate in family outings. The occupational therapist also worked with Maria to write letters and make video recordings and other remembrances so that Maria would be able to leave something for each of her children as they went through milestones of life, such as high school graduation, entering college, marriage, and the birth of a child. This occupational therapy intervention supported Maria's desire to maintain her role as mother until her death and then to leave something behind so she could still have a presence in the lives of her children, even after her death.

- Peter was a 5-year-old boy who received hospice care. Both of his parents and two older siblings lived with Peter and were involved in his care. Occupational therapy was included in the hospice plan of care to maintain Peter's ability to play and engage socially with his family despite declining physical and cognitive abilities. The occupational therapist involved Peter and his family in interventions. The occupational therapist recommended modifications to current games that Peter enjoyed playing and also taught the family to position him in appropriate positions for different activities. The occupational therapist instructed Peter's parents to adapt other games and activities so that Peter would be able to successfully maintain the ability to engage in play and family interaction even as his condition deteriorated.

- Ethel was an older woman who lived with her husband. After being informed by her physicians that her cancer had metastasized, Ethel made the decision to terminate planned interventions and to elect hospice care. Initially, Ethel's ability to engage in daily routines and roles was unchanged, but she gradually experienced significant fatigue and had difficulty performing valued activities, such as cooking and cleaning her house. Occupational therapy was referred to address her concerns. The occupational therapist taught Ethel how to use energy conservation strategies to reduce fatigue and accommodate her limited tolerance. The outcome of this intervention was Ethel's continued ability to perform valued activities. However, Ethel's disease progressed, and her ability to perform these occupations subsequently declined. Occupational therapy was referred again. Intervention now focused on interdependence. The occupational therapist educated Ethel and her husband regarding modifications to activities so they could do them together. Ethel still could participate actively in valued activities, but her husband would perform some components of the activities to reduce her stress and fatigue.

  Later, Ethel's condition deteriorated to the point that she could no longer actively participate in activities such as cooking and cleaning. The hospice team again referred for occupational therapy. Intervention focused on strategies for Ethel to continue to participate in valued activities. Although Ethel no longer had the physical skills needed to perform meal preparation activities, the occupational therapist identified strategies for her to use her knowledge of the activities to plan meals and help her husband to prepare a grocery list.

  At all three stages the occupational therapist worked with Ethel to help her to begin to plan for her death. These involved occupations such as passing on recipes to family members, teaching family members how to make specific foods and recipes, and bequeathing a favorite cooking utensil to a particular family member.

An occupational therapy practitioner's personal awareness and deep understanding of the meaning of occupation make a powerful contribution to the process of caring for the dying person. To this end, occupational therapists and occupational therapy assistants function across the continuum of hospice care to help support the roles of the client with terminal illness. Although a client's body systems and skills may deteriorate, occupational therapy interventions can support the client's ability to maintain important roles and relationships, and to engage in the occupations related to those roles. Having choices and being able to participate in daily activities of self-care can support a sense of self-efficacy and control during the dying process. Continuation of important rituals of everyday activity can support meaningfulness in the dying person's final days (Thompson, 1991).

By its philosophy, hospice incorporates a team approach to client care. Occupational therapy practitioners are an important part of the care team, either as direct care providers or as consultants. As consultants to the hospice team, occupational therapy practitioners educate other team members on the meaning and importance of occupation in a person's life and in the dying process. Occupational therapy practitioners also can instruct team members in specific skills and strategies, such as helping volunteers learn safe ways to provide support for specific clients and teaching the use of adaptive equipment to caregivers assisting with personal care, such as bathing. An occupational therapy practitioner's expertise, personal awareness, and deep understanding of the meaning of occupation make a powerful contribution to the process of caring for the dying person. The ability to identify a person's occupational roles and values, and to address these roles and needs through appropriate intervention to ensure a quality life in the dying process, makes occupational therapy an important contributor to hospice care.

References

American Occupational Therapy Association. (2004). Guidelines for supervision, roles, and responsibilities during the delivery of occupational therapy services. *American Journal of Occupational Therapy, 58,* 663–667.

Bye, R. A. (1998). When clients are dying: Occupational therapists' perspectives. *Occupational Therapy Journal of Research, 18*(1), 3–24.

Hasselkus, B. R. (1993). Death in very old age: A personal journey of caregiving. *American Journal of Occupational Therapy, 47,* 717–723.

Hasselkus, B. R., & Jacques, N. D. (1998). Occupational therapy and hospice. *American Journal of Occupational Therapy, 52,* 872–873.

Jacques, N. D., & Hasselkus, B. R. (2004). The nature of occupation surrounding dying and death. *OTJR: Occupation, Participation and Health, 24,* 44–53.

Moustakas, C. (1977). *Creative life.* New York: Van Nostrand.

National Hospice and Palliative Care Organization. (2002). *Standards of practice for hospice programs.* Arlington, VA: Author.

Thompson, B. (1991). Occupational therapy with the terminally ill. In J. Kiernat (Ed.), *Occupational therapy and the older adult* (pp. 324–337). Gaithersburg, MD: Aspen.

Trump, S. M. (2001). Occupational therapy and hospice: A natural fit. *OT Practice, 6*(20).

Related Readings

Albom, M. (1997). *Tuesdays with Morrie.* New York: Doubleday.

Byock, I. (1997). *Dying well: The prospect for growth at the end of life.* New York: Riverhead Books.

Callahan, M., & Kelley, P. (1992). *Final gifts.* New York: Bantam.

Jacques, N. D., & Thompson, B. (2001). Occupational therapy. In National Hospice and Palliative Care Organization (Ed.), *Complementary therapies in end-of-life care* (pp. 69–82). Arlington, VA: Author.

Levine, S. (1982). *Who dies?* Garden City, NY: Anchor Press/Doubleday.

Nuland, S. (1993). *How we die.* New York: Random House.

Rahman, H. (2000). Journey of providing care in hospice: Perspectives of occupational therapists. *Qualitative Health Research, 10,* 806–818.

Trump, S. M. (2000). The role of occupational therapy in hospice. *Home & Community Health Special Interest Section Quarterly, 7*(2), 1–4.

Authors
Suzanne M. Trump, MDiv, MA, OTR/L
Missi Zahoransky, MSHS, OTR/L
Carol Siebert, MS, OTR/L

for

The Commission on Practice
Sara Brayman, PhD, OTR/L, FAOTA, *Chairperson*

Adopted by the Representative Assembly 2004C0162

Note: This Statement replaces the 1998 Statement *Occupational Therapy and Hospice.*

Occupational Therapy in the Promotion of Health and the Prevention of Disease and Disability

Introduction

The purpose of this paper is to describe occupational therapy's contribution in the areas of health promotion and prevention and is intended for internal and external audiences. The American Occupational Therapy Association (AOTA) supports and promotes involvement of occupational therapists and occupational therapy assistants in the development and provision of health promotion and disease or disability prevention programs and services.

It is important to frame the discussion of occupational therapy's role in health promotion and disease or disability prevention by defining these terms as they are used in this paper. The World Health Organization (WHO) provides the following definition in the Ottawa Charter for Health Promotion:

> *Health promotion* is the process of enabling people to increase control over, and to improve, their health. To reach a state of complete physical, mental, and social well-being, an individual or group must be able to identify and realize aspirations, to satisfy needs, and to change or cope with the environment. Health is, therefore, seen as a resource for everyday life, not the objective of living. Health is a positive concept emphasizing social and personal resources, as well as physical capacities. Therefore, health promotion is not just the responsibility of the health sector, but goes beyond healthy lifestyles to well-being. (WHO, 1986, italics added)

Trentham and Cockburn (2005) expand on this definition by stating that

> Health promotion is equally and essentially concerned with creating the conditions necessary for health at individual, structural, social, and environmental levels through an understanding of the determinants of health: peace, shelter, education, food, income, a stable ecosystem, sustainable resources, *social justice,*[1] and equity. (p. 441, italics added)

For the past two decades, the U.S. Department of Health and Human Services (DHHS) has used health promotion and disease prevention objectives to improve the health of the American people. The primary goal of *Healthy People 2010* (DHHS, 1998), the national prevention initiative, is to increase the quality as well as the number of years of healthy life. It emphasizes health status and not just longevity. From an individual perspective, healthy life means a full range of functional capacities across the life span, allowing one to enter into satisfying relationships with others, to work, and to play. From a national perspective, healthy life means a vital, creative, and productive citizenry contributing to thriving communities and a thriving nation.

The second goal of *Healthy People 2010* is to eliminate health disparities (DHHS, 2000). The Health Resources and Services Administration (HRSA) defines health disparities as "population-specific differences in the presence of disease, health outcomes, or access to health care" (HRSA, 2000). Addressing health disparities is consistent with the occupational therapy profession's official document on nondiscrimination and inclusion, which states "inclusion requires that we ensure not only that everyone is treated fairly and equitably but also that all individuals have the same opportunities to participate in the naturally occurring activities of society" (AOTA, 2004b, p. 668). Population health focuses on *aggregates,* or communities of

---

[1]Some italicized terms in this statement are defined in the glossary.

people, and the many factors that influence their health. A population health approach strives to identify and reduce health disparities as well as enhance the overall health and well-being of a population (Finlayson & Edwards, 1997).

Health promotion programs and services may target individuals, organizations, communities and populations, and policymakers. The focus of these programs is to

- Prevent or reduce the incidence of illness or disease, accidents, injuries, and disabilities in the population;

- Reduce health disparities among racial and ethnic minorities and other underserved populations;

- Enhance mental health, resiliency, and quality of life;

- Prevent secondary conditions and improve the overall health and well-being of people with chronic conditions or disabilities and their caregivers; and

- Promote healthy living practices, social participation, *occupational justice,* and healthy communities, with respect for cross-cultural issues and concerns.

A key purpose of health promotion is the prevention of disease and disability in individuals and populations. Prevention is generally categorized into three levels: primary, secondary, and tertiary. *Primary prevention* is defined as education or health promotion strategies designed to help people avoid the onset and reduce the incidence of unhealthy conditions, diseases, or injuries. Primary prevention attempts to identify and eliminate risk factors for disease, injury, and disability. *Secondary prevention* includes early detection and intervention after disease has occurred and is designed to prevent or disrupt the disabling process. *Tertiary prevention* refers to treatment and services designed to arrest the progression of a condition, prevent further disability, and promote social opportunity (Patrick, Richardson, Starks, Rose, & Kinne, 1997).

Occupational Therapy and Health Promotion

Healthy People 2010 and the Ottawa Chapter of Health Promotion parallel occupational therapy's belief that engagement in meaningful occupations supports health and leads to a productive and satisfying life. Wilcock (2006) states that

> Following an occupation-focused health promotion approach to well-being embraces a belief that the potential range of what people can do, be, and strive to become is the primary concern and that health is a by-product. A varied and full occupational lifestyle will coincidentally maintain and improve health and well-being if it enables people to be creative and adventurous physically, mentally, and socially. (p. 315)

According to Christiansen (1999), "Health enables people to pursue the tasks of everyday living that provide them with the life meaning necessary for their well-being" (p. 547).

The Guide to Occupational Therapy Practice (Moyers & Dale, 2006) affirms the profession's participation in disability prevention and health promotion at both the individual and population levels. Occupational therapy services are provided to clients of all age groups, infants through older adults, from a variety of socioeconomic, cultural, and ethnic backgrounds, who possess or who are at risk for impairments, activity limitations, or participation restrictions. According to the *Occupational Therapy Practice Framework* (AOTA, 2002), occupational therapy practitioners[2] recognize that health is supported when individuals are able to engage in occupations and activities that allow them to achieve the desired outcome of participation in their chosen environments. This focus on the outcome of "engagement in occupation to support participation" (p. 611) is interwoven through the delivery of service, beginning with the evaluation and continuing through the intervention phase. Health management and maintenance are included within the domain of occupational therapy as an instrumental activity of daily living; health promotion and prevention are listed

---

[2]When the term *occupational therapy practitioner* is used in this document, it refers to both occupational therapists and occupational therapy assistants (AOTA, 2006).

as occupational therapy intervention approaches; and health, wellness, and quality of life are potential outcomes of occupational therapy services (AOTA, 2002).

Occupations are purposeful and meaningful daily activities that fill a person's time and are typically categorized as self-care, work, play or leisure, and rest (AOTA, 1995; Meyer, 1922). *Occupational health and wellness* includes the elements of choice, meaning, balance, satisfaction, opportunity, and self-actualization (Wilcock, 1998). A natural, balanced pattern of occupations is believed to be health enhancing and fulfills both the needs of the individual and the demands of the environment (Kielhofner, 2004; Meyer, 1922). This belief has been supported in studies with well elderly individuals (Clark et al., 1997).

Occupational imbalance, deprivation, and *alienation* are risk factors for health problems in and of themselves. They also may result from or lead to the development of other risk factors, which in turn can result in larger health and social problems. Causes are varied (e.g., unanticipated caregiving responsibilities, losses in employment or housing) and can lead to occupational imbalance, deprivation, and alienation, which can then lead to individual health problems (e.g., stress, sleep disturbance, depression). People who experience these health problems may be at greater risk for suicide; elder, spousal, and child abuse; substance use disorders; and so forth (Wilcock, 1998). Belle et al. (2006) demonstrated that caregivers of people with dementia experienced significant improvement in quality of life and a decrease in depression after intervention that included stress management; strategies for engaging in pleasant events; and teaching of healthy behaviors, communication skills, and problem-solving skills regarding behavior management of care recipients' difficult behaviors. Occupational therapy practitioners are in a prime position to recognize these occupational health problems and offer interventions to alleviate them through task analysis and modification.

Role of Occupational Therapy

There are three critical roles for occupational therapy practitioners in health promotion and disease or disability prevention: to promote healthy lifestyles; to emphasize occupation as an essential element of health promotion strategies; and to provide interventions, not only with individuals but also with populations. It is important that occupational therapy practitioners promote a healthy lifestyle for all individuals and their families, including people with physical, mental, or cognitive impairments. An occupation-focused approach to prevention of illness and disability is defined by Wilcock (2006) as

> The application of medical, behavioral, social, and *occupational science* to prevent physiological, psychological, social, and occupational illness; accidents; and disability; and to prolong quality of life for all people through advocacy and mediation and through occupation-focused programs aimed at enabling people to do, be, and become according to their natural health needs. (p. 282, italics added)

The following are some examples of occupation-based primary prevention intervention that target individuals:

- Musculoskeletal injury prevention and management programs;

- Anger management and conflict resolution training for parents, teachers, and school-aged youth to reduce the incidence of violence;

- Parenting skills training for adolescent mothers;

- Fall prevention programs for community-dwelling seniors.

Examples of secondary prevention carried out by occupational therapy practitioners may include

- Education and training regarding eating habits, activity levels, and prevention of secondary disability subsequent to obesity;

- Education and training on stress management and adaptive coping strategies for people with mood disorders and post traumatic stress disorder;

- Osteoporosis prevention and management classes for individuals recently diagnosed or at high risk for this condition.

Examples of occupation-based tertiary prevention intervention may include

- Transitional or independent-living skills training for people who have mental illness and those with cognitive impairments;

- Groups for older adults with dementia to prevent depression, enhance socialization, and improve quality of life;

- A program of leisure and educational activities for a drop-in center for adults with severe mental illness;

- Stroke support groups.

Occupational therapy practitioners have an opportunity to complement existing health promotion efforts by adding the contribution of occupation to programs developed by experts in health education, nutrition, exercise, and so forth. For example, when working with a person with a lower-extremity amputation due to diabetes, the occupational therapy practitioner may focus on the occupation of meal preparation using foods and preparation methods recommended in the nutritionist's health promotion program. This enables achievement of the occupational therapy goal of functional independence in the kitchen and reinforces the importance of proper nutrition for the prevention of further disability (Scaffa, 2001).

To be effective, health promotion efforts cannot focus only on intervention at the individual level. Because of the inextricable and reciprocal links between people and their environments, larger groups, organizations, communities, populations, and government policymakers must also be considered for intervention (Law, 1991; Wilcock, 2006). The function of occupational therapy at these levels uses the knowledge and perspective of occupational science in a variety of roles and settings (Baum & Law, 1997; Brownson, 1998).

Organizational-level interventions may include

- Providing consultation to businesses to promote emotional well-being through identification of problems and solutions for balance among work, leisure, and family life;

- Consulting to schools regarding implementation of Americans With Disabilities Act (ADA) requirements;

- Providing education for day care staff regarding normal growth and development, handling behavior problems, and identifying children at risk for developmental delays; and

- Promoting ergonomically correct work stations in schools and offices.

Community or population-level interventions may include

- Consulting on accessible public transportation;

- Consulting with contractors, architects, and city planners regarding accessibility and universal design;

- Implementing a community-wide screening program for depression at nursing homes, assisted-living facilities, and senior centers for the purpose of developing group and individual prevention and intervention programs addressing depression;

- Conducting needs assessments and implementing intervention strategies to reduce health disparities in communities with high rates of disease or injury; intervention strategies may include lifestyle management programs addressing issues such as hypertension, diabetes, and obesity;

- Addressing the health and occupation needs of the homeless population by eliminating barriers and enhancing opportunities for occupational engagement; and

- Training volunteers to function effectively in special needs shelters during disasters.

Governmental or policy-level interventions may include

- Promoting policies that offer affordable, accessible health care to everyone, including people with disabilities;

- Promoting policies that support economic self-sufficiency for all people;

- Supporting full inclusion of children with disabilities in schools and day care programs;

- Lobbying for public funds to support research and program development in areas related to improvement in quality of life for people at risk and those with disabilities; and

- Promoting policies that establish opportunities for rehabilitation in the community for people discharged from inpatient psychiatric programs.

Occupational Therapy's Contributions

Occupational therapy has an important role in health promotion and disease or disability prevention due to its focus on the health effects of purposeful, productive, and meaningful occupation. It is the profession's focus and associated knowledge base that is occupational therapy's contribution to the health and well-being of Americans. Occupational therapy practitioners can

- Evaluate occupational capabilities, values, and performance;

- Provide education regarding occupational role performance and balance;

- Reduce risk factors and symptoms through engagement in occupation;

- Provide skill development training in the context of everyday occupations;

- Provide self-management training to prevent illness and manage health;

- Modify environments for healthy and safe occupational performance;

- Consult and collaborate with health care professionals, organizations, communities, and policymakers regarding the occupational perspective of health promotion and disease or disability prevention;

- Promote the development and maintenance of mental functioning abilities through engagement in productive and meaningful activities and relationships (adapted from DHHS, 1999, p. 4); and

- Provide training in adaptation to change and in coping with adversity to promote mental health (adapted from DHHS, 1999, p. 4).

While recognizing the role of occupational therapy in health promotion and disease and disability prevention, it is important to acknowledge and respect the contributions of other health care professions in this important arena. Occupational therapy practitioners should operate within their scope of practice and training and partner with other health promotion disciplines with specialized expertise such as in the areas of public health, health education, nutrition, and exercise physiology. The roles of the occupational therapist and the occupational therapy assistant in evaluation and intervention in health promotion practice are based on the *Guidelines for Supervision, Roles, and Responsibilities During the Delivery of Occupational Therapy Services* (AOTA, 2004a). Occupational therapists and occupational therapy assistants possess the basic knowledge to carry out health promotion and interventions to prevent disability and disease. However, this is a very broad area of practice, and practitioners need to continually expand their knowledge in health promotion to be effective and competent members of the team.

As in all other areas of practice, health promotion services should be evidence based. Law, Steinwender, and LeClair (1998) conducted an extensive review of the literature on the relationship between occupation and health. The longitudinal studies that were reviewed found that activity participation had a significant effect on perceived health. Maintenance of everyday activities, social interactions, and community mobility influenced self-reported quality of life. A long-term benefit attributable to preventive occupational therapy was demonstrated by Clark et al. (2001) when they re-evaluated participants from the Well Elderly Study and found that 90% of therapeutic gain observed following intervention was retained at the 6-month follow-up.

Funding for health promotion programs can come from governmental agencies, foundations, nonprofit organizations, insurance companies, and large corporations, among others. In addition, fee for service is an option. Typically, health promotion and prevention programs do not rely on a single source of funding (Brownson, 1998; Scaffa, 2001).

The following case studies provide examples of the role of occupational therapy in health promotion and prevention of disease and disability.

Case Study: Primary Prevention—Individual Level

A retired husband and wife consult an occupational therapist regarding a home safety assessment for the purpose of remaining in their home as they age.

Assessment: The occupational therapist uses a semi-structured interview format to gather information about the clients' health, occupational performance, and satisfaction level within the various performance areas, as well as social connectedness and overall life satisfaction. Both the husband and wife are healthy and able to perform daily tasks with a high level of satisfaction. They have a strong social support network and report being very satisfied with their life. The occupational therapist also explores the health history of their parents and learns of a history of Alzheimer's disease and diabetes. The environment (i.e., home, yard, neighborhood) is assessed regarding accessibility and safety.

The occupational therapist notes that the living area is on three levels (several steps have no railings); rooms and hallways are generally poorly lit; and too much furniture is in each room, leaving narrow or obstructed passageways. The yard has uneven and poorly defined walkways. The couple lives in a residential neighborhood with a distance of 3 miles to shopping. No public transportation is available (even for people with mobility impairments).

Intervention: For immediate consideration, the occupational therapist recommends that the couple install railings by all steps, increase the level of lighting, and decrease the amount of furniture. She works with them to find the best configuration of furniture placement to maximize safety when walking in a room. She recommends that they consider changing the landscape to include clearly defined and level walkways that also will accommodate wheeled mobility, should that ever be needed.

A second set of recommendations includes how to retrofit the house if mobility impairments preclude climbing stairs in the future. Optimal placement of an elevator from the first to the second floor is described. There is not an easy placement of an elevator from the basement to the first floor, so the occupational therapist describes how the occupations now performed in the basement (exercise, laundry, and computer use) may be transferred to the other two floors. The occupational therapist works with the couple on problem solving around transportation, should driving become difficult.

Case Study: Primary Prevention—Organizational Level

A commercial bakery contacts an occupational therapist to assess the various work stations in the bakery and make recommendations for improvements. Management goals are to increase productivity and to decrease sick days and worker compensation claims.

Assessment: The occupational therapist observes the work performed at the various work stations and interviews the workers. She notes body mechanics, repetitive motions, machine design, layout of work stations with travel distances, weights lifted and number of lifts per time unit, work speed and load, noise, temperature, air quality, clothing comfort, and length and frequency of rest breaks. Worker-to-worker interaction and interaction among workers, supervisors, and management also are noted. In general, the supervisors and management seem approachable and open to suggestions from the workers.

The occupational therapist finds much lifting and repetitive motion done by the workers. Work stations require much static standing, which contributes to many musculoskeletal problems. Travel distances are long, work speed is rapid, noise level is high in certain parts of the factory, and the temperature is uncomfortably warm.

Intervention: The occupational therapist recommends ergonomically designed work stations with decreased amount of static work, time standing, travel, or lifting and improved working positions. Because some jobs involve repetitive motions that may not be avoided, the occupational therapist instructs the managers in the benefits of rest breaks and instructs the workers in stretching exercises. Each worker also is instructed in proper body mechanics at his or her work station. The occupational therapist works with the management on designing a daily schedule that allows for an even workflow to decrease times of high stress. The occupational therapist is asked to return every 6 months to reassess and instruct new employees.

Case Study: Primary Prevention—Community/Population Level

An elementary school is planning a new playground, which must be accessible to every child in the school. An occupational therapist is consulted for input on design features that will make the playground aesthetically pleasing, fun, and challenging to use for children of all abilities.

Assessment: The occupational therapist surveys the area where the school is planning to locate the playground. He uses the guidelines for play areas developed by the U.S. Access Board (2005) to make sure the minimum requirements are met. He then researches commercially available playground equipment to find equipment that will be fun and challenging to use for all populations in the school as well as encourage interactions among the children.

Intervention: The occupational therapist provides the school with a report detailing his recommendations for important features in the playground equipment and the layout of the playground. He is careful to identify all the safety issues and suggests ways to make the playground as safe as possible. The report also includes recommendations for landscaping so that children using wheeled mobility can easily navigate around the playground. The occupational therapist remains on the design team for consultation until the playground is completed.

Case Study: Primary Prevention—Governmental/Policy Level

An occupational therapist working in home health has noticed that her elderly clients who no longer drive have no other means of transportation to go grocery shopping, run errands, and visit friends. The occupational therapist contacts the Occupational Science Department at the local university to collaborate on a grant proposal asking for start-up money to research the need for and develop a system of transportation for non-drivers in the community.

Case Study: Tertiary Prevention—Individual Level

A rehabilitation unit in a hospital decides to offer health promotion classes to former patients with chronic conditions. An occupational therapy assistant is chosen to lead a class for patients with chronic obstructive pulmonary disease.

Assessment: The occupational therapy assistant researches information on the disease, existing programs, and their content and outcomes. She researches optimal group size, length of each session frequency, and number of sessions.

Intervention: Using the assessment information, the supervising occupational therapist works with the occupational therapy assistant to develop the health promotion class, including number of participants, length of session, and topics offered. It is decided that a maximum of 15 participants will meet monthly for 1.5 hours for a total of 12 sessions. Topics include self-management, assertive communication, information seeking, and problem-solving skills. The group also will function as a support group.

Appendix: Glossary

Occupational alienation: "Sense of isolation, powerlessness, frustration, loss of control, and estrangement from society or self as a result of engagement in occupation that does not satisfy inner needs" (Wilcock, 2006, p. 343).

Occupational deprivation: "Deprivation of occupational choice and diversity because of circumstances beyond the control of individuals or communities" (Wilcock, 2006, p. 343).

Occupational imbalance: "A lack of balance or disproportion of occupation resulting in decreased well-being" (Wilcock, 2006, p. 343).

Occupational justice: To experience meaning and enrichment in one's occupations; to participate in a range of occupations for health and social inclusion; to make choices and share decision-making power in daily life; and to receive equal privileges for diverse participation in occupations (Townsend & Wilcock, 2004).

Occupational science: "An interdisciplinary academic discipline in the social and behavioral sciences dedicated to the study of the form, the function, and the meaning of human occupations" (Zemke & Clark, 1996, p. vii).

Social justice: "The promotion of social and economic change to increase individual, community, and political awareness, resources, and opportunity for health and well-being" (Wilcock, 2006, p. 344).

References

American Occupational Therapy Association. (1995). Occupation: A position paper. *American Journal of Occupational Therapy, 49,* 1015–1018.

American Occupational Therapy Association. (2002). Occupational therapy practice framework: Domain and process. *American Journal of Occupational Therapy, 56,* 609–639.

American Occupational Therapy Association. (2004a). Guidelines for supervision, roles, and responsibilities during the delivery of occupational therapy services. *American Journal of Occupational Therapy, 58,* 663–667.

American Occupational Therapy Association. (2004b). Occupational therapy's commitment to nondiscrimination and inclusion. *American Journal of Occupational Therapy, 58,* 668.

American Occupational Therapy Association (2006). Policy 1.44: Categories of occupational therapy personnel. *American Journal of Occupational Therapy, 60,* 683–684.

Baum, C. M., & Law, M. (1997). Occupational therapy practice: Focusing on occupational performance. *American Journal of Occupational Therapy, 51,* 277–287.

Belle, S. H., Burgio, L., Burns, R., Coon, D., Czaja, S. J., Gallagher-Thompson, D., et al. (2006). Enhancing the quality of life of dementia caregivers from different ethnic or racial groups. *Annals of Internal Medicine, 145,* 727–738.

Brownson, C. A. (1998). Funding community practice: Stage 1. *American Journal of Occupational Therapy, 52,* 60–64.

Christiansen, C. H. (1999). Defining lives: Occupation as identity: An essay on competence, coherence, and the creation of meaning. *American Journal of Occupational Therapy, 53,* 547–558.

Clark, F., Azen, S. P., Zemke, R., Jackson, J., Carlson, M., Mandel, D., et al. (1997). Occupational therapy for independent-living older adults: A randomized controlled trial. *Journal of the American Medical Association, 278,* 1321–1326.

Clark, F., Azen, S. P., Carlson, M., Mandel, D., LaBree, L., Hay, J., et al. (2001). Embedding health-promoting changes into the daily lives of independent-living older adults: Long-term follow-up of occupational therapy intervention. *Journal of Gerontology: Psychological Sciences, 56,* 60–63.

Finlayson, M., & Edwards, J. (1997). Evolving health environments and occupational therapy: Definitions, descriptions, and opportunities. *British Journal of Occupational Therapy, 60,* 456–460.

Health Resources and Services Administration. (2000). *Eliminating health disparities in the United States.* Retrieved June 12, 2006, from http://newsroom.hrsa.gov/NewsBriefs/2001/eliminatingdisparities.htm

Kielhofner, G. (2004). *Conceptual foundation of occupational therapy* (3rd ed.). Philadelphia: F. A. Davis.

Law, M. (1991). The environment: A focus for occupational therapy [Murial Driver Memorial Lecture]. *Canadian Journal of Occupational Therapy, 58,* 171–179.

Law, M., Steinwender, S., & LeClair, L. (1998). Occupation, health, and well-being. *Canadian Journal of Occupational Therapy, 65,* 81–91.

Meyer, A. (1922). The philosophy of occupation therapy. *Archives of Occupational Therapy, 1,* 1–10.

Moyers, P., & Dale, L. (2006). *The guide to occupational therapy practice* (2nd ed.). Bethesda, MD: AOTA Press.

Patrick, D. L., Richardson, M., Starks, H. E., Rose, M. A., & Kinne, S. (1997). Rethinking prevention for people with disabilities part II: A framework for designing interventions. *American Journal of Health Promotion, 11,* 261–263.

Scaffa, M. E. (2001). *Occupational therapy in community-based practice settings.* Philadelphia: F. A. Davis.

Townsend, E., & Wilcock, A. A. (2004). Occupational justice and client-centered practice: A dialogue in progress. *Canadian Journal of Occupational Therapy, 71,* 75–87.

Trentham, B., & Cockburn, L. (2005). Participatory action research: Creating new knowledge and opportunities for occupational engagement. In F. Kronenberg, S. Simó Algado, & N. Pollard (Eds.), *Occupational therapy without borders: Learning from the spirit of survivors* (pp. 440–453). Philadelphia: Elsevier/Churchill Livingstone.

U.S. Access Board. (2005). *Accessible play areas: A summary of accessibility guidelines for play areas.* Retrieved August 8, 2007, from http://www.access-board.gov/play/guide/guide.pdf

U.S. Department of Health and Human Services. (1998). *Healthy People 2010 objectives: Draft for public comment.* Washington, DC: Author.

U.S. Department of Health and Human Services. (1999). *Mental health: A report of the Surgeon General.* Rockville, MD: Author.

U.S. Department of Health and Human Services. (2000). *Healthy People 2010: Understanding and improving health* (2nd ed.). Washington, DC: U.S. Government Printing Office.

Wilcock, A. A. (1998). *An occupational perspective of health.* Thorofare, NJ: Slack.

Wilcock, A. A. (2006). *An occupational perspective of health* (2nd ed.). Thorofare, NJ: Slack.

World Health Organization. (1986). The Ottawa charter for health promotion. *Health Promotion, 1,* iii–v.

Zemke, R., & Clark, F. (1996). *Occupational science: The evolving discipline.* Philadelphia: F. A. Davis.

Authors

Marjorie E. Scaffa, PhD, OTR, FAOTA
Nancy Van Slyke, EdD, OTR, FAOTA
Carol A. Brownson, MSPH

for

The Commission on Practice
Susanne Smith Roley, MS, OTR/L, FAOTA, *Chairperson*

Adopted by the Representative Assembly 2007CO146

This document replaces the 2000 Statement *Occupational Therapy in the Promotion of Health and the Prevention of Disease and Disability.*

Occupational Therapy Services for Individuals Who Have Experienced Domestic Violence

Purpose

The primary purpose of this paper is to define the role of occupational therapy and the scope of services available for survivors and families who have experienced domestic violence. This document is intended for use by occupational therapists, occupational therapy assistants, and individuals interested in this topic as it relates to the occupational therapy profession.

Introduction to Domestic Violence

Domestic violence is a societal problem in the United States and abroad that affects not only the survivor of the violence but also the children witnessing it, the family and friends of the survivor, and the communities in which it occurs. Domestic violence affects 1,500,000 women and 835,000 men in the United States each year (National Institute of Justice [NIJ], 2000). In the United States it is estimated that 1 in 3 women have experienced domestic violence in an intimate relationship (Heise, Ellsberg, & Gottemoeller, 1999; Helfrich, 2001). These statistics do not account for those men and women who have not spoken up and admitted that they are survivors of domestic violence or for the lasting effects that violence has on children and families. The term *victim* is sometimes used to describe individuals who are currently in an abusive relationship. The term *survivor* is used to describe individuals who are currently in the abusive relationship or who have overcome the abuse. The term survivor is viewed as more empowering and denotes the great strength and courage needed to endure and survive domestic violence.

There are numerous definitions of domestic violence depending on the state and organization. This document defines *domestic violence* as a pattern of "coercive behavior designed to exert power and control over a person in an intimate relationship through the use of intimidating, threatening, harmful, or harassing behavior" (Office for Victims of Crime [OVC], 2002). Domestic violence therefore focuses on *intimate partners*. Child and sibling abuse also may occur concurrently with or as a consequence of living in a domestic violence situation. Although women are abused in 85% to 95% of the reported domestic violence cases (Fisher & Shelton, 2006), men also are abused. New research suggests that women may be abusers in intimate relationships more often than previously thought (OVC, 2002). Therefore, it is important to view domestic violence as an issue of obtaining power and control over a partner rather than as a gender issue. Domestic violence occurs in both heterosexual and homosexual relationships at nearly the same rate. Survivors of domestic violence in a homosexual relationship, however, may have more difficulty accessing services and may face further oppression.

Additionally, women with disabilities who are abused may face additional barriers that make it more difficult to leave the abusive relationship and access services. Although there are inconsistent findings regarding the incidence of abuse of women with disabilities, several sources indicate that they are assaulted, raped, and abused at a rate twice that of women without disabilities (Helfrich, 2001; Helfrich, Lafata, MacDonald, Aviles, & Collins, 2001). These studies indicate that women with disabilities may be dependent on their partners for financial, physical, or medical support, and thus may stay in abusive relationships for longer periods of time (Helfrich et al., 2001; NIJ, 2000). Their abusers may withhold necessary equipment such as wheelchairs, braces, medications, and transportation as a means to control them (NIJ, 2000).

Domestic violence also affects older adults. The National Coalition Against Domestic Violence (NCADV) defines *elder abuse* as abuse by an intimate partner rather than by a caregiver (NCADV, n.d.). Domestic violence in older adults has unique considerations that include the chronic effects of abuse over many years, guilt mixed with a sense of responsibility to be the caregiver for the abusive partner, and conditions such as Alzheimer's that may mask signs of abuse or exacerbate behaviors (NCADV, n.d.).

The effects of domestic violence on children can be devastating as well. In addition to experiencing the abuse between their parents or a parent and partner, it is estimated that child abuse occurs in 30% to 60% of domestic violence cases (Appel & Holden, 1998; McKibben, DeVos, & Newberger, 1998). These children often have low self-esteem, psychosomatic complaints, nightmares, impaired social skills, and poor academic performance. They may be aggressive, withdrawn, anxious, depressed, and even suicidal (OVC, 2002). In families of domestic violence, young boys may model their father's behavior, while girls may model their mother's behavior and show more signs of withdrawal and isolation (Cummings, Peplar, & Moore, 1999; Huth-Beck, Levendosky, & Semel, 2001; Stiles, 2002). According to the OVC (2002), some children will begin to disrespect the victim of domestic violence and identify more with the abuser, modeling the manipulating power that the abuser has over the victim and the children living in the household where domestic violence is occurring. Domestic violence knows no boundaries; it crosses into all socioeconomic classes, races, societies, and ages, regardless of the sexual orientation that defines the relationships. The key issue in domestic violence is the use of a pattern of abusive behavior by the abuser to establish fear, power, and control over an intimate or formerly intimate partner.

Abuse in domestic violence comes in many forms. It may be physical, psychological, or sexual. *Physical violence* may include such behaviors as hitting, slapping, punching, or stabbing. *Psychological violence* may take the form of verbal abuse, harassment, possessiveness, destruction of personal property, cruelty to pets, and isolation (NCADV, n.d.; OVC, 2002). *Sexual abuse* can occur between two intimate partners when the abuser forces or coerces the victim into a sexual act. The abuser often isolates the victim from family and friends, thus limiting access to support systems. The abuser may control the finances, leaving the victim with no money or a limited allowance. It is particularly difficult for a woman to leave her abuser when she has no financial means to support herself and her children.

Research indicates that women who are survivors of domestic violence may struggle when performing a number of their daily life occupations or activities, particularly in the areas of work performance, educational participation, home management, parenting, and leisure participation (Gallew, Krabacher, Andriacco, & German, in press; Gorde, Helfrich, & Finlayson, 2004). They may have difficulty with cognitive functioning, including decision making, judgment, problem solving, and following directions. They may experience problems with money management, task initiation, self-confidence, coping skills, stress management, and interpersonal relationships (Carlson, 1997; D'Ardenne & Balakrishna, 2001; Levendosky & Graham-Bermann, 2001; Monahan & O'Leary, 1999).

Studies of children exposed to domestic violence indicate that they may have difficulties with self-calming, sleeping, and eating activities; may demonstrate developmental delays or maladaptive behaviors; and may have poor verbal and social skills that negatively affect their academic performance. They also may have higher rates of somatic complaints and interpersonal problems (Cummings et al., 1999; Huth-Beck et al., 2001; Norwood, Swank, Stephens, Ware, & Buzy, 2001; Sternberg et al., 1993; Stiles, 2002).

Occupational Therapy and Domestic Violence

In its broadest sense, the domain of occupational therapy is the facilitation of the ability of people to engage in their daily life activities—occupations—in a manner that supports their full participation in various contexts and that positively affects health, well-being, and life satisfaction (American Occupational Therapy Association [AOTA], 2002). Occupational therapists and occupational therapy assistants view occupations as central to a person's identity and competence, influencing how a person spends time and makes decisions (AOTA, 2002). Because domestic violence negatively affects the ability of the survivors and their families to engage in their daily life occupations in a competent, healthy, and satisfying manner, occupational therapy practitioners[1] focus on developing or restoring these abilities. Specifically, occupational therapy practitioners focus on enhancing the ability of the survivors and their families to participate in activities of daily living (ADLs), instrumental activities of daily living (IADLs), education, work, leisure, play, and social participation for the purpose of gaining skills and abilities needed to take control of their lives and develop healthy independent lifestyles.

Occupational therapy practitioners work directly and indirectly with survivors of domestic violence and their families in a variety of settings such as hospitals, rehabilitation centers, outpatient therapy clinics, school systems, and community programs. Occupational therapy practitioners may work with survivors and family members who have

- Sustained injuries or disabilities as a result of domestic violence,

- Chosen to remain in and rebuild a relationship in which abuse has occurred, or

- Decided to leave the abusive relationship and reconstruct their lives.

In the course of their practice, occupational therapy practitioners also may work with individuals whom they suspect or discover are victims or survivors of domestic violence but who have not reported the domestic violence. In such cases, occupational therapy practitioners have a professional and ethical responsibility to take action that promotes the health and safety of these individuals. Occupational therapy practitioners are mandated to report suspected child abuse. Some states also mandate that they report suspected abuse in adults. Occupational therapy practitioners need to consult their state regulatory acts and facility guidelines regarding procedures they are to follow when they suspect or know that domestic violence has occurred. Actions that practitioners may take include

- Filing a report to the local law enforcement agency or children's protective services;

- Interviewing, evaluating, and providing interventions without the abuser present to allow the client the opportunity to discuss the situation in relative safety;

- Identifying and assessing injuries and their potential cause;

- Talking to the client about healthy relationships, and addressing areas of occupation and performance patterns and skills that may have been affected by the abusive relationship such as leisure, IADLs, work, and ADLs;

- Respecting the client's perception of the relative danger of the situation to his or her life and the well-being of other family members, and remaining empathetic and nonjudgmental about the client's decision to remain in or leave the abusive situation;

- Providing the client with the phone number for the area domestic violence hotline; and

- Abiding by practice setting safety precautions to determine if it is appropriate to conduct home visits.

---

[1]When the term *occupational therapy practitioner* is used in this document, it refers to both occupational therapists and occupational therapy assistants (AOTA, 2006). *Occupational therapists* are responsible for all aspects of occupational therapy service delivery and are accountable for the safety and effectiveness of the occupational therapy service delivery process. *Occupational therapy assistants* deliver occupational therapy services under the supervision of and in partnership with an occupational therapist (AOTA, 2004).

Occupational Therapy Services

The occupational therapy service delivery process occurs in collaboration with the survivors of domestic violence, their family members, and other service providers. Throughout the occupational therapy evaluation, intervention, and assessment of outcomes, occupational therapy practitioners value and consider the desires, choices, needs, personal and spiritual values, and sociocultural backgrounds of the survivors and their family members. Occupational therapy practitioners also consider the service delivery context. Important outcomes of occupational therapy service provision include, but are not limited to, facilitating the ability of the survivors and their family members to consistently engage in and perform their daily activities, achieving personal satisfaction and role competence, developing a healthy lifestyle, and improving their quality of life.

The occupational therapy evaluation process is focused on finding out what the survivors and their family members want and need to do and identifying the factors that act as supports or barriers to performance of desired occupations (AOTA, 2002). Current occupational performance; routines and habits; activity demands; sociocultural beliefs/expectations; and physical, cognitive, and psychosocial factors are addressed during the evaluation process.

The occupational therapy intervention process is based on findings from the evaluation and the survivors' and the family members' stated priorities. It is the process of "effecting change in the client's occupational performance, leading to engagement in occupations or in activities to support participation" (AOTA, 2002, p. 618). Interventions with adults who are survivors of domestic violence focus on empowerment and active participation in healthy occupations or daily life activities. These may include working on the development of a realistic budget, facilitating the use of effective decision-making skills regarding employment opportunities, learning calming techniques to use with their children, learning assertiveness skills, and teaching stress management and relaxation techniques to improve sleep patterns. Interventions with children who have witnessed domestic violence may include facilitation of developmentally appropriate play skills, social skills training, the use of techniques for improving concentration and attention span during school activities, and assistance with the organization of study habits and school materials.

Occupational therapy practitioners focus on outcomes throughout the occupational therapy service delivery process. Assessing outcome results assists occupational therapy practitioners with making decisions about future directions of interventions at the individual as well as at the systems level (AOTA, 2002). At the individual level, the selection of outcomes is based on the survivors' priorities and may be modified based on changing needs, contexts, and performance abilities (AOTA, 2002). For example, an occupational therapy practitioner may work with a woman who is a survivor of domestic violence on her goal of obtaining housing. After the woman moves into the new living situation, the occupational therapy practitioner may help the woman work on her goal of maintaining a healthy home environment for herself and her children. At the systems level, data about targeted outcomes can be aggregated and reported to boards of directors of community agencies, state and federal regulators, and funding agencies. An example of this type of outcome assessment would be the reporting of the number of children who demonstrated difficulty participating in their daily life activities at home, school, and in their communities because of exposure to domestic violence and the progress they made during the occupational therapy intervention to increase their level of healthy participation.

Occupational therapy practitioners also may work with the abusers in collaboration with other professionals such as psychologists, social workers, and pastoral counselors. Sometimes the judicial system issues a court order for the abuser to participate in a formal program to address the violent behaviors. These programs are generally based on six principles: (a) the abuser is responsible for the behavior, (b) provocation does not justify violence, (c) violent behavior is a choice, (d) there are nonviolent alternatives, (e) violence is a learned behavior, and (f) domestic violence affects the entire family whether it is directly or indirectly witnessed (OVC, 2002). Occupational therapy interventions with the abuser may include social skills training, assertiveness training, anger management, stress management, and spiritual exploration as related to daily life occupations.

Education, Training, and Competencies

Occupational therapists and occupational therapy assistants are educationally prepared to address the various occupation-related concerns of survivors of domestic violence. The Accreditation Council for Occupational Therapy Education (ACOTE) standards for educational programs require content related to daily life occupations, human development, human behavior, sociocultural issues, diversity factors, medical conditions, theory, models of practice, evaluation, and techniques for the development and implementation of intervention plans under the scope of occupational therapy (ACOTE, 2006). Occupational therapy practitioners are competent to address life skills, lifestyle management, adaptive coping strategies, adaptation, time management, and values clarification that affect the ability of survivors of domestic violence to participate in their ADLs, IADLs, education, work, play, leisure, and social participation activities. In addition, occupational therapy practitioners have the expertise to work with individuals and groups. Occupational therapists, and occupational therapy assistants who are supervised by an occupational therapist, are competent in the following areas:

- Establishing and maintaining therapeutic relationships

- Conducting interviews

- Administering functional assessments to determine occupational performance needs and to develop an intervention plan

- Utilizing interpersonal communication skills

- Designing and facilitating therapeutic groups

- Developing individualized teaching and learning processes with clients, family, and significant others

- Coordinating program interventions in collaboration with clients, caregivers, families, and communities grounded in evidence-based practice

- Developing therapeutic programs

- Promoting health and wellness through engagement in meaningful occupations

- Understanding the effects of health, disability, and social conditions on the individual within the context of family and society (ACOTE, 2006).

Participating in continuing education initiatives advances occupational therapy practitioners' understanding of and capacity to provide interventions that address domestic violence.

Supervision of Other Personnel

When provided as part of an occupational therapy program, the occupational therapist is responsible for all aspects of the service delivery and is accountable for the safety and effectiveness of the service delivery process. The occupational therapy assistant delivers occupational therapy services under the supervision of and in partnership with the occupational therapist (AOTA, 2004). The education and knowledge of occupational therapy practitioners also prepares them for employment in arenas other than those related to traditional delivery of occupational therapy. In these circumstances, the occupational therapy practitioner should determine whether the services they provide are related to the delivery of occupational therapy by referring to their state practice acts, the regulatory agency standards and rules, the domain of occupational therapy practice, and the written or verbal agreement with the agency or payer about the services provided (AOTA, 2004). Occupational therapy practitioners should obtain and use credentials and a job title commensurate with their roles in the specific arena. In such arenas, nonoccupational therapy professionals may provide the supervision of occupational therapy assistants.

The following case studies provide examples of the role of occupational therapy in domestic violence.

Adult Case Study

An occupational therapist working in a shelter for survivors of domestic violence was asked to assess Maria, a 28-year-old woman who has two children.

Assessment

Using the *Canadian Occupational Performance Measure*, Maria indicates that the following occupational performance areas are the most important to her. She feels competent in her ability to take care of a house, parent her children, and keep them safe. She wants to work with the occupational therapist on finding and maintaining a job, budgeting, and completing her GED. Maria rates her performance as 1—*unable to do it*, and her satisfaction levels as 1—*not satisfied at all*, for these performance areas. When budgeting is discussed, Maria states that she had never been responsible for money management. She went straight from her parent's home into her marriage at the age of 17, and her husband would not allow her to have anything to do with the money. He constantly told her that she was "too stupid" to take care of money. She was not allowed to work outside the home, so she was dependent on her husband for money.

Intervention

The occupational therapist helps Maria to procure and fill out job applications and practice job interviewing skills. After Maria finds a steady job, she and her children move into the shelter's transitional living program. To stay in this program, Maria needs to put a certain amount of money into a savings account on a monthly basis to secure a home for her and her children. Following her first paycheck, the occupational therapist meets with Maria to project a budget for her expenses and savings. Maria asks the occupational therapist to develop her budget for her because she "isn't smart enough to do it herself." She states that math was her worst subject in school. The occupational therapist grades the complexity of the task to enable Maria to develop problem-solving skills and reasoning abilities for budgeting. The occupational therapist then models for Maria how to contact community agencies to obtain information about GED programs. They determine a daily schedule and identify support networks so that Maria can work, complete her studies, and care for her children.

Adult Case Study

An occupational therapist in an outpatient clinic receives a referral to provide occupational therapy services to Mr. Lee, a 72-year-old man with a right distal radius fracture and a boxer's fracture. Mr. Lee has chronic obstructive pulmonary disease (COPD) and uses a wheelchair for mobility. He has been living with his current partner for the past 10 years. During the evaluation the occupational therapist asks Mr. Lee to explain how the injury occurred. He is vague in his responses and simply states that he became weak and fell out of his wheelchair. Over the next few sessions, while providing interventions to address Mr. Lee's hand injuries and COPD, the occupational therapist notices additional bruises on his arms and suspects that he is involved in an abusive relationship.

Assessment and Intervention

Because the occupational therapist lives in a state that mandates reporting of abuse in adults, she files a report to the appropriate law enforcement agency. She lets Mr. Lee know that law requires such action. The occupational therapist then initiates conversation about domestic violence. Research (Bacchus, 2003;

McCauley, 1998) has shown that victims of domestic violence want their health care provider to ask them about domestic violence, thereby creating a venue for them to open up as they feel able. While continuing to provide interventions related to hand function and energy management, the occupational therapist also reassesses Mr. Lee's areas of occupation, performance skills, and performance patterns to identify additional home and community supports he may need because of the domestic violence. She provides Mr. Lee with resources on domestic violence and the local crisis number. She includes interventions to focus on building self-esteem and empowerment.

Adolescent Case Study

Heong is a 16-year-old girl in 10th grade. For the past 2 months she has dated a popular young man who is in the 11th grade. Heong initially thought that his frequent phone calls throughout the day were very romantic. He started telling her that he didn't want her to go out with her friends and got into several fights with Heong's male classmates. After dating for about 1 month, he began to slap and punch her. The next day he would bring her flowers. Rather than tell anyone, Heong withdrew from her friends and after-school activities; she did not socialize with other boys at school or work.

A representative from the local women's shelter spoke to Heong's 10th-grade class about teen dating violence. Realizing that she was a victim of teen dating violence, Heong spoke to her guidance counselor. The counselor referred her to a teen dating violence group run by the school occupational therapist.

Assessment

The occupational therapist administers an initial assessment to evaluate Heong's occupational needs, problems, and concerns. The therapist analyzes Heong's occupational performance skills, performance patterns, context, and activity demands (AOTA, 2002). After reviewing the results of the initial assessment, the occupational therapist develops collaborative goals with Heong related to her job, leisure activities, and social participation in after-school activities.

Intervention

Utilizing a cognitive–behavioral approach, the occupational therapist helps Heong to explore the impact the dating violence had on her work performance, social participation, and her sense of identity. She encourages Heong to identify the importance of leisure occupations in the development of self-esteem, friendships, health, and identity. Together they develop a plan for Heong to participate again in familiar leisure occupations as well as in new ones.

Infant Case Study

Jonella brought her 4-month-old daughter, Kia, to an occupational therapist, as part of an early intervention service for infants and toddlers. Jonella tells the occupational therapist that she is concerned about Kia, who sleeps only 30 minutes at a time and consistently wakes up screaming. Jonella explains that she and Kia have just left an abusive relationship and now live with some friends. Since infancy, Kia has been awakened many times because of the shouting and physical violence. In addition, Jonella could not establish a daily nap and sleep routine for Kia because she frequently had to rush Kia out of the house to keep her safe.

Assessment and Intervention

The occupational therapist administers the *Test of Sensory Functions in Infants* and the *Transdisciplinary Play Based Assessment* to Kia to assess for sensory issues focusing on self-regulation and for potential developmental complications. The occupational therapist and Jonella collaborate to identify strategies for establishing a consistent nap and sleep routine for Kia. The occupational therapist models strategies that

Jonella can use to help calm Kia and modulate the amount of sensory input she receives. They also identify strategies for modifying the environment in the room where Kia sleeps and for helping Jonella relax with Kia before putting her to bed.

Toddler Case Study

A school system occupational therapist is asked to assess Daniel, a 5-year-old boy. His teacher states that Daniel is having extreme problems with manipulating crayons and performing gross motor activities. The teacher informs the therapist that the mother has just gotten out of a very abusive situation. The mother stated that Daniel's father would not let her place Daniel in a preschool or a Mother's Morning Out program. She was not allowed to take Daniel outside to play. In addition, when the father was home, Daniel was expected to sit quietly and was not allowed to play with toys. In spite of these restrictions, Daniel's mother did her best to expose her son to books and songs and teach him ways to play with household materials.

Assessment

The occupational therapist performs the *Quick Neurological Screening Test II* (QNST II) and sends the *Sensory Profile* home with Daniel for his mother to complete. Daniel scores within the "Definite Difference" range on the following factors on the Sensory Profile: Emotionally Reactive, Oral Sensory Sensitivity, Inattention/Distractibility, Auditory Processing, Vestibular Processing, and Multisensory Processing. As measured by the QNST II, Daniel also has difficulty with gross motor skills, balance, tactile processing, visual tracking, motor planning, impulsivity, and anxiety.

Intervention

The occupational therapist observes Daniel in the classroom and makes recommendations for strategies that the teacher can use to decrease Daniel's distractibility and to increase his attention and participation at school. The occupational therapy assistant works with Daniel for 45 minutes twice a week with time divided between intervention in the classroom to address cutting and drawing activities and outside the classroom to increase his motor control, sensory awareness, and problem-solving skills.

Teen Case Study

An occupational therapist is part of a diabetic program treatment team. The physician wants the therapist to assess and provide services to Herminie, a 34-year-old woman who is not routinely checking her glucose levels or taking her insulin. Because Herminie speaks limited English, her sister accompanies her to the session and translates for her.

Assessment

During the interview, Herminie shares that her 13-year-old daughter has taken on the responsibility for prompting Herminie to perform the techniques necessary to keep the diabetes under control. The 13-year-old daughter also takes care of her 7-year-old brother while Herminie works. Herminie left home with her children a year ago because her husband was physically and emotionally abusive to her. According to Herminie's sister, as a result of witnessing the abuse, the daughter is continually afraid that something is going to happen to her mother and brother. She is afraid to leave the house, except to go to school, and does not socialize with friends.

Intervention

With the aid of Herminie's sister who provides verbal and written translation, the occupational therapist develops a daily check sheet that Herminie can use to prompt herself to independently check her glucose levels and take her insulin. She discusses with Herminie how important it is for her, rather than her daughter, to be responsible for managing her diabetes. The occupational therapist meets with Herminie and her daughter on a weekly basis for several weeks to reinforce and monitor the progress that Herminie is making and to assist the daughter with reducing her anxiety. With Herminie's and her daughter's permission, the therapist called the daughter's school guidance counselor to discuss the situation and request help with decreasing the daughter's anxiety while facilitating increased socialization. In addition, the occupational therapist recommends that Herminie participate in a domestic violence counseling program.

References

Accreditation Council for Occupational Therapy Education. (2006). *ACOTE standards and interpretive guidelines.* Retrieved September 19, 2006, from http://www.aota.org/nonmembers/area13/docs/acotestandards806.pdf

American Occupational Therapy Association. (2002). Occupational therapy practice framework: Domain and process. *American Journal of Occupational Therapy, 56,* 609–639.

American Occupational Therapy Association. (2004). Guidelines for supervision, roles, and responsibilities during the delivery of occupational therapy services. *American Journal of Occupational Therapy, 58,* 663–667.

American Occupational Therapy Association. (2006). Policy 1.44: Categories of occupational therapy personnel. In *Policy manual* (2005 ed.). Bethesda, MD: Author. Retrieved from http://www.aota.org/members/area6/docs/pm-1205.pdf

Appel, A., & Holden, G. (1998). The co-occurrence of spouse and physical child abuse: A review and appraisal. *Journal of Family Psychology, 12,* 578–599.

Bacchus, L. (2003). Experiences of seeking help from health professionals in a sample of women who experienced domestic violence. *Health and Social Care in the Community, 11*(1), 10–18.

Carlson, B. (1997). A stress and coping approach to intervention with abused women. *Family Relations, 46,* 291–298.

Cummings, J., Peplar, D., & Moore, T. (1999). Behavior problems in children exposed to wife abuse: Gender differences. *Journal of Family Violence, 14,* 133–156.

D'Ardenne, P., & Balakrishna, J. (2001). Domestic violence and intimacy: What the relationship therapist needs to know. *Sexual and Relationship Therapy, 16,* 229–246.

Fisher, J., & Shelton, A. (2006). Survivors of domestic violence demographics and disparities in visitors to an interdisciplinary specialty clinic. *Community Health, 29,* 118–130.

Gallew, H., Krabacher, V., Andriacco, K., & German, D. (in press). Surviving domestic violence: Rebuilding one's life. *Occupational Therapy in Health Care.*

Gorde, M. W., Helfrich, C. A., & Finlayson, M. L. (2004). Trauma symptoms and life skills needs of domestic violence victims. *Journal of Interpersonal Violence, 19,* 691–708.

Heise, L., Ellsberg, M., & Gottemoeller, M. (1999, December). Ending violence against women. *Population Reports,* Series L(11), 1–43.

Helfrich, C. A. (Ed.). (2001). *Domestic violence across the lifespan. The role of occupational therapy.* Binghamton, NY: Haworth Press.

Helfrich, C. A., Lafata, M. J., MacDonald, S. L., Aviles, A., & Collins, L. (2001). Domestic abuse across the lifespan: Definitions, identification, and risk factors for occupational therapists. In C. A. Helfrich (Ed.), *Domestic violence across the lifespan. The role of occupational therapy* (pp. 5–34). Binghamton, NY: Haworth Press.

Huth-Beck, A., Levendosky, A., & Semel, M. (2001). The direct and indirect effects of domestic violence on young children's intellectual functioning. *Journal of Family Violence, 16,* 269–290.

Levendosky, A., & Graham-Bermann, S. (2001). Parenting in battered women: The effects of domestic violence on women and their children. *Journal of Family Violence, 16,* 171–192.

McCauley, J. (1998). Abused women's experiences with clinicians and health services. *Journal of General Internal Medicine, 13,* 549–555.

McKibben, L., DeVos, E., & Newberger, E. (1998). Victimization of mothers of abused children: A controlled study. *Pediatrics, 84,* 531–535.

Monahan, K., & O'Leary, K. D. (1999). Health injury and battered women: An initial inquiry. *Health and Social Work, 24,* 269–279.

National Coalition Against Domestic Violence. (n.d.). *What is battering?* Retrieved November 20, 2003, from http://www.ncadv.org

National Institute of Justice. (2000). *Extent, nature, and consequences of intimate partner violence.* Washington, DC: U.S. Department of Justice.

Norwood, W., Swank, P., Stephens, N., Ware, H., & Buzy, W. (2001). Reducing conduct problems among children of battered women. *Journal of Counseling and Clinical Psychology, 69,* 774–785.

Office for Victims of Crime. (2002). *National Victim Assistance Academy: Foundations in victimology and victims' rights and services* (Chapter 9: Domestic Violence). Retrieved June 8, 2006, from http://www.ojp.gov/ovc/assist/nvaa2002/chapter9.html

Sternberg, K., Lamb, M., Greenbaum, C., Cicchetti, D., Dawud, S., Cortes, R., et al. (1993). Effects of domestic violence on children's behavior problems and depression. *Developmental Psychology, 29,* 44–52.

Stiles, M. (2002). Witnessing domestic violence: The effect on children. *American Family Physician, 66,* 2052–2058.

Authors

Heather A. Javaherian, OTD, OTR/L
Robin T. Underwood, MS, OTR/L
Janet V. DeLany, DEd, OTR/L, FAOTA

for

The Commission on Practice
Susanne Smith Roley, MS, OTR/L, FAOTA, *Chairperson*

Adopted by the Representative Assembly 2006CO446

Occupational Therapy Services in Early Intervention and School-Based Programs

Occupational therapy plays an important role in early intervention and school-based programs. This document is written to explain that role to persons outside the occupational therapy profession.

Occupational therapists and occupational therapy assistants work in early intervention and school-based programs with children, parents, caregivers, educators, and other team members to facilitate the child's ability to engage in meaningful occupations. These occupations are activities that are meaningful for the child and are based on social or cultural expectations or peer performance. For example, a middle-school-aged child with physical limitations may have difficulty completing written work. The occupational therapist or the occupational therapy assistant under the supervision of the therapist collaborates with the student, parents, and educators to identify the skills of the student, the demands of the environment, and appropriate solutions for interventions. Another example is the family of a newborn baby with poor feeding skills. The occupational therapist may provide training and support for the family to enhance the baby's ability to drink from a bottle. Occupational therapy practitioners provide services that enable people to organize, manage, and perform their daily life occupations and activities. Occupational therapy services support a child's participation in activities of daily living, education, work, play, leisure, and social interactions.

Federal Legislative Influence on Service Delivery

Although the Individuals With Disabilities Education Act (IDEA) is the key federal law supporting occupational therapy services in early intervention and school-based settings, there are several other federal laws that influence occupational therapists and occupational therapy assistants working in these settings (see Table 1). The American Occupational Therapy Association (AOTA, 1999b) provides further information about these laws.

Occupational Therapy Domain and Process

Occupational therapy addresses engagement in occupations to support participation in context(s) (AOTA, 2002). *Occupations* are "activities . . . of everyday life, named, organized and given value and meaning by individuals and a culture" (Law, Polatajiko, Baptiste, & Townsend, 1997, p. 34). Occupational therapists and occupational therapy assistants focus on the following occupations: activities of daily living, instrumental activities of daily living, education, leisure, play, social participation, and work. The occupational therapy service delivery process includes evaluation, intervention, and outcomes. During the evaluation, the occupational therapist must gain an understanding of the client's priorities and his or her problems engaging in occupations and activities. Evaluation and intervention address factors that influence occupational performance, including

- Performance skills (e.g., motor, process, and communication/interaction skills);

- Performance patterns (e.g., habits, routines, and roles);

- Context (e.g., physical and social environments);

Table 1. Summary of Federal Laws and Their Influence on Occupational Therapy Services

Law	Influence on Occupational Therapy Services
Individuals With Disabilities Education Act—Part B (IDEA)	Mandates occupational therapy as a related service for those children with disabilities, 3–21 years old, who need it to benefit from special education.
Individuals With Disabilities Education Act—Part C (IDEA)	Allows for occupational therapy as a primary early intervention service for children up to 3 years of age who are experiencing developmental delays or who are at risk of having a delay.
Section 504 of the Rehabilitation Act of 1973, as amended (504)	Prohibits discrimination on the basis of disability by programs receiving federal funds. Disability here is defined more broadly than in IDEA. Children who are not IDEA-eligible may be eligible for 504 services, such as environmental adaptations to help them access the learning environment.
Americans With Disabilities Act of 1990 (ADA)	Extends Section 504's anti-discrimination provisions to all services and activities of state and local governments (which provide education and early intervention programs), whether or not they receive federal funds. As with Section 504, children who are not IDEA-eligible may be eligible for services as a reasonable accommodation to help them access the learning environment.
No Child Left Behind Act of 2001 (NCLB)	Requires public schools to raise the educational achievement of all students, particularly those from disadvantaged backgrounds, students with disabilities, and those with limited English proficiency. Holds states and local education agencies accountable for high standards for teaching and student learning.
Head Start Act, as amended	Provides comprehensive health, education, and social services to infants, toddlers, and preschoolers and their family members, including children with disabilities. Occupational therapy may be provided in these settings under the Head Start requirements or under IDEA.
Assistive Technology Act of 1998 (Tech Act)	State grant program that promotes access to assistive technology for persons with disabilities and universal design of information technology for persons with disabilities.
National School Lunch Program (NSLP)—USDA Regulations 2003	Provides free and reduced meals for income-eligible children. Any school receiving monies through this program must provide food substitutions at no extra charge for a child with a disability when the disability prevents the child from eating the regular school meal, as determined by a doctor.

- Activity demands (e.g., required actions and body functions); and

- Client factors (e.g., the mental, neuromuscular, sensory, visual, perceptual, digestive, cardiovascular, and integumentary systems).

Desired outcomes are identified to determine future actions with the client and as a means for evaluating the effectiveness of occupational therapy services.

> The occupational therapist is responsible for all aspects of occupational therapy service delivery and is accountable for the safety and effectiveness of the occupational therapy service delivery process . . . The occupational therapy assistant delivers occupational therapy services under the supervision of and in partnership with the occupational therapist. (AOTA, 2004, p. 6)

Service Provision

Early Intervention (IDEA Part C; Birth Through 2 Years Old)

Early intervention occupational therapy services may be provided to infants and toddlers with diagnoses of physical or mental conditions, with developmental delays, or who are at risk for having a developmental delay. Part C of IDEA focuses on five areas of development: physical, cognitive, communication, social–emotional, and adaptive. When evaluating infants or toddlers, the occupational therapist considers their strengths and needs with respect to these areas of development and their ability to participate in the environment at home, school, day care, and community. IDEA requires that services be developed in collaboration with the child's caregivers, educators, and community agencies. These services become part of the individualized family service plan (IFSP). Some examples of occupational therapy services for each of the five specified areas of Part C are listed below:

- *Physical development*—promoting movement for environmental exploration, facilitating use of the hands, designing and modifying technology to enhance interaction with environment, training family and caregivers in handling and positioning techniques, fostering the ability of the child to tolerate and use sensory information to perform daily life tasks

- *Cognitive development*—introducing activities that promote attention to tasks, teaching sorting and classifying of objects, promoting skills for listening and following directions, and modifying the environment so that distractions are minimized

- *Communication development*—facilitating oral–motor skills for sound production and for efficient intake of food and teaching operation of communication devices or sign language

- *Social–emotional development*—fostering self-regulation and social play skills, promoting interactions with peers and adults, training family and caregivers on methods for eliciting positive interactions and decreasing inappropriate behaviors, and modifying environments to promote positive interactions

- *Adaptive development*—helping the child develop skills for eating and drinking independently, teaching dressing and grooming tasks, training parents in safe positioning techniques, and modifying food textures to enhance eating.

In early intervention programs, occupational therapists may also act as service coordinators to monitor the implementation of the IFSP and coordinate services with other agencies. Occupational therapists and occupational therapy assistants also are important members of the team when the transition plan is developed for children as they approach 3 years of age.

School-Age Children (IDEA Part B; 3–21 Years Old)

The local school district is responsible for determining whether children with disabilities between the ages of 3 and 21 qualify under IDEA Part B as a "child with a disability . . . and [who] needs special education and related services" [IDEA, Section 602 (3)(A)(ii)]. A full and individual evaluation is conducted, and an individualized education program (IEP) is developed if the student is eligible for services. There are 10 disability categories by which a student with a disability might be eligible for IDEA services. They include the following:

- Mental retardation

- Hearing impairments (including deafness)

- Speech or language impairments

- Visual impairments (including blindness)

- Serious emotional disturbance

- Orthopedic impairment

- Autism

- Traumatic brain injury

- Other health impairment

- Specific learning disabilities [IDEA, Section 602(3)(A)].

Occupational therapy is one of the related services that may be provided to an IDEA-eligible student who is receiving special education in schools, homes, hospitals, and other types of settings, including juvenile justice and alternative education settings. When an occupational therapy assessment is required under IDEA, data collection is focused on identifying student strengths as well as what may be interfering with learning and participation in the context of his or her educational activities, routines, and environments. Observations are made where difficulties are occurring at school at times and in the location in which the student would normally be engaged in the activities or evidencing the behaviors that are of concern. These locations include the classroom, hallways, cafeteria, restrooms, gym, and playground. The student's work, participation, and behaviors are compared with other students in the same environments and situations. Curricular demands and existing task and environmental modifications are reviewed. Interviews with instructional personnel, the student, and family members are conducted to determine their impressions of the student's performance. Cultural differences that may exist between home and school are explored. Existing special education supports and services, including strategies utilized to improve performance, are reviewed. Standardized testing may be conducted when needed to gather additional data.

Occupational therapists collaborate with the IEP team regarding the educational need for occupational therapy services. Based on assessment data, the student's skills and abilities, the therapist's professional judgment, and the student's goals and objectives to be achieved, the IEP team decides whether occupational therapy services are needed. The development of the IEP is a collaborative process with participation from all team members. The IEP team determines when the student goals and objectives need the expertise of occupational therapy, as well as the time, frequency, duration, and location of those services. According to Nolet and McLaughlin (2000), the IEP indicates needed accommodations, modifications, and instructional strategies to access the general education curriculum and other educational supports for behavior skills, social skills, or skills needed for activities of daily living.

Intervention can be targeted toward individuals (including teachers and other adults working with the child), groups and environmental factors, and programmatic needs. According to Brannen et al. (2002), "consultation, collaboration, and teamwork are essential to effective implementation." Education and training of other team members is essential. Interventions provided in natural settings during daily routines are most likely to be applied consistently. Intervention methodologies using curriculum content and classroom materials are most likely to achieve maximum contextual integration and replication.

Outcomes are measured by student achievement of the IEP goals and other educational objectives, including participation on state and district-wide assessments that are supported by services from the occupational therapist and occupational therapy assistants. Data collected on targeted outcomes is reviewed by the IEP team and is important to the required annual IEP review.

Occupational Therapy Services Under Section 504

Section 504 of the Rehabilitation Act of 1973 (Section 504) prohibits discrimination on the basis of disability for any program receiving federal funds. Children with disabilities who do not qualify for services under IDEA may qualify under Section 504. Examples include children who have AIDS, asthma, arthritis, attention-deficit disorder, traumatic brain disorder, conduct disorder, or depression. Occupational therapists may be asked to help local school district teams determine student eligibility under 504 and to assist in the identification of services and development of the 504 plan. Occupational therapy services may be provided directly to a child or as a necessary accommodation.

Pre-Referral Services and Supports

As a member of a school's student support or resource team, occupational therapists may assist in the identification and provision of appropriate pre-referral services and supports to support a student's learning and behavior in the general education environment. These preventative, early intervention strategies are designed to minimize the occurrence of behavior and learning problems and reduce the need for more intensive services later. Occupational therapists can be significant contributors to this team-based problem-solving model. A brief, informal meeting may be held, attended by the child's teacher and any other professionals who may be able to offer general suggestions for overcoming difficulties with learning and participation. Occupational therapy suggestions might include the use of wide-lined paper or a pencil grip to support improvements in handwriting, modification of the classroom environment to increase accessibility, use of elastic-waist pants for a child unable to fasten clothing after toileting, strategies to deal with a child who hits others on the playground when he or she becomes frustrated, or general strategies for breaking down steps for jumping rope so that a child struggling with this skill can be successful in physical education.

Supervision of Other Personnel

Many early intervention programs, schools, or community agencies employ paraprofessionals to assist in the classroom or to provide direct support to some children. The occupational therapist may utilize these individuals, as allowed by state law and regulation. The paraprofessionals must be properly trained and supervised to assist with the provision of selected exercises or programming that will enhance the student's ability to achieve his or her IEP goals or IFSP outcomes. Paraprofessionals should perform only those tasks that can be safely performed within the child's routine and do not require the expertise of an occupational therapist. The tasks delegated to a paraprofessional should be documented. A plan to train and supervise the paraprofessional must be developed by the occupational therapist. An occupational therapy assistant may train and supervise a paraprofessional in specifically delegated tasks; however, the occupational therapist is ultimately responsible for monitoring programs carried out by paraprofessionals and occupational therapy assistants.

Conclusion

Occupational therapists and occupational therapy assistants provide services to children, families, caregivers, and educational staff within a variety of programs and settings. Regardless of where the evaluation and intervention services are provided, the ultimate outcome is to enable the child to participate in activities of daily living, education, work, play, leisure, and social interactions.

References

Americans With Disabilities Act of 1990, P. L. 101–336, 42 U.S.C. §12101.

American Occupational Therapy Association. (1999a). Guidelines for the use of aides in occupational therapy practice. *American Journal of Occupational Therapy, 53*, 595–597.

American Occupational Therapy Association. (1999b). *Occupational therapy services for children and youth under the Individuals With Disabilities Education Act* (2nd ed). Bethesda, MD: Author.

American Occupational Therapy Association. (2002). Occupational therapy practice framework: Domain and process. *American Journal of Occupational Therapy, 56*, 609–639.

American Occupational Therapy Association. (2004). Guidelines for supervision, roles, and responsibilities during the delivery of occupational therapy. *American Journal of Occupational Therapy, 58*.

Assistive Technology Act of 1998, P. L. 105–394.

Brannen, S. J., Cooper, E. B., Dellegrotto, J. T., Disney, S. T., Eger, D. L., Ehren, B. J., et al. (2002). *Developing educationally relevant IEPs: A technical assistance document for speech-language pathologists*. Reston, VA: Council for Exceptional Children.

Head Start Amendments of 1998, P. L. 105–285.

Individuals With Disabilities Education Act Reauthorization of 1997, P. L. 105–17, 20 U.S.C. §1400 *et seq.*

Law, M., Polatajiko, H., Baptiste, W., & Townsend E. (1997). Core concepts of occupational therapy. In E. Townsend (Ed.), *Enabling occupation: An occupational therapy perspective* (pp. 29–56). Ottawa, ON: Canadian Association of Occupational Therapists.

National School Lunch Program, 7 CFR, Part 210.10(g)(1)(2003).

No Child Left Behind Act of 2001, P. L. 107–110.

Nolet, V., & McLaughlin, M. J. (2000). *Accessing the general curriculum.* Thousand Oaks, CA: Corwin Press.

Rehabilitation Act Amendments of 1998, Pub. L. 105–220, 29 U.S.C. §794.

U.S. Department of Agriculture. (2001). *Accommodating children with special dietary needs in the school nutrition programs: Guidance for school food service staff.* Washington, DC: Author.

Authors

Gloria Frolek Clark, OTR/L, MS, FAOTA, *COP Member*
Jean Polichino, MS, OTR, *Chair, School System Special Interest Section*
Leslie Jackson, MEd, OT, *AOTA Federal Affairs Representative*

for

The Commission on Practice
Sara Jane Brayman, PhD, OTR/L, FAOTA, *Chairperson*

Adopted by the Representative Assembly 2004C26

This document replaces the 1998 Statement *Occupational Therapy for Individuals With Learning Disabilities* (previously published and copyrighted by the American Occupational Therapy Association in the *American Journal of Occupational Therapy, 52,* 874–880).

Occupational Therapy Services in Facilitating Work Performance

Introduction

The purpose of this statement is to describe for external audiences the role of the occupational therapist and the occupational therapy assistant in assisting people to successfully engage in work tasks and satisfactorily participate in meaningful work roles. The *Occupational Therapy Practice Framework* defines work as "activities needed for engaging in remunerative employment or volunteer activities" (AOTA, 2002, p. 620). Work performance supports participation and productivity, which are essential to the health and well-being of each individual.

Occupational therapists and occupational therapy assistants provide services to individuals or populations with deficits or problems in the area of work performance. The occupational therapist focuses on problem identification and analysis and the selection and/or design of appropriate evaluations and interventions for problem solution. The occupational therapy assistant may carry out the intervention plan, including reporting and documenting client responses, participation, and progress toward goals. The occupational therapy assistant works under the supervision of the occupational therapist in accordance with relevant agency, state, and federal regulations (AOTA, 2004).

Problems in work performance can arise from physical, sensory, cognitive, perceptual, psychological, social, or developmental changes. Therefore, occupational therapy practitioners[1] provide work-related services in a variety of settings, including, but not limited to, acute care and rehabilitation facilities, industrial sites and office environments, psychiatric treatment centers, and in the community. Within these settings, occupational therapy practitioners provide services in occupational rehabilitation, sheltered work, supported employment, and community mental health programs. Occupational therapy practitioners provide two key services in these settings: evaluation and intervention (including consultative, preventive, restorative, and compensatory services).

Occupational Therapy Evaluation in Work Programs

Through skilled observation, interviews, and evaluation of a client's performance skills and patterns, the occupational therapist can identify a person's interests, abilities, and needs as they relate to general work performance and specific job requirements. In addition, when providing work-related services, such as workplace redesign, worker disability prevention, and management programs, the occupational therapy evaluation may involve data collection in the following areas:

- Job analysis to identify the required activity demands of an individual's work tasks.

- Evaluation of contextual factors, including work and productive tasks, work routines, tools and equipment, ergonomic stressors, and accessibility. In the employment setting, analysis of essential job functions may be provided as part of this strategy.

---

[1]*Occupational therapy practitioner:* An individual initially certified to practice as an occupational therapist or occupational therapy assistant or licensed or regulated by a state, district, commonwealth, or territory of the United States to practice as an occupational therapist or occupational therapy assistant and who has not had that certification, license, or regulation revoked due to disciplinary action (AOTA, 1998).

Occupational Therapy Intervention in Work Programs

Occupational therapists and occupational therapy assistants deliver services to promote and manage productive occupations as well as to prevent and treat work-related disability. Using the evaluation data, the occupational therapist and the occupational therapy assistant collaborate with the worker, other team members (e.g., employers, case managers), or agencies (e.g., educational, local/state mental health, local/state mental retardation, vocational rehabilitation, social services) to plan and implement intervention strategies. When developing these intervention strategies, occupational therapy practitioners consider a client's age, interests, values, culture, skills and abilities, motivation, and psychological and psychosocial status, as well as work role, task demands, work context, and available resources. The intervention strategies are designed to explore and expand work options, enhance or develop work-related capabilities (e.g., improve physical capacities, improve safety of performance, develop skills), and obtain or retain employment. Intervention strategies may include direct services or consultation to individuals and groups. The following are some examples of occupational therapy intervention aimed at improving work performance:

- Education related to injury prevention, stress management, safety, proper body mechanics, postural awareness, pain management strategies, joint protection, and symptom awareness as applied to work and productive activities.

- Development of graded activities that allow the individual to perform physical work tasks essential for his or her worker role.

- Development of occupational activities to increase or improve productive behaviors and skills.

- Development of individualized work transition programs, job modifications, or job adaptations to facilitate successful work performance.

- Provision of recommendations about adaptation of work tasks, tools and equipment, or the work environment for the worker and/or the employer.

- Consultation with the employer on injury management and prevention services to reduce the incidence of disability related to injury.

- Collaboration with other team members, employers, services, and agencies in coordinating services provided to the worker.

- Case management services to assist in the coordination and planning for transition or return to work.

Table 1 provides examples of how performance patterns related to work may be compromised and how occupational therapy practitioners may assist individuals and/or populations in participating in meaningful productive activities.

Funding Sources

Reimbursement for services in the occupational performance area of work depend on the setting in which the services are provided. Reimbursement entities include, but may not be limited to,

- Direct reimbursement;

- State and or federally related programs, such as workers' compensation, Social Security Disability Insurance, and Medicare or medical assistance (see Appendix for an overview of relevant legislation impacting rehabilitation services for the worker); and

- Community agency resources, where funding may be secured through federal or state monies, community or private grants, or philanthropic donations.

Table 1.

Case Description	Work-Related Activity or Deficit	OT Role or Intervention
Mark, a 16-year-old high school student with developmental disabilities	Mark wants to seek employment after graduation. He lacks well-developed work behaviors and skills and is not able to independently initiate job seeking.	Assist in the development of a transition plan. Work with education staff to develop Mark's work behavior and skills, identify possible community work opportunities, assist in environmental adaptation, and provide job coaching. Educate Mark about the Americans With Disabilities Act.
Natalie, a 27-year-old woman with a history of schizophrenia who is a consumer at a community support program	Based on recent positive response to antipsychotic medication and success in volunteer work at the day program, Natalie has identified a goal of acquiring part-time work.	Assist Natalie with experiential exploration of potential jobs of interest. Collaborate with vocational counselor to set up a job-coaching program. Educate employer and job coach regarding Natalie's abilities and provide specific strategies related to job duties and organization to compensate for limitations.
Donna, a 36-year-old carpenter with a work-related back injury	Due to restricted activity from back injury, Donna is unable to safely perform the physical tasks required in her job. She has been off work for 3 months.	Perform a job analysis to identify essential functions, critical physical demands, and psychological factors. Identify possible job modifications and work with the employer to implement the changes. Perform a functional capacity evaluation to determine physical deficits related to performing job tasks. Based on the results, design a return-to-work program using graded activities and simulated job tasks, education, cardiovascular conditioning, and exercise. Educate in proper lifting, handling, and positioning to prevent further injury. Address stress management, work behaviors, and attitudes.
Sarah, a 45-year-old woman with rheumatoid arthritis, employed as a housekeeper at a hotel	Sarah is unable to perform her work tasks due to exacerbation of her rheumatoid symptoms.	Work with Sarah and her employer to identify priority tasks. Observe performance and analyze activities to determine points of difficulty. Suggest ergonomic modifications in process, tools, materials, approach, and context of housekeeping tasks to support improved performance. Train in work simplification and adapted techniques. Explore alternative jobs.
Ned, a 70-year-old retired civil engineer	Ned is experiencing difficulty in identifying satisfying productive volunteer activities to replace structured employment.	Explore Ned's interests. Identify interest areas and related volunteer opportunities. Expose to new activities. Connect with community socialization and interest groups.
Industrial site—a large factory that manufactures cartons	Workers are at risk for work-related injury.	Observe the workers performing their jobs. Provide consultation to employer regarding potential ergonomic stressors. Educate supervisors and worker groups regarding proper posture and body mechanics when performing work tasks. Work with employer on implementing ergonomic changes.
Large office setting	Workers are at risk for low back pain, carpal tunnel syndrome, and visual strain.	Provide consultation to employer. Identify and recommend environmental changes. Observe and evaluate individual office workstations and recommend changes based on individual needs. Engage the employees in the process. Educate supervisors and workers on early reporting, prevention techniques, and proper use of computers and office equipment.
Homeless shelter	Clients have expressed need to increase self-sufficiency and to seek support in developing realistic career objectives/goals.	Evaluate individual clients' work skills and assist in development of realistic career plans. Assist in development of work behaviors and skills, identify possible work opportunities, and provide job coaching.

References

American Occupational Therapy Association. (1998). Policy 1.44: Categories of occupational therapy personnel. In *AOTA policy manual*. Bethesda, MD: Author.

American Occupational Therapy Association. (2002). Occupational therapy practice framework: Domain and process. *American Journal of Occupational Therapy, 56,* 609–639.

American Occupational Therapy Association. (2004). Guidelines for supervision, roles, and responsibilities during the delivery of occupational therapy services. *American Journal of Occupational Therapy, 58,* 663–667.

Additional Reading

Aja, D. (1996, July). Finding a niche in job-site analysis. *OT Practice, 1*(7), 36–41.

Aja, D. (2004, March). Using a functional capacity evaluation as a successful benchmark in the life care plan process. *Work Programs Special Interest Section Quarterly, 18*(1), 1–4.

American Occupational Therapy Association. (1995). Concept paper: Service delivery in occupational therapy. *American Journal of Occupational Therapy, 49,* 1029–1031.

Fisher, T. F. (1994). Industrial rehabilitation: A natural environment for occupational therapy practitioners. *Work: A Journal of Prevention, Assessment, and Rehabilitation, 4*(4), 259–263.

Hanson, C. S. (1992). The history of work in physical dysfunction. *American Journal of Occupational Therapy, 46,* 56–62.

Harvey-Krefting, L. (1985). The concept of work in occupational therapy: A historical review. *American Journal of Occupational Therapy, 39,* 301–307.

Jeong, G. (1996, September). Enabling people with cognitive disabilities to join the workforce. *OT Practice, 1*(9), 40–45.

Johnson, J. (1993). Role of the occupational therapist in an on-site occupational rehabilitation program: A case study. *Work: A Journal of Prevention, Assessment, and Rehabilitation, 3*(3), 73–76.

King, P. M. (Ed). (1998). *Sourcebook of occupational rehabilitation.* New York: Plenum.

Kornblau, B. L., & Ellexson, M. (1995). Reasonable accommodation and the ADA. In S. J. Isernhagen (Ed.), *A comprehensive guide to work injury management* (pp. 781–798). Gaithersburg, MD: Aspen.

Larson, B. A. (2001). Work injury activities. In K. Sladyk & S. E. Ryan (Eds.), *Ryan's occupational therapy assistant: Principles, practice issues, and techniques* (3rd ed., pp. 393–398). Thorofare, NJ: Slack.

Mackinnon, J. R. (1992). Occupational profiles: Individuals with rheumatoid arthritis and a matched comparison sample. *Work: A Journal of Prevention, Assessment, and Rehabilitation, 2*(3), 39–49.

Maloney, C. C. (2003, September). Work simulation strategies in work programs. *Work Programs Special Interest Section Quarterly, 17*(3), 1–3.

Miller, D. M. (2004, February 9). Psychosocial issues and the return-to-work process. *OT Practice, 9*(3), 16–20.

Siporin, S., & Lysack, C. (2004). Quality of life and supported employment: A case study of three women with developmental disabilities. *American Journal of Occupational Therapy, 58,* 455–465.

Thiers, N. (1995, February 23). What happens after high school? *OT Week, 9*(8), 16–18.

Wright, M. (1997, May). Early return to work and occupational therapy. *OT Practice, 2*(5), 36–42.

Authors
Barbara Larson, MA, OTR, FAOTA
Melanie Ellexson, MBA, OTR/L, FAOTA

for

The Commission on Practice
Sara Jane Brayman, PhD, OTR/L, FAOTA, *Chairperson*

Adopted by the Representative Assembly 2005C257

Note: This replaces the 2000 document *Occupational Therapy Services in Facilitating Work Performance*.

Copyright © 2005, by the American Occupational Therapy Association. Previously published in the *American Journal of Occupational Therapy, 59, 676–679.*

Appendix. Selected Work Legislation

Name of Legislation	Scope of Legislation
Workers' Compensation Act, 1908 (35 Stat. 556)	No-fault insurance system that pays benefits to employees for accidental injuries or diseases that are work related.
Vocational Rehabilitation Act, 1943 (PL 78–113)	Changed the original provision of PL 66–236. Added physically disabled, blind, developmentally delayed, and psychiatrically disabled to those served. Established the office of vocational rehabilitation. Put a new emphasis on activities of daily living and adaptation. Removed ceiling on appropriation.
Hill Burton Act, 1954 (Vocational Rehab Act Amendments, PL 86–565)	Authorized greater financial support, research and demonstration grants, professional preparation grants, state agency expansion and improvements grants, and grants to expand rehabilitation facilities.
Vocational Rehabilitation Act Amendments of 1965 (PL 89–333)	Increased services for several types of people with disabilities and social handicaps. Made construction money available for rehabilitation centers and workshops.
Architectural Barriers Act, 1968 (PL 90–48)	Led the way to changes in access for people with disabilities.
Developmental Disabilities Services and Facilities Construction Act, 1970 (PL 91–517)	Gave states broad responsibility for planning and implementing a comprehensive program of services to people with developmental delays, epilepsy, cerebral palsy, and other neurological impairments.
Occupational Safety and Health Act, 1970 (PL 91–596)	Mandated that the employer provide employment free from recognized hazards that are likely to cause death or serious harm to workers.
Rehabilitation Act of 1973 (PL 93–112)	Expanded services to the more severely disabled. Provided for affirmative action in employment (Section 503) and nondiscrimination in facilities (Section 504) by federal contractors and grantees.
Rehabilitation Act Amendments of 1986 (PL 99–506)	Clarifications included that in evaluating rehabilitation potential, one must consider recreation, employability, and rehabilitation engineering needs.
Education of the Deaf Act of 1986 (PL 99–371)	Extended statutory authority of the National Technical Institute of the Deaf to provide technical training and education to prepare deaf people for employment.
Omnibus Budget Reconciliation Act of 1987 (PL 100–203)	Permitted states to offer prevocational, educational, and supported employment services to people deinstitutionalized at any time before the waiver program.
Americans with Disabilities Act of 1990 (PL 101–336)	Prevented discrimination against individuals with disabilities. Guaranteed equal protection for the individual with disabilities in employment, public accommodations, transportation, state and local government, and telecommunications.
Ticket-to-Work and Work Incentives Improvement Act of 1999 (PL 106–170)	Established to increase opportunities and choices for Social Security disability beneficiaries to obtain employment, vocational rehabilitation, and other support services from public and private providers, employers, and other organizations.

Philosophy of Occupational Therapy Education

Occupational therapy education is grounded in the belief that humans are complex beings engaged in a dynamic process of interaction with the physical, social, temporal, cultural, psychological, spiritual, and virtual environments. Through active engagement within the internal and external environments, humans evolve, change, and adapt. Occupational therapy educators advocate the use of occupation to facilitate health promoting growth, change, and/or adaptation with the goal of participation in meaningful occupation that supports survival, self-actualization, occupational balance, and quality of life.

The profession of occupational therapy is unique and dynamic, grounded in core principles of occupation, and is influenced by emerging knowledge and technologies. Thus, the education of future occupational therapists and occupational therapy assistants must consistently reinforce the development of new knowledge supporting the use of occupation, the application of clinical reasoning based on evidence, the necessity for lifelong learning, and the improvement of professional knowledge and skills.

Occupational therapy education promotes competence through educational experiences that foster the occupational therapists' and occupational therapy assistants' practice potential and scholarship development. Occupational therapy educators use active learning that engages the learner in a collaborative process that builds on prior knowledge and experience and integrates professional academic knowledge, experiential learning, clinical reasoning, and self-reflection. Occupational therapy education promotes integration of philosophical and theoretical knowledge, values, beliefs, ethics, and technical skills for broad application to practice in order to improve human participation and quality of life for those individuals with and without impairments and limitations.

The occupational therapy education process emphasizes continuing critical inquiry in order that occupational therapists and occupational therapy assistants be well prepared to function and thrive in the dynamic environments of a diverse and multicultural society, using the power of occupation as the primary method of evaluation, intervention, and health promotion.

Authors
The Commission on Education:
David A. Haynes, MBA, OTR/L, *OTA Program Director*
Terrianne Jones, MA, OTR/L, *OTA Academic Educator*

for

The Commission on Education
Linda S. Fazio, PhD, OTR/L, FAOTA, *Chairperson*

Adopted by the Representative Assembly 2007C9

Note: This document replaces the 2003 *Philosophy of Professional Education* (previously published and copyrighted in 2003 by the American Occupational Therapy Association in the *American Journal of Occupational Therapy, 57,* 640).

The Philosophical Base of Occupational Therapy

Man is an active being whose development is influenced by the use of purposeful activity. Using their capacity for intrinsic motivation, human beings are able to influence their physical and mental health and their social and physical environment through purposeful activity. Human life includes a process of continuous adaptation. Adaptation is a change in function that promotes survival and self-actualization. Biological, psychological, and environmental factors may interrupt the adaptation process at any time throughout the life cycle. Dysfunction may occur when adaptation is impaired. Purposeful activity facilitates the adaptive process.

Occupational therapy is based on the belief that purposeful activity (occupation), including its interpersonal and environmental components, may be used to prevent and mediate dysfunction and to elicit maximum adaptation. Activity as used by the occupational therapist includes both an intrinsic and a therapeutic purpose.

This statement was adopted by the April 1979 Representative Assembly of the American Occupational Therapy Association, Inc. as Resolution C #531–79. The text can be found as noted below.

American Occupational Therapy Association. (1979). The philosophical base of occupational therapy. *American Journal of Occupational Therapy, 33*, 785. (Reprinted in 1995 in the *American Journal of Occupational Therapy, 49*, 1026.) Reviewed by COE and COP in 2004.

American Occupational Therapy Association. (1979). Policy 1.11. The philosophical base of occupational therapy. In *Policy manual of the American Occupational Therapy Association, Inc.* Bethesda, MD: Author.

Providing Occupational Therapy Using Sensory Integration Theory and Methods in School-Based Practice

The American Occupational Therapy Association (AOTA) recognizes sensory integration (SI) as one of several theories and methods used by occupational therapists and occupational therapy assistants[1] working with children in public and private schools to improve a child's ability to access the general education curriculum and to participate in school-related activities. These methods are used to achieve the overarching goal of occupational therapy to improve the client's health and participation through engagement in everyday activities or "occupations" (AOTA, 2008). SI methods are used within occupational therapy when sensory-related issues are suspected to affect a child's ability to access the general and special education curriculum, behave adaptively, and participate in activities at school. It is estimated that, within the general population, approximately 5–10 percent of children may have SI dysfunction (Ahn, Miller, Milberger, & McIntosh, 2004).

Operating Within State and Federal Mandates in Public and Private Education

According to AOTA's (2009b) *Scope of Practice,*

> Occupational therapists and occupational therapy assistants are required to abide by statutes and regulations when providing occupational therapy services. State laws and other regulatory requirements typically include statements about educational requirements to practice occupational therapy, procedures to practice occupational therapy legally within the defined area of jurisdiction, the definition and scope of occupational therapy practice, and supervision requirements (p. 283).

Specific to public schools are parameters established by federal law such as the Individuals with Disabilities Education Improvement Act (IDEA, 2004), No Child Left Behind (NCLB) of 2001, and Section 504 of the Rehabilitation Act of 1973 mandating a child's right to a free, appropriate public education that includes occupational therapy as a related service. General education initiatives such as early intervening services and special education criteria for eligibility and related services are determined by each state on the basis of federal code. Local education agencies must provide, at a minimum, services mandated by federal and state levels and are able to provide a creative range of services at their own discretion.

Occupational therapists and occupational therapy assistants working in public schools may provide intervention to students in general education under early intervening services (e.g., using a response-to-intervention approach) and to students who are eligible under IDEA or Section 504 of the Rehabilitation Act of 1973. A child determined by the educational team to have a disability under IDEA must have an individualized education program (IEP). This includes a statement of the child's present level of functioning and the impact of the disability on the child's involvement and progress in the general education curriculum (§300.320(a)(1)(i)). The IEP must contain "a statement of the special education and related services...based on peer-reviewed research to the extent practicable, to be provided to the child, or on behalf of the child"

---

[1]*Occupational therapists* are responsible for all aspects of occupational therapy service delivery and are accountable for the safety and effectiveness of the occupational therapy service delivery process. *Occupational therapy assistants* deliver occupational therapy services under the supervision of and in partnership with an occupational therapist (AOTA, 2009a). When the term *occupational therapy practitioner* is used in this document, it refers to both occupational therapists and occupational therapy assistants (AOTA, 2006).

(§300.320(4)) in order for the child to progress on annual IEP goals, to be involved and make progress in the general education curriculum, and to be educated and participate with other children. A child determined by the school district to be a "qualified student with a disability" under Section 504 must have a 504 Plan that identifies the accommodations, modifications, and services needed. Occupational therapists and occupational therapy assistants may be participants in the development of the 504 Plan.

Application of SI Theory and Methods in Schools

Clinical and Professional Reasoning

Clinical reasoning based on professional training, evidence, and expertise guides the occupational therapist's selection of the use of one or more frames of reference such as SI (Burke, 2001; Parham, 1987; Schaaf & Smith Roley, 2006; Schell & Schell, 2008). While concepts of SI theory are included in the entry-level education of occupational therapists (Jacobs, Koomar, Mailloux, & Smith Roley, 1999), comprehensive assessment and intervention focused on SI is considered advanced-level practice (Smith Roley & Jacobs, 2008). Opportunities for additional knowledge and skills are available to therapists through workshops, publications, mentoring, and post-graduate certification in SI, including administering and interpreting the Sensory Integration and Praxis Tests (SIPT).[2]

SI theory describes information processing as a neurobiological process requiring the detection, assimilation, organization, interpretation, and use of sensory information that allows an individual to interact adaptively within the environment in daily activities at home, at school, and in other settings (Ayres, 1972b). The theory of SI is grounded on research in neuroscience (Ayres, 1972a; Bundy, Lane, & Murray, 2002; Smith Roley, Blanche, & Schaaf, 2001) and occupational science (Blanche & Parham, 2001; Parham, 2002; Smith Roley & Jacobs, 2008). Occupational therapy provides evaluation and interventions designed to identify, prevent, and remediate deficits related to the child's sensory sensitivities, sensory–perceptual skills, motor and praxis skills, and related patterns of performance (Ayres, 1972b, 1975; Bundy et al., 2002; Dunn, 2001; Mulligan, 1998a, 1998b, 2000; Schaaf & Smith Roley, 2006; Smith Roley et al., 2001; Smith Roley, Mailloux, Miller-Kuhaneck, & Glennon, 2007). The outcome of occupational therapy using SI theory is to improve function in various daily occupations (Ayres, 1979; Bundy et al., 2002; Dunn, 2001; Parham & Mailloux, 2004; Roley, Blanche, & Schaaf, 2001; Spitzer, Roley, Clark, & Parham, 1996).

Evaluations

Occupational therapy practitioners working in schools consider existing academic and nonacademic expectations when determining the child's academic, adaptive, and functional needs. Services are recommended as a result of the findings to support success in reaching positive yearly and long-term outcomes in education. Evaluations in the educational setting must include a review of educational information including (1) information and evaluation results provided by the parents, (2) assessment or observation results related to performance in the current classroom or on local or state assessments, and (3) teacher and other service provider observations (§300.305). In addition, therapists may review pertinent medical information; interview teachers, parents, and the student; observe in natural settings to observe performance; and use various assessments, including standardized tests (Clark & Coster, 1998). Multiple

---

[2]It is important to note occupational therapy's use of the term *sensory integration*. A. Jean Ayres developed her sensory integration theory originating from the work of Sherrington (1906, cited in Ayres, 1972a). Using supportive evidence from neuroscience and applied science, this theoretical model supports its application in occupational therapy practice. The trademarked term *Ayres Sensory Integration™* is used to describe the use of sensory processing and sensory-related methods as guided by Ayres's sensory integration theory. Occupational therapy practitioners are the key professionals using this sensory integration therapy founded on principles of neuroscience (Reeves, 2007).

sources of information must be used when determining educational disabilities. The occupational therapist selects a variety of measures that include developmental and skill-based observations in addition to those that identify occupational and sensory strengths and weaknesses. The occupational therapist interprets the test findings relative to the child's performance skills, patterns of engagement, and ability to participate.

The evaluation specific to SI includes performance measures of the child's ability to adapt, organize, and integrate sensory information in the environment that affects participation in academic and nonacademic activities at school. Sensory deficits are complex and include various patterns of perceptual, motor, and praxis difficulties (Parham & Mailloux, 2004) affecting the speed and accuracy of learning as well as variations in sensory responsiveness (Ayres & Tickle, 1980; Dunn, 1999) affecting emotional well-being (Ayres, 1979) and social competencies, including play (Mailloux & Burke, 2008).

Structured and unstructured assessments of sensory responsiveness, sensory perception, motor skills, and praxis are essential features of the evaluation (Windsor, Smith Roley, & Szklut, 2001). Multiple data sources should be used when evaluating skills and performance in SI.

Several structured screenings and assessments have been developed for children:

- *DeGangi Berk Test of Sensory Integration* (DeGangi & Berk, 1983) is a preschool screening focused on sensory-based postural and motor functions.

- *Sensory Integration and Praxis Tests (SIPT)* (Ayres, 1989, 1998) is a standardized performance measure used to diagnose sensory integrative dysfunction related to learning and behavior. Professionals using this tool must complete postgraduate training leading to certification in the administration and interpretation of the SIPT and related measures. The SIPT (Ayres, 1989, 1998) is a series of 17 individual tests that provide information on visual perception, visual–motor and fine-motor performance, construction, tactile discrimination, tactile sensitivity, kinesthesia, vestibular functions including post-rotary nystagmus and balance, bilateral motor control, and praxis, including following verbal instructions, sequencing, oral–facial imitation, and imitation of body gestures. This test is predictive of academic function especially math and reading abilities (Parham, 1998).

- *Sensory Processing Measure (SPM)* (Miller-Kuhaneck, Henry, Glennon, Parham, & Ecker, 2007), for home and school, is an integrated system of rating scales that enables assessment based on parent and educational staff report of sensory processing issues, planning and ideas, and social participation in elementary school-age children.

- *Sensory Profile* (Dunn, 1999), *Infant/Toddler Sensory Profile* (Dunn, 2002), and the *Sensory Profile School Companion* (Dunn, 2006) are standardized questionnaires that focus on the student's sensory processing performance patterns within the natural context.

Unstructured assessments may include direct observation of the child's performance in a variety of tasks to analyze the sensory–motor and cognitive demands of the activities, the social and physical characteristics of the environment(s), the effectiveness of the student's performance skills and patterns in those activities and environments, and assessments of neuromotor functions via clinical observations (Blanche, 2002; Wilson, Pollock, Kaplan, & Law, 1994) and play performance (Knox, 2008; Skard & Bundy, 2008).

Intervention and Service Delivery

The team determines services necessary for the child to access general education and benefit from special education on the basis of the child's educationally related needs. Guided by the identified needs and IEP goals of the child, the occupational therapist working in collaboration with the student and the IEP team determines the most appropriate and effective interventions and service delivery models to address the goals. By definition, occupational therapy services are a collaborative process used for the benefit of individuals, populations, and organizations (AOTA, 2008). Related to a child's classroom placement, IDEA requires that "removal of children with disabilities from the regular educational environment occurs only if the nature or severity of the disability is such that education in regular classes...cannot be achieved satisfactorily" (34 C.F.R. 300.114(a)(i)).

Occupational therapy interventions can occur in a variety of settings to support the child's success within the least restrictive environment (LRE). The context of service delivery can include locations at the school such as the classroom, playground, lunchroom, bathroom, or therapy room and off-site locations within the community. Interventions may include one or more of the following types of occupational therapy interventions, preparatory methods, purposeful activities, and occupation-based interventions, depending on the needs of the child and identified outcomes.

Occupational therapy services in schools include the application of specialized knowledge and skills to facilitate adaptive responses the children need to support their learning and behavior. Consultation and direct intervention are both aspects of the service. As related to the use of SI interventions, this may include education that reframes the understanding of the sensory-related concerns; recommendations that incorporate sensory–motor activities throughout the day such as before, during, and after school; and environmental modifications that assist the student's school-related performance. Sensory activities directed by the occupational therapist can be embedded into the classroom routine that can be carried out by the teacher, instructional aides, or parent volunteers. It also may include direct intervention that address the underlying sensory, motor, and praxis concerns through therapeutic use of environment affordances such as mats and swings that provide opportunities for moving through space; climbing in, over, and under large equipment; falling safely onto matted areas; and rearranging the equipment.

Characteristics of the SI approach are outlined in the work conducted by several researchers on adherence to fidelity to the intervention (Parham et al., 2007). Table 1 provides examples of OT intervention approaches using a SI frame of reference. Table 2 provides case examples. The choice of interventions is guided by research regarding the effectiveness of the intervention related to the identified goals for the child.

Outcomes

The federal NCLB and IDEA are two of the most important federal laws relating to the outcomes of education for children with and without disabilities. NCLB seeks to improve accountability for the outcomes of education for all children, and IDEA ensures that children with disabilities will have individualized services to meet unique needs in order to benefit from and appreciate positive outcomes of public education. Both NCLB and IDEA endorse the need for an evidence-based education approach. NCLB stresses accountability as measured by the "use of effective methods and instructional strategies that are based on evidence-based practice" (Sec. 1114 (b)(1)(B)(ii)). IDEA 2004 states that the child's IEP will provide "a statement of the special education and related services and supplementary aids and services, based on peer-reviewed research to the extent practicable" (Sec. 614(d)(1)(A)(i)(IV)).

Occupational therapy using SI theory and methods is designed to improve a person's ability to interact adaptively in the environment, learn, behave, and to prevent future adaptive difficulties and thus improve quality of life. The efficacy of occupational therapy's use of SI has been investigated by several researchers over the past 35 years. Critical review of the literature has provided evidence of efficacy as well as limitations in the design of several studies. Examples of studies supporting occupational therapy using SI theory and methods are provided in Table 3.

Through accurate functional baseline data, measurable student goals, and data collection to monitor a child's successful participation in the natural environment, occupational therapists provide accountability for a child's progress in occupational therapy intervention as it relates to education. Goal attainment scaling

Table 1. Approaches and Sensory Strategies for Occupational Therapy Intervention

Occupational Therapy Approaches	Examples of Sensory-Related Strategies
Create, Promote Health and Participation	• Create a class for parents and/or educational staff to teach the relationships among sensory processing, learning, and behavior • Promote increased physical activity for students to improve physical and mental health and cognitive and social performance • Support installment of a variety of equipment available at schools and public playgrounds to promote a diversity of sensory play experiences • Design sensory-enriched classrooms with a variety of seating options, as well as opportunity for tactile, movement, and proprioceptive experiences throughout the day
Establish/Restore Performance Skills and Performance Patterns	• Design activities rich in tactile, vestibular, and proprioceptive information that increase body awareness needed during activities of daily living • Facilitate the development of appropriate SI and motor-planning skills needed for organizing materials, completing tasks within an appropriate time frame, and adapting to transitions • Establish/restore mobility needed for social and object play • Provide controlled sensory input through activities that require increasingly more complex adaptive responses to novel activity to support ability to engage in group activities with peers
Maintain Student Ability to Engage in and Cope With School-Related Activities	• Structure sensory environment to meet the student's needs such as reducing distractions and improving attention to salient auditory and visual information • Teach sensory strategies for emotional, physiological, behavioral, motor, and social self-regulation • Maintain ability to organize behavior by providing scheduled sensory breaks and sensory accommodations such as changing the size, texture, and location of the desk • Maintain peer relationships by supporting and compensating for motor planning needs in age-appropriate games and sports • Maintain student productivity by providing compensation techniques for sensory and motor-planning deficits using study carrels, visual timers, weighted vests, alternate seating arrangements, modified writing tools, paper, and other assistive technology
Modify Activity to Help Student Compensate for Sensory, Motor, and Praxis Deficits	• Through collaborative consultation with education staff and parents, develop strategies for modifying the sensory, motor, or praxis demands of assignments to increase student productivity • Support student participation in general curriculum by modifying sensory and motor-planning (praxis) demands of activity • Structure or modify the environment to support the student's sensory, motor, motor-planning, and self-regulatory capacities and needs
Prevent Barriers to Participation and Improve Safety	• Prevent inattention, poor posture, and restlessness when sitting for prolonged periods by modifying seating options, allowing sensory breaks, and allowing student to work in various positions • Prevent social isolation by providing motor-planning and social strategies to participate with peers • Prevent socially inappropriate behaviors and behavioral distress or disruption by detecting and meeting sensory and self-regulatory needs • Prevent injury by providing ergonomic seating and safety strategies for students whose nervous systems fail to register sensory information • Prevent barriers to child participation by increasing the understanding of the school district staff regarding of the role that SI and praxis play in influencing learning and behavior

Note. SI = sensory integration.

Table 2. Case Examples

The following vignettes are outlined relative to the *Occupational Therapy Practice Framework: Domain and Process,* 2nd Edition (AOTA, 2008) to illustrate occupational therapy using sensory integrative theory and methods in schools.

Case No. 1 Natasha: Preschool-Age Child

Evaluation

Referral: Natasha is a 3-year-old child enrolled in a special education preschool. The IEP team recommended an OT evaluation because Natasha has difficulty with classroom transitions and social interactions.

Occupational Profile

Natasha's family and educational team are seeking OT services due to her difficulty with transitioning and coping in the classroom. Natasha is sensitive to noise, cries, and clings to the aide in the classroom. She performs well at skilled tasks. Additional information was gathered from her medical, developmental, educational, and occupational histories. The priorities listed by the teacher and parents include social interactions (friendships) and performance within the flow of the classroom (transitioning).

Evaluation and Analysis of Occupational Performance

Interview data:
- *Speech and language therapist report:* Receptive language is below average and decreases when there is noise in the room.
- *Teacher report:* Natasha has difficulty adapting to the flow of classroom activities. She needs an exceptional amount of attention from adults in order to stay calm. Natasha is able to cognitively perform the tasks but is overwhelmed with the noise and movement in the room.
- *Parent report:* Natasha's mother is concerned about her unhappiness at school and her inability to play and make friends.

Observation data:
- Natasha prefers to sit alone or next to an adult.
- Natasha needs extra cues to pay attention. Although physically capable, she does not complete the fine-motor preschool activity without adult direction.
- She does not initiate social interaction with other children and becomes irritable when children come near her.
- She cries when entering the lunchroom or when a group of noisy children run past her during recess.
- She does not like to go to lunch and refuses to eat anything but chips.

Test data:
- Infant/Toddler Sensory Profile demonstrates inefficient sensory self-regulation and sensory modulation, poor tactile discrimination, poor motor planning, and increased auditory sensitivity.
- Beery Visual Motor Integration suggests poor visual–motor integration.
- Knox Preschool Play Scale shows immature play patterns.
- Adequate cognitive performance (from IQ measures).
- Adequate fine-motor performance.
- Miller Function and Participation Scales demonstrates delays in gross-motor and visual–motor skills.

Intervention (includes, but not limited to, the following ideas)

IEP Goals:
Natasha:
- Will transition between classroom activities independently 4 out of 5 transitions for 3 days.
- Will sustain adult-facilitated interaction with her peers during free play for 5 minutes during a 15-minute observation 4 out of 5 free play periods.
- Will carry out verbal instructions with visual cues 4 out of 5 opportunities with 80% accuracy.

OT Intervention Plan Includes the Following Goals:
OT is provided within the classroom setting during routine activities. Natasha's response to intervention in relation to learning, behavior, and adjustment to preschool will be monitored closely for progress and signs of a disorder in SI. Changes to the service delivery may be recommended, as needed, to the IEP team.
Natasha:
- Will regulate her responses to environmental stimuli to remain calm during routine class transitions.

OT Intervention Process and Strategies:
The OT practitioner will facilitate and enhance performance through these interventions:
Client Level:
- Increase sensory modulation through the use of heavy work activities.
- Improve vestibular spatial body awareness through moving on swings and locating visual and auditory targets.
- Improve adaptive responses and motor planning to increase competence when faced with dynamic activities and overall repertoire of play skills.

Table 2. Case Examples *(cont.)*

Case No. 1 Natasha: Preschool-Age Child *(cont.)*

Intervention (includes, but not limited to, the following ideas) *(cont.)*

- Will self-regulate her responses to tactile stimuli to sit next to several peers and focus on the activity during playground and eating activities.
- Will motor plan her body movements to engage in preschool play.
- Will improve spatial location of sound relative to the position of her body in the classroom with and without background noise.

Activity Level:
- Increase texture and weight of materials used during class activities.
- Use visual cues for improved independence during familiar sequences and routines.

Environmental Level:
- Before class, Natasha will arrive early and will enter classroom prior to other children to gradually adjust to the increased noise and pace of the day.
- Natasha will receive visual cues and tangible transition prompts such as a visual schedule to provide advanced notice of classroom activity changes.
- Natasha will be provided with a variety of seating options during circle time such as a bean bag chair, rocking chair, ball chair, or cube seat.
- Seating will be arranged near an adult.

Natasha:
- Will regulate her responses to environmental stimuli to remain calm during routine class transitions.
- Will self-regulate her responses to tactile stimuli to sit next to several peers and focus on the activity during playground and eating activities.
- Will motor plan her body movements to engage in preschool play.
- Will improve spatial location of sound relative to the position of her body in the classroom with and without background noise.

Outcomes

Outcomes were reported by members of the IEP team:

Performance Skills:
- Improvement noted in all skill areas: sensory–perceptual skills, motor and praxis skills, emotional regulation skills, cognitive skills, and social communication skills.

Performance Patterns:
- Easier transitions.
- Increased attention.
- Developed friendships.
- Sustained participation during classroom activities without withdrawing.
- Teacher and parent are pleased that Natasha is able to participate in her preschool program and appears happier at school.

Adaptation:
- Improved self-regulation and adaptation in the preschool routine.

(continued)

Table 2. Case Examples *(cont.)*

Case No. 2 Billy: Elementary School-Age Student

Evaluation

Referral: Billy is a 7-year-old student in a general education classroom environment. An OT evaluation was requested due to Billy's extremely poor handwriting.

Occupational Profile

Billy's guardians and educational team requested an OT evaluation due to his difficulty with writing, attention, and peer relationships. Information was obtained from the medical, developmental, educational, and occupational histories. Priorities include improving Billy's ability to meet state standards in Language Arts, that is, complete written work legibly, and to adapt to the social and prevocational expectations in first grade by engaging with peers and staying on task at school.

Evaluation and Analysis of Occupational Performance

Interview data:

Teacher report:

- Billy has above-average academic ability but completes less than half of his assignments in the proper amount of time.
- Billy does not interact with his peers.
- He expressed concerns that as the demands of school increased, Billy was going to fall further and further behind.
- Billy has poor use of his hands for tasks, such as opening his lunch containers and managing classroom tools.
- Billy's writing is illegible.

Parent report:

- He has no friends.
- He has difficulty comprehending simple verbal instructions.
- He has unusual habits and rituals.
- He has poorly established patterns of daily activities, such as getting ready to go to bed or mealtimes.

Test data:

Sensory Integration and Praxis Tests and clinical observations results:

- Visual–perception tests within normal limits.
- Visual–motor tests fall 1–2 standard deviations below the mean.
- Visual construction test scores fall in the high average range.
- Poor bilateral motor control.
- Poor oral praxis and postural praxis.
- Poor tactile discrimination.
- Poor posture and eye control.
- Decreased prone extension and supine flexion.

Sensory Processing Measure–Home Form (Miller-Kuhaneck et al., 2007) revealed definite differences in social participation, movement, tactile functions, body awareness, and ideas and planning.

Sensory Processing Measure–Main Classroom Form revealed definite differences in response to movement and body awareness; he is easily overwhelmed with auditory and visual activity in the environment.

Classroom handwriting portfolio was compared with peers to determine discrepancy.

Intervention (includes, but not limited to, the following ideas)

IEP Goals:

Billy:

- Will be able to write 3 legible sentences in his journal during a 20-minute writing period 4 out of 5 opportunities.
- Will stay on topic and remain in his seat for the duration of a 15-minute social studies lesson 4 out of 5 opportunities.
- Will participate appropriately in a structured playground activity with

OT Intervention Plan Includes the Following Goals:

OT was recommended to improve visual–motor control and improve overall attention.

OT to be provided to student in a specially equipped environment, and consultation to be provided to the IEP team members

Billy:

- Will organize visual–motor information in order to write legible words.

OT Intervention Process and Strategies:

The OT will facilitate adaptive responses through provision of sensory and motor challenges through the following interventions:

Client Level:

- Use weight-bearing and heavy work activities to increase strength of Billy's trunk and upper extremities.
- Increase exploration of multiple textures, sizes, and shapes to improve sensitivity and stereognosis in his hands.

Table 2. Case Examples *(cont.)*

Case No. 2 Billy: Elementary School-Age Student *(cont.)*

Intervention (includes, but not limited to, the following ideas) *(continued)*		
one other child without leaving the activity or arguing with the child for 10 minutes during the recess or lunch break 2 out of 3 opportunities.	• Will organize somatosensory input from his body to imitate and follow visual directions during structured playground activities. • Will remain comfortably seated and regulate his attention during instruction so that he remains focused and on task during social studies. • Will confidently access playground equipment and perform in recess and physical education games with peers.	*Activity Level:* • Instruct teacher in kinesthetic and visual support method to re-teach fundamentals of handwriting. • Use weighted pencils, pencil grips, and paper with highlighted areas. • Allow Billy to do some of his work while standing, ball-sitting, or lying on his stomach. *Environmental Level:* • Provide written text to copy rather than copying from blackboard. • Provide written instructions and pictures of daily sequences of activities, with times and locations. • Allow structured time for movement throughout the day as needed.

Outcomes

Outcomes that were reported by IEP team members:

Occupational Performance:
- Improved penmanship and Language Arts skills.
- Increased attention to topic.
- Increased amount of time spent focused and ready to learn, sitting still and upright in the chair.
- Increased self-determination and independent engagement in structured activities.
- Improved participation and organization of behavior in daily routines.
- Increased spontaneous peer interaction during academic tasks, lunchtime, and playground activities.

(continued)

Table 2. Case Examples (cont.)

Case No. 3 John: Middle-School Student

Evaluation

Referral: John is 12 years old and entering middle school. The IEP team requested an OT evaluation because he cannot organize his belongings and schedule or find his way around the middle school campus and is experiencing high anxiety, refusing to go to his new school. While psycho-educational assessments reveal adequate cognitive abilities, the IEP team members report escalating concerns related to his ability to keep up with his peers academically and physically.

Occupational Profile

John's family and the educational team requested an OT evaluation due to his difficulty finding his way around his school and his resulting in anxiety and depression. Additional information from medical, developmental, educational, and occupational histories was reviewed. Team priorities include increasing John's confidence and independence in performing school curriculum activities and ability to navigate around school without getting lost.

Evaluation and Analysis of Occupational Performance

Interview Data:

Parent reports that John:

1. Gets lost easily.
2. Works best in a self-contained classroom with group transitions; however, the middle school is not structured this way.
3. Demonstrates poor spatial abilities such as when aligning numbers in math.
4. Talks his way out of anything he finds difficult.

John reports that he:

- Has anxiety attacks.
- Feels sick during rides in the car.
- Feels stupid.
- Wants to be home-schooled.
- Spends most of his day in sedentary activities.
- Cannot tolerate backward movement of his head.
- Cannot play desired team sports at the skill level of his peers and as a result feels rejected and humiliated by other children.

Data From Record Review:

The elementary school file indicates that John is good in academics but rarely finishes written work on time in a legible or organized manner. He is well behaved and liked by peers.

- Teacher noted that John did not volunteer for classroom errands on the school grounds unless he could go with a peer.
- John often lost his completed assignments in the classroom, later to be found lost in his messy desk or in unlikely places in the classroom.

Observation Data:

- Below-age level on Beery Visual Motor Integration and Visual Perception Within normal limits on Beery (fine) Motor Coordination in tracing precision.
- Poor 2- and 3-dimensional construction ability.
- Poor balance with eyes closed.
- Self-reports of dizziness on playground swings.
- Poor disassociation of his head, neck, and body.
- Excessive talking to avoid performing during the evaluation observation.
- Inability to locate familiar landmarks such as office.

Intervention (includes, but not limited to, the following ideas)

IEP Goals:

John:

- Will arrive at all of his classes independently and on time, for 2 weeks.
- Will attend school and for 8 of 10 days with low levels of anxiety as noted by self-report.
- Will show increased tolerance for bus

OT was recommended for this student in his school setting.

OT Intervention Plan Includes the Following Goals:

John:

- Will identify a strategy out of 3 options (map, written sequence, or self-instruction) that works best for him to get to familiar places.

OT Intervention Process and Strategies:
The OT will facilitate and enhance performance through these interventions:

Client:

- Practice various strategies developed by the OT to improve awareness of the geography of the campus.
- Provide strategies to help John

Table 2. Case Examples *(cont.)*

Case No. 3 John: Middle-School Student *(cont.)*

Intervention (includes, but not limited to, the following ideas) *(cont.)*		
rides as reported by child, guardian, and bus driver 4 of 5 days. • Will identify age-appropriate leisure time options that are within his ability and interest level such as individually oriented community sports and lessons (e.g., karate, yoga, swimming, chess, arts and crafts). • Will explore junior high extracurricular activities and clubs	• Will identify, select, and participate in leisure and extracurricular physical activities. • Will learn to identify antecedents to the periods of his increased anxiety and utilize relaxation techniques to remain calm when transitioning from home to school and between classes.	become aware of and identify his own sensory strengths, sensitivities, and preferences. • Increase proprioceptive "heavy work" activities to improve sense of body in space. • Avoid intense vestibular activities. *Activity Level:* • Provide cues, landmarks, and signs that John can record as he walks to his class. • Enroll John in extracurricular activities such as karate, yoga, swimming, or rock climbing *Environmental Level:* • Pair John initially with a peer to walk to class. • Make a list of visual details as landmarks, take pictures, or put room numbers on an index card color-coded for each of John's classes to enable him to get to different classes.

Outcomes

Outcomes that were reported by IFP team members.

Participation:
- *Self-confidence in his own ability to adapt to and meet the everyday spatial demands of school activities, greatly reducing stress at school.*
- *Self-awareness and self-determination to seek advice in devising strategies to compensate for things that are uncomfortable or intimidating.*
- *Arrives at class on time.*
- *Able to finish and find 75% of his assignments independently.*
- *No longer resists going to school.*
- *Initiates participation in leisure activities with peers, such as school clubs.*

Client Satisfaction:
- *John is confident that he can travel between classes without assistance.*
- *Parents report that John is much happier at home and at school.*
- *There are no further reports of depression or anxiety.*

Note. IEP = individualized education program; OT = occupational therapy; SI = sensory integration.

Table 3. Occupational Therapy Service Continuum and Curriculum-Related Outcomes

The following table provides samples of studies supporting various SI-related methods and outcomes in school-based practice. It is not an exhaustive list of the available evidence.

Examples of OT Focus Areas Using SI Theory in School-Based Practice	Projected Educational Outcomes	Examples of Resources and Evidence
Participation in education Emotional regulation, sensory–perceptual, motor, praxis, and cognitive skills	Students will access general education curriculum and attend to classroom instruction for longer periods of time prior to identification for special education eligibility and formal OT evaluation.	Schilling, D. L., Washington, K., Billingsley, F. F., & Deitz, J. (2003). Classroom seating for children with attention deficit hyperactivity disorder: Therapy balls versus chairs. *American Journal of Occupational Therapy, 57,* 534–541.
School readiness for education participation Play and leisure Communication and social skills	Students access general education standards and learn adaptive behavior and social skills.	Jarrett, O. S., & Maxwell, D. M. (2000). What research says about the need for recess. In R. Clements (Ed.), *Elementary school recess: Selected readings, games, and activities for teachers and parents* (pp. 12–23). Lake Charles, LA: American Press. Pellegrini, A. D., & Smith, P. K. (1993). School recess: Implications for education and development. *Review of Educational Research, 63,* 51–67. Pellegrini, A. D., & Smith, P. K. (1998). Physical activity play: The nature and function of a neglected aspect of play. *Child Development, 69,* 577–598.
Self-regulation, including the development of emotional regulation, cognitive, and sensory–perceptual skills	Students build sensory self-awareness and self-regulatory strategies to increase focus of attention and completion of school work.	Williams, M. S., & Shellenberger, S. (1994). *How does your engine run? A leader's guide to the Alert Program for Self-regulation.* Albuquerque, NM: TherapyWorks.
Attention/on-task behavior to improve participation in education	Students increase on-task behavior through sensory strategies, sensory breaks, and sensory diets integrated into the school routine.	VandenBerg, N. L. (2001). The use of a weighted vest to increase on-task behavior in children with attention difficulties. *American Journal of Occupational Therapy, 55,* 621–628.
Cognitive, sensory–perceptual, and motor and praxis skills that enhance academic learning	Academic scores are improved through SI methods focusing on eliciting adaptive responses during OT.	Ayres, A. J. (1972a). Improving academic scores through sensory integration. *Journal of Learning Disabilities, 5,* 338–343.
Cognitive, sensory–perceptual, and motor and praxis skills that enhance academic learning	Gains in language comprehension and on expressive language measures are noted after OT using SI methods.	Ayres, J., & Mailloux, Z. (1981). Influence of sensory integration procedures on language development. *American Journal of Occupational Therapy, 35,* 383–390.

Table 3. Occupational Therapy Service Continuum and Curriculum-Related Outcomes *(cont.)*

Examples of OT Focus Areas Using SI Theory in School-Based Practice	Projected Educational Outcomes	Examples of Resources and Evidence
Sensory functions and sensory–perceptual skills influencing the readiness to learn Adaptation	This study analyzed which sensory test variable predicted response to therapy. Participants with hyper-responsiveness such as tactile defensiveness and gravitational insecurity and orienting to an air puff responded better than those with under-responsiveness or who failed to orient to sensory input.	Ayres, A. J., & Tickle, L. S. (1980). Hyper-responsivity to touch and vestibular stimuli as a predictor of positive response to sensory integration procedures by autistic children. *American Journal of Occupational Therapy, 34,* 375–381.
Cognitive, sensory–perceptual, and motor and praxis skills that enhance academic learning and communication and social skills	Following sensory-based intervention, children with decreased cognitive function showed improved spontaneous language, indicating that vestibular activities are effective nonverbal strategies for increasing spontaneous language.	Magrun, W. M., Ottenbacher, S. M., & Keefe, R. (1981). Effects of vestibular stimulation on spontaneous use of verbal language in developmentally delayed children. *American Journal of Occupational Therapy, 35,* 101–104.
Participation in activities of daily living and availability to engage in a variety of functional activities	Group who received SI intervention showed reduced self-stimulating behaviors that interfere with participation in functional activities. Study compared an SI approach with tabletop activities in children with pervasive developmental disorder and mental retardation.	Smith, S. A., Press, B., Koenig, K. P., & Kinnealey M. (2005). Effects of sensory integration intervention on self-stimulating and self-injurious behaviors. *American Journal of Occupational Therapy, 59,* 418–425.
Sensory–perceptual and fine-motor skills affecting penmanship and handwriting	Implementing interventions related to sensory processing improved visual–motor skills, which support penmanship, and writing skills using sensory strategies via classroom consultation and direct intervention.	Hall, L., & Case-Smith, J. (2007). The effect of sound-based intervention on children with sensory processing disorder and visual–motor delays. *American Journal of Occupational Therapy, 61,* 209–215.
Participation in play and leisure, including curiosity and independent learning	SI approaches improved play and interactions with others and with toys and other objects, as well as tolerance for vestibular and proprioceptive sensations, and led to greater sensory exploration of the environment. Sensory exploration improves as a key feature of independent learning intervention when OT with a SI approach was used to address symptoms related to learning disorders.	Schaaf, R., Merrill, S., & Kinsella, N. (1987). Sensory integration and play behavior: A case study of the effectiveness of occupational therapy using sensory integrative techniques. *Occupational Therapy in Health Care, 4*(2), 61–75.

(continued)

Table 3. Occupational Therapy Service Continuum and Curriculum-Related Outcomes *(cont.)*

Examples of OT Focus Areas Using SI Theory in School-Based Practice	Projected Educational Outcomes	Examples of Resources and Evidence
Reading	Smooth eye pursuits, which are important in developing reading skills, improved in this study, which demonstrated a reduction in the number of saccades for the intervention cohort and reduced time necessary to accomplish smooth pursuits.	Horowitz, L. J., Oosterveld, W. J., & Adrichem, R. (1993). Effectiveness of sensory integration therapy on smooth pursuits and organization time in children. *Pediatrie und Grenzgebiet, 31*, 331–344.
Academic skills Motor skills	SI intervention methods proved equally as effective as tutoring in improving academic and motor skills with maintenance of gains in motor-skills development. This randomized clinical trial compared OT using SI with tutoring to improve academic and motor skills. Although the SI group did not make greater gains in the initial study, at follow-up 2 years later only the SI group maintained their gross-motor skills.	Wilson, B., Kaplan, B., Fellowes, S., Gruchy, C., & Faris, P. (1992). The efficacy of sensory integration intervention compared to tutoring. *Physical and Occupational Therapy in Pediatrics, 12*, 1–37.
Emotional regulation skills resulting in positive behavior Health and wellness Quality of life	A decrease in disruptive behaviors was noted with improved speech, play, attention, and social dialogue. This single-case study of 2 children demonstrated improvements in social interaction, approach to novel activities, response to affection, and response to movement.	Linderman, T. M., & Stewart, K. B. (1999). Sensory integrative–based occupational therapy and functional outcomes in young children with pervasive developmental disorders: A single-subject study. *American Journal of Occupational Therapy, 53*, 207–213.
Self-advocacy and parent advocacy Quality of life	Parents reported increased ability to advocate for their child based on improved understanding of their child's behavior and validation of their parenting efforts. At the clinic site, waiting room interactions allowed parents time to share experiences and resources with others and expand their understanding of their children.	Cohn, E. S. (2001). Parent perspectives of occupational therapy using a sensory integration approach. *American Journal of Occupational Therapy, 55*, 285–294. Cohn, E. S., Miller, L. J., & Tickle-Degnan, L. (2000). Parental hopes for therapy outcomes: Children with sensory modulation disorders. *American Journal of Occupational Therapy, 54*, 36–43.
Positive behavior Increased engagement Independent work	Supporting behavior in preschool-age child, including increased engagement, decreased aggression, less need for intense teacher direction, and decreased mouthing of objects. Using a single-case-study design, the researchers found that the child benefited from classic Ayres Sensory Integration, affecting his preschool performance.	Roberts, J. E., King-Thomas, L., & Boccia, M. L. (2007). Behavioral indices of the efficacy of sensory integration. *American Journal of Occupational Therapy, 61*, 555–562.

Table 3. Occupational Therapy Service Continuum and Curriculum-Related Outcomes *(cont.)*

Examples of OT Focus Areas Using SI Theory in School-Based Practice	Projected Educational Outcomes	Examples of Resources and Evidence
Participation at school	Supporting occupational performance and behavior in a school-age child, improving participation at school, at home, and in the community. Using a single-case-study design, the researchers found that the child benefited from classic Ayres Sensory Integration, affecting his occupational performance and behavior.	Schaaf, R. C., & Nightlinger, K. M. (2007). Occupational therapy using a sensory integrative approach: A case study of effectiveness. *American Journal of Occupational Therapy, 61*, 239–246.
Play Learning	Research suggests that learning is enhanced by emotion, spontaneity, and play, which are the essential ingredients in a SI approach used within OT. Physiological data shows increased cortical blood volume during performance of novel integration activities in a spontaneous, playful manner.	Peyton, J. L., Bass, W. T., Burke, B. L., & Frank, M. (2005). Novel motor and somatosensory activity is associated with increased cerebral cortical blood volume measured by near-infrared optical topography. *Journal of Child Neurology, 20*, 817–821.
Occupational performance in educational settings observed via academic achievement	Measures of SI in elementary students are significantly related to school achievement both concurrently and predicatively over a 4-year period, even when controlling for intelligence. A particularly strong link between praxis and math achievement is evident.	Parham, L. D. (1998). The relationship of sensory integrative development to achievement in elementary students: Four-year longitudinal patterns. *Occupational Therapy Journal of Research, 18*, 105–127.

Note. OT = occupational therapy; SI = sensory integration.

is a promising method providing therapists the possibility to measure achievement towards customized goals (Mailloux et.al., 2007).

Summary

AOTA recognizes SI as one of several theories and methods used by occupational therapists and occupational therapy assistants working with children in public and private schools. Regardless of the theories and methods utilized, occupational therapy practitioners work within the framework of occupational therapy toward the desired outcome of health and participation through engagement in occupations that allow participation in a child's daily life (AOTA, 2008). When children demonstrate sensory-related deficits that interfere with their ability to access the general education curriculum, occupational therapy using a sensory integrative approach is appropriate.

References

Ahn, R. R., Miller, L. J., Milberger, S., & McIntosh, D. N. (2004). Prevalence of parents' perception of sensory processing disorders among kindergarten children. *American Journal of Occupational Therapy, 58,* 287–293.

American Occupational Therapy Association. (2006). Policy 1.44: Categories of occupational therapy personnel. In *Policy manual* (2008 ed., p. 10). Bethesda, MD: Author

American Occupational Therapy Association. (2008). Occupational therapy practice framework: Domain and process (2nd ed.). *American Journal of Occupational Therapy, 62,* 625–688.

American Occupational Therapy Association. (2009a). Guidelines for supervision, roles, and responsibilities during the delivery of occupational therapy services. *American Journal of Occupational Therapy, 63.*

American Occupational Therapy Association. (2009b). Scope of practice. *American Journal of Occupational Therapy, 63.*

Ayres, A. J. (1972a). Improving academic scores through sensory integration. *Journal of Learning Disabilities, 5,* 336–343.

Ayres, A. J. (1972b). Types of sensory integrative dysfunction among disabled learners. *American Journal of Occupational Therapy, 26,* 13–18.

Ayres, A. J. (1975). Sensorimotor foundations of academic ability. In W. M. Cruickshank & D. P. Hallahan (Eds.), *Perceptual and learning disabilities in children* (Vol. 2, pp. 301–358). Syracuse, NY: Syracuse University Press.

Ayres, A. J. (1979). *Sensory integration and the child.* Los Angeles: Western Psychological Services.

Ayres, A. J. (1989). *Sensory integration and praxis tests manual.* Los Angeles: Western Psychological Services.

Ayres, A. J. (1998). *Sensory integration and praxis tests manual* (rev. ed.). Los Angeles: Western Psychological Services.

Ayres, A. J., & Mailloux, Z. (1981). Influence of sensory integration procedures on language development. *American Journal of Occupational Therapy, 35,* 383–390.

Ayres, A. J., & Tickle, L. S. (1980). Hyper-responsivity to touch and vestibular stimuli as a predictor of positive response to sensory integration procedures by autistic children. *American Journal of Occupational Therapy, 34,* 375–381.

Blanche, E. I. (2002). *Observations based on sensory integration theory.* Torrance, CA: Pediatric Therapy Network.

Blanche, E. I., & Parham, L. D. (2001). Praxis and organization of behavior in time and space. In S. Smith Roley, E. I. Blanche, & R. Schaaf (Eds.), *Understanding the nature of sensory integration with diverse populations* (pp. 183–200). San Antonio, TX: Therapy Skill Builders.

Bundy, A. C., Lane, S. J., & Murray, E. A. (2002). *Sensory integration: Theory and practice* (2nd ed.). Philadelphia: F. A. Davis.

Burke, J. (2001). Clinical reasoning and the use of narrative in sensory integration assessment and intervention. In S. Roley, E. Blanche, & R. Schaaf (Eds.), *Understanding the nature of sensory integration with diverse populations* (pp. 203–214). San Antonio, TX: Therapy Skill Builders.

Clark, G. F., & Coster, W. (1998). Evaluation/problem solving and program evaluation. In J. Case-Smith (Ed.), *Making a difference in school practice* (pp. 1–36). Bethesda, MD: American Occupational Therapy Association.

Cohn, E. S. (2001). Parent perspectives of occupational therapy using a sensory integration approach. *American Journal of Occupational Therapy, 55,* 285–294.

Cohn, E. S., Miller, L. J., & Tickle-Degnan, L. (2000). Parental hopes for therapy outcomes: Children with sensory modulation disorders. *American Journal of Occupational Therapy, 54,* 36–43.

DeGangi, G. A., & Berk, R. A. (1983). *DeGangi–Berk Test of Sensory Integration manual.* Los Angeles: Western Psychological Services.

Dunn, W. (1999). *The Sensory Profile.* San Antonio, TX: Psychological Corporation.

Dunn, W. (2001). The sensations of everyday life: Empirical, theoretical, and pragmatic considerations. *American Journal of Occupational Therapy, 55,* 608–620.

Dunn, W. (2002). *Infant/Toddler Sensory Profile.* San Antonio, TX: Psychological Corporation.

Dunn, W. (2006). *The Sensory Profile School Companion.* San Antonio, TX: Psychological Corporation.

Hall, L., & Case-Smith, J. (2007). The effect of sound-based intervention on children with sensory processing disorder and visual–motor delays. *American Journal of Occupational Therapy, 61,* 209–215.

Horowitz, L. J., Oosterveld, W. J., & Adrichem, R. (1993). Effectiveness of sensory integration therapy on smooth pursuits and organization time in children. *Pediatrie und Grenzgebiet, 31,* 331–344.

Individuals with Disabilities Education Improvement Act, P.L. 108–446, 118 Stat. 2647 (2004).

Jacobs, S. E., Koomar, J., Mailloux, Z., & Smith Roley, S. S. (1999). Entry-level curriculum content for sensory integration: Survey results and proposed teaching modules. *Sensory Integration Special Interest Section Quarterly, 2*(3), 1–3.

Jarrett, O. S., & Maxwell, D. M. (2000). What research says about the need for recess. In R. Clements (Ed.), *Elementary school recess: Selected readings, games, and activities for teachers and parents* (pp. 12–23). Lake Charles, LA: American Press.

Linderman, T. M., & Stewart, K. B. (1999). Sensory integrative–based occupational therapy and functional outcomes in young children with pervasive developmental disorders: A single-subject study. *American Journal of Occupational Therapy, 53,* 207–213.

Knox, S. (2008). Development and current use of the revised Knox Preschool Play Scale. In L. D. Parham & L. S. Fazio (Eds.), *Play in occupational therapy for children* (2nd ed., pp. 55–70). St. Louis, MO: Mosby/Elsevier.

Magrun, W. M., Ottenbacher, S. M., & Keefe, R. (1981). Effects of vestibular stimulation on spontaneous use of verbal language in developmentally delayed children. *American Journal of Occupational Therapy, 35,* 101–104.

Mailloux, Z., & Burke, J. P. (2008). Play and the sensory integrative approach. In L. D. Parham & L. S. Fazio (Eds.), *Play in occupational therapy for children* (2nd ed., pp. 263–278). St. Louis, MO: Mosby/Elsevier.

Mailloux, Z. K., May-Benson, T. A., Summers, C. A., Miller, L. J., Burke, J. P., Brett-Green, B., et al. (2007). Goal attainment scaling as a measure of meaningful outcomes for children with sensory integration disorders. *American Journal of Occupational Therapy, 61,* 254–259.

Miller-Kuhaneck, H., Henry, D., Glennon, T., Parham, D., & Ecker, C. (2007). *Sensory Processing Measure: Home form, main classroom form, and school environments form.* Los Angeles: Western Psychological Services.

Mulligan, S. (1998a). Application of structural equation modeling in occupational therapy research. *American Journal of Occupational Therapy, 52,* 829–834.

Mulligan, S. (1998b). Patterns of sensory integration dysfunction: A confirmatory factor analysis. *American Journal of Occupational Therapy, 52,* 819–828.

Mulligan, S. (2000). Cluster analysis of scores of children on the Sensory Integration and Praxis Tests. *Occupational Therapy Journal of Research, 20,* 256–262.

No Child Left Behind Act of 2001, P.L. 107–110, [20, USC §6301].

Parham, L. D. (1987). Toward professionalism: The reflective therapist. *American Journal of Occupational Therapy, 41,* 555–561.

Parham, L. D. (1998). The relationship of sensory integrative development to achievement in elementary students: Four-year longitudinal patterns. *Occupational Therapy Journal of Research, 18,* 105–127.

Parham, L. D. (2002). Sensory integration and occupation. In A. C. Bundy, S. J. Lane, & E. A. Murray (Eds.), *Sensory integration theory and practice* (2nd ed., pp. 413–434). Philadelphia: F. A. Davis.

Parham, L. D., Cohn, E. S., Spitzer, S., Koomar, J. A., Miller, L. J., Burke, J. P., et al. (2007). Fidelity in sensory integration intervention research. *American Journal of Occupational Therapy, 61,* 216–227.

Parham, L. D., Ecker, C., Miller- Kuhaneck, H., Henry, D. A., & Glennon, T. J. (2007). *Sensory Processing Measure.* Los Angeles: Western Psychological Services.

Parham, L. D., & Mailloux, A. (2004). Sensory integration. In. J. Case- Smith (Ed.), *Occupational therapy for children* (5th ed., pp. 356–411). St. Louis, MO: Mosby.

Pellegrini, A. D., & Smith, P. K. (1993). School recess: Implications for education and development. *Review of Educational Research, 63,* 51–67.

Pellegrini, A. D., & Smith, P. K. (1998). Physical activity play: The nature and function of a neglected aspect of play. *Child Development, 69,* 577–598.

Peyton, J. L., Bass, W. T., Burke, B. L., & Frank, M. (2005). Novel motor and somatosensory activity is associated with increased cerebral cortical blood volume measured by near-infrared optical topography. *Journal of Child Neurology, 20*(1), 817–821.

Reeves, G. (2007). Looking back on 30 years of the Sensory Integration Special Interest Section. *Sensory Integration Special Interest Section Quarterly 30*(4), 1–4.

Roberts, J. E., King-Thomas, L., & Boccia, M. L. (2007). Behavioral indices of the efficacy of sensory integration. *American Journal of Occupational Therapy, 61,* 555–562.

Roley, S., Blanche, E., & Schaaf, R. (Eds.). (2001). *Understanding the nature of sensory integration with diverse populations.* San Antonio, TX: Therapy Skill Builders.

Schaaf, R. C., Merrill, S., & Kinsella, N. (1987). Sensory integration and play behavior: A case study of the effectiveness of occupational therapy using sensory integrative techniques. *Occupational Therapy in Health Care, 4*(2), 61–75.

Schaaf, R., & Smith Roley, S. (2006). *Sensory integration: Applying clinical reasoning to practice with diverse populations.* San Antonio, TX: ProEd.

Schaaf, R. C., & Nightlinger, K. M. (2007). Occupational therapy using a sensory integrative approach: A case study of effectiveness. *American Journal of Occupational Therapy, 61,* 239–246.

Schell, B. A. B., & Schell, J. W. (2008). *Clinical and professional reasoning in occupational therapy.* Baltimore: Lippincott Williams & Wilkins.

Schilling, D. L., Washington, K., Billingsley, F. F., & Deitz, J. (2003). Classroom seating for children with attention deficit hyperactivity disorder: Therapy balls versus chairs. *American Journal of Occupational Therapy, 57,* 534–541.

Section 504 of the Rehabilitation Act of 1973, 29 U.S.C. 706(8) and 794.

Skard, G., & Bundy, A.C. (2008). Test of playfulness. In L. D. Parham & L. Fazio (Eds.), *Play in occupational therapy for children* (2nd ed., pp. 71–93). St. Louis, MO: Mosby / Elsevier.

Smith, S. A., Press, B., Koenig, K. P., & Kinnealey, M. (2005). Effects of sensory integration intervention on self-stimulating and self-injurious behaviors. *American Journal of Occupational Therapy, 59,* 418–425.

Smith Roley, S., Blanche, E. I., & Schaaf, R. C. (Eds.). (2001). *Understanding the nature of sensory integration with diverse populations.* San Antonio, TX: Therapy Skill Builders.

Smith Roley, S., & Jacobs, S. (2008). Sensory integration. In E. B. Crepeau, E. S. Cohn, & B. A. B. Schell (Eds.), *Willard and Spackman's occupational therapy* (11th ed., pp. 792–817). Philadelphia: Lippincott Williams & Wilkins.

Smith Roley, S., Mailloux, Z., Miller-Kuhaneck, H., & Glennon, T. (2007). Understanding Ayres Sensory Integration.® *OT Practice, 12*(17), CE1–CE8.

Spitzer, S., Roley, S. S., Clark, F., & Parham, D. (1996). Sensory integration: Current trends in the United States. *Scandinavian Journal of Occupational Therapy, 3,* 123–138.

VandenBerg, N. L. (2001). The use of a weighted vest to increase on-task behavior in children with attention difficulties. *American Journal of Occupational Therapy, 55,* 621–628.

Williams, M. S., & Shellenberger, S. (1994). *How does your engine run? A leader's guide to the Alert Program for Self-Regulation.* Albuquerque, NM: TherapyWorks.

Wilson, B., Kaplan, B., Fellowes, S., Gruchy, C., & Faris, P. (1992). The efficacy of sensory integration intervention compared to tutoring. *Physical and Occupational Therapy in Pediatrics, 12,* 1–37.

Wilson, B. N., Pollock, N., Kaplan, B. J., & Law, M. (1994). *Clinical observations of motor and postural skills.* Tucson, AZ: Therapy Skill Builders.

Windsor, M., Smith Roley, S., & Szklut, S. (2001).Assessment of Sensory Integration and Praxis. In S. Roley, E. Blanche, & R. Schaaf. (Eds.), *Understanding the nature of sensory integration with diverse populations* (pp. 215–245). San Antonio, TX: Therapy Skill Builders.

Authors

Susanne Smith Roley, MS, OTR/L, FAOTA

Julie Bissell, MA, OTR/L

Gloria Frolek Clark, MS, OTR/L, FAOTA

for

The Commission on Practice

Janet V. DeLany, DEd, OTR/L, FAOTA, *Chairperson*

Adopted by the Representative Assembly 2009FebCS110

This document replaces the 1997 *Sensory Integration Evaluation and Intervention in School-Based Occupational Therapy* and the 2003 *Applying Sensory Integration Framework in Educationally Related Occupational Therapy Practice* (previously published and copyrighted by the American Occupational Therapy Association in 2003 in the *American Journal of Occupational Therapy, 57* (652–659).

The Scope of Occupational Therapy Services for Individuals With Autism Spectrum Disorders Across the Life Span

Introduction

Occupational therapy is important in both assessment and intervention services for individuals with autism spectrum disorder (ASD). Autism currently affects 16.8/10,000 children, while another 45.8/10,000 children are affected by other pervasive developmental disorders (Fombonne, 2003). These numbers reflect a dramatic increase in the number of children diagnosed with ASD in the United States over the past 10 years. The primary purpose of this paper is to define the role of occupational therapy and the scope of services available for individuals with ASD to persons outside of the occupational therapy profession. In addition, this document is intended to clarify the role of occupational therapy with this population for occupational therapy practitioners.[1]

Pervasive developmental disorders (PDD) is the diagnosis used in the *Diagnostic and Statistical Manual of Mental Disorders, 4th edition, text revision* (DSM-IV-TR; American Psychiatric Association [APA], 2000) and in the *International Classification of Diseases* (ICD-10; World Health Organization, 1993) to describe children with a cluster of symptoms that vary widely in type and severity. The symptoms are grouped into three broad categories: (1) qualitative impairment in social interaction; (2) communication disorders; and (3) stereotyped, repetitive patterns of behaviors or a restricted range of interests. Depending on the level and distribution of impairment across these categories, a child can be diagnosed with autistic disorder, Asperger's disorder, or pervasive developmental disorder–not otherwise specified (PDD–NOS). All three of these diagnoses are usually included under the umbrella term "autism spectrum disorders." This practice statement addresses occupational therapy service provision for individuals with autistic disorder, Asperger's disorder, and PDD–NOS. These are considered medical classifications of the ASDs.

The Individuals with Disabilities Education Act (IDEA, Pub. L. 108–446) also includes autism as a disability category under which children might be eligible for special education and related services. The IDEA regulations define *autism* as "a developmental disability significantly affecting verbal and nonverbal communication and social interaction generally evident before age 3 that adversely affects a child's educational performance. Other characteristics often associated with autism are engagement in repetitive activities and stereotyped movements, resistance to environmental change or change in daily routines, and unusual responses to sensory experiences" (34 C.F.R., §300.7[c][1][i]). Under IDEA, occupational therapy is a related service and must be provided to students with autism if those services will help the student to benefit from special education (P. L. 108–446, §602[a][6]). Because educational classification and identification criteria vary considerably from state to state, the reader is referred to the particular state policies and requirements.

Occupational therapy practitioners work with individuals with autism as well as parents, caregivers, educators, and other team members in a variety of settings, including the home, school, clinic, and community to assist the individual with ASD to engage in meaningful occupations.

---

[1]The term *practitioner* refers to an individual initially certified to practice as an occupational therapist or occupational therapy assistant or licensed or regulated by a state, district, commonwealth, or territory of the United States to practice as an occupational therapist or occupational therapy assistant and who has not had that certification, license, or regulation revoked due to disciplinary action (AOTA, 2004b).

Occupational Therapy Domain and Process

The domain of occupational therapy addresses engagement in occupations to support participation in context (American Occupational Therapy Association [AOTA], 2002). *Occupations* are defined as "activities . . . of everyday life, named, organized, and given value and meaning by individuals and a culture" (Law, Polatajko, Baptiste, & Townsend, 1997, p. 34). Occupational therapy services focus on enhancing participation in and performance of activities of daily living, instrumental activities of daily living, education, work, leisure, play, and social participation. For an individual with ASD, the domain of occupational therapy services is defined according to that individual's goals and priorities for participation. Some examples of skills addressed by the occupational therapy practitioner are included in Table 1.

The process of occupational therapy service delivery for individuals with ASD includes evaluation, intervention, and assessment of outcomes. Throughout the process, collaboration with family, caregivers, teachers, and other team members is essential in understanding the daily life experiences of the individual and those with whom the individual interacts. Occupational therapy service provision focuses on salient outcomes that include, but are not limited to, the individual's engagement in and performance of daily activities, personal satisfaction, adaptation, role competence, and quality of life. The needs of the family are also addressed.

The evaluation process is designed to gain an understanding of the individual's challenges with engagement in occupations and activities. Research shows that individuals with autism may have difficulties in the areas of self-care, sensory modulation, self-regulation, praxis, motor imitation, functional and pretend play, social participation, education participation, and work performance (Baranek, 2002; Case-Smith & Bryan, 1999; Dawson & Watling, 2000; Kientz & Dunn, 1997; Libby, Powell, Messer, & Jordan, 1998; Rutherford & Rogers, 2003; Watson, Baranek, & DiLavore, 2003). These performance skills and patterns, client factors, and activity demands impacting occupational performance should be evaluated by an occupational therapist when working with an individual with ASD (Filipek et al., 2000). In addition, given

Table 1. Examples of Skills Addressed by an Occupational Therapy Practitioner

Domain of Occupational Therapy	Examples of Skills That May Be Impaired in Individuals With ASD
Self-care (activities of daily living/ instrumental activities of daily living)	Dressing, eating, toileting, hygiene, sleep/rest, communication device use, community mobility, meal preparation, fiscal management, shopping
Education	Written language skills, computer use, assistive technology, skills needed to access the curriculum, participation in classroom, and other school activities
Leisure and Play	Identifying desired play or leisure activities, participating in play and leisure activities, making choices for free time
Social Participation	Appropriate interactions with others (e.g., peers, adults, neighbors), social skills awareness, behavior management
Work	Identifying and selecting work opportunities, preparing for interviews, developing skills related to job performance (e.g., punctuality, completion of work)

the well-documented difficulties that individuals with ASD have with generalization of skills, the environments in which occupational performance occurs is a vital consideration in evaluation. Recent textbooks have been developed to help guide the practice of occupational therapy with this population and include comprehensive chapters on evaluation of individuals with ASD (Frolek Clark, Miller-Kuhanek, & Watling, 2004; Tomchek, 2001).

The occupational therapy intervention process is based on the results of the evaluation and is individualized to foster occupational engagement and social participation through techniques and procedures directed at the client, the activity, and the environment. When providing services to clients with ASD, occupational therapy practitioners routinely include intervention in the areas of attention, behavior, social skills, sensory processing, motor function, play, and self-care skills (Case-Smith & Miller, 1999; Watling, Deitz, Kanny, & McLaughlin, 1999). Occupational therapy practitioners may use a variety of intervention approaches when working with children with ASD, all aimed at improving participation and performance in those areas identified as problematic for the individual. Effective programs for individuals with ASD described in the literature emphasize active engagement in activity (Dawson & Osterling, 1997; Dunlap, 1999; Hurth, Shaw, Izeman, Whaley, & Rogers, 1999; National Research Council [NRC], 2001; Strain, Wolery, & Izeman, 1998). The physical, social, and cultural environments in which an individual with ASD functions are considered in planning intervention.

Assessing the outcomes of service is an integral part of the occupational therapy process and is important for determining future actions with the client and to evaluate occupational therapy services. This involves monitoring the client's responses to intervention, re-evaluating and modifying the intervention plan, and measuring intervention success through outcomes that are important to the individual within the dynamic physical, social, and cultural contexts where functioning occurs. Progress is noted through improved occupational performance, client satisfaction, role competence, improved health and wellness, prevention of further difficulties, and improved quality of life. Occupational therapy practice for individuals with ASD is consistent with the World Health Organization's (WHO, 2001) framework (i.e., the *International Classification of Functioning, Disability, and Health [ICF]*; WHO, 2001) and the National Research Council's (NRC's) recommended practices for educating individuals with ASD (NRC, 2001).

Supervision of Other Personnel

The occupational therapist is responsible for all aspects of occupational therapy service delivery and is accountable for the safety and effectiveness of occupational therapy service delivery process. The occupational therapy assistant delivers occupational therapy services under the supervision of and in partnership with the occupational therapist (AOTA, 2004a).

Case Studies

The following chart provides examples of how the occupational therapy process can be applied to individuals with ASD across the life span.

Case Description	Occupational Therapy Process
Quentin, a 2½-year-old nonverbal boy with autistic disorder. He receives weekly occupational therapy as part of the statewide early intervention system in his home with parent present. *Play:* Quentin's play is repetitive and non-interactive. His mother would like him to be able to play with others on the playground. *Behavior:* Quentin has frequent temper tantrums when changes occur in his routine or he does not get what he wants.	• Assess Quentin's self-regulation, play skills, and social interaction skills during daily routines in the natural environment. Screen self-care and gross motor abilities. • Identify triggers for temper tantrums and the function of these behaviors (e.g., escape, attention) based on observation and parent input. • Explore, identify, and implement calming strategies incorporating parental input, sensory strategies, environmental modification, and behavioral methods, as appropriate. • Assist parent in identifying triggers for temper tantrums and incorporating behavior management and calming strategies into the family's daily life activities. Include strategies for Quentin to self-regulate so he can calm or arouse himself, as appropriate. • Provide direct/hands-on intervention to address difficulties in play and peer interaction. Consult with parent regarding methods for supporting Quentin in his daily play activities (e.g., peer play, independent play). • Address development of gross motor skills, including coordination, motor planning, initiation, execution, and completion of activities for success while playing on playground.
Michael is a 5-year-old boy with PDD–NOS. He is receiving occupational therapy and speech therapy services in a clinic setting and a behavioral program in the home. *Self-Care:* Michael has difficulty with self-care skills (eating, dressing, and toileting) and selecting and engaging with play materials. *Sensory Functions and Social Participation:* Michael has many sensory issues, including tactile, auditory, and oral sensitivities. When overstimulated, he rocks back and forth and hums. His parents would like him to be able to go with them to restaurants and to attend neighborhood social functions such as children's birthday parties. *Motor Performance:* Gross and fine motor skills are delayed.	• Assess Michael's self-care abilities, play skills, self-regulation, sensory processing abilities, and motor skills during his daily routine and in his natural environments. Screen social interaction. • Identify circumstances related to Michael's overstimulation, develop hypotheses about relationship between overstimulation and performance delays, test hypotheses, identify and implement strategies to prevent overstimulation and support performance. • Explore, identify, and implement strategies to regulate arousal and improve underlying sensory processing. Teach Michael strategies to self-regulate. • Work with Michael's parents to prevent episodes of overstimulation and to implement strategies that support self-regulation when overstimulation does occur. • Provide direct intervention to address deficits in self-care, motor skills, and play abilities. • Collaborate with speech–language pathologist and parents to expand repertoire of food textures and thicknesses. • Consult with and train the behavioral therapist in the appropriate use of sensory and behavioral strategies for regulation and developmentally appropriate gross and fine motor activities for Michael. • Work with parents on strategies to prepare Michael for community outings and social events.

Case Studies *(cont.)*

Case Description	Occupational Therapy Process
Jackson is an 8-year-old boy with Asperger's disorder. He is in the second grade at his neighborhood elementary school and receives school-based occupational therapy services to support his written school work and peer interaction. *Social Participation:* Jackson has difficulty making friends and interacting socially with peers. He talks non-stop about computers. He has difficulty playing with other children. He is very literal about rules and does not read social cues well. His teacher would like to see him participate in school-related activities with his classmates. His parents would like him to participate in T-ball and Cub Scouts with his peers. *Sensory/Motor:* Jackson is experiencing difficulty with handwriting.	• Provide Jackson's teacher with strategies for helping him to identify and practice appropriate behavior and topics for discussion with Jackson's classmates. • Support the teacher in establishing a peer buddy system to build social–communication skills during naturally reinforcing activities in the lunchroom, in corridors, and on the playground. • Train in classroom computer use as an alternative to handwriting. Jackson can also continue to practice handwriting skills, and a decision can be made as to which system works best for him. • Initiate a "computer club" with two other boys in the second grade to talk about computers, practice computer skills, and play games. • Work with Jackson and one other child on T-ball skills during recess. • Consult with the Cub Scout den mother and parent to provide training and support as necessary.
Luke is an 18-year-old male with autism. He is in a self-contained high school class for adolescents with moderate developmental disabilities. Luke receives occupational therapy services to support his transition program in the areas of prevocational skills, behavior skills, community mobility, and independent living skills. *Cognition and Leisure:* Luke is able to do some basic reading and math and is very interested in sports. *Motor Skills:* Luke's body awareness and coordination are poor. *Social Participation:* Luke has difficulty with social interactions. *Work:* Luke, his teacher, and his parents are beginning to plan for the transition from school to supported work and living after high school.	• Assist teacher or speech pathologist with a weekly social skills group to help Luke identify and develop socially appropriate behavior, recognize social cues, and develop strategies for managing social situations. • Consult with the owner of sporting goods store where Luke will work in the coming semester regarding motor difficulties and strategies for avoiding handling of fragile items or working in high-traffic areas. • Identify job skills Luke will need. Provide direct intervention to facilitate development of these skills. Collaborate with the educational team to facilitate further development of job skills and self-management related to employment. • Work with Luke to develop skills in using a hand-held electronic cueing device with digital pictures and auditory cues to guide him through his job routine. • Train the employer in how to use visual supports to show Luke what to do rather than rely on verbal communication. • Provide training in how to use public transportation. • Meet with Luke and his parents regarding transition to adult living situation and lifestyle choices.
Louise is a 32-year-old female with autism. She recently began living in a group home that provides 24-hour supervision. An occupational therapy consults bimonthly. *Communication:* Louise is verbal but difficult to understand. *Mental Functions, Behavior, and Leisure:* Louise has anxiety and poor behavioral regulation that often results in aggressive behaviors. These behaviors have increased since the move to the group home. Her caregivers would like her to be at ease in her new home and participate with the other residents in leisure activities and community outings.	• Consult with the residential staff and provide training in the following areas: sensory strategies to reduce the high arousal associated with anxiety; behavioral strategies to help reinforce positive behavior and compliance; educational strategies such as forward and backward chaining, visual supports, and environmental structure to support success during everyday activities, leisure, and community outings. • Identify leisure activities in which Louise expresses interest. Monitor Louise's participation in these activities through weekly consultations with the staff and provide training, as needed, to facilitate further engagement and participation.

References

American Occupational Therapy Association. (2002). Occupational therapy practice framework: Domain and process. *American Journal of Occupational Therapy, 56*, 609–639.

American Occupational Therapy Association. (2004a). Guidelines for supervision, roles, and responsibilities during the delivery of occupational therapy services. *American Journal of Occupational Therapy, 58*, 663–667.

American Occupational Therapy Association. (2004b). Policy 1.44: Categories of occupational therapy personnel. In *Policy manual* (2004 ed.). Bethesda, MD: Author.

American Psychiatric Association. (2000). *Diagnostic and statistical manual of mental disorders* (4th ed., text rev.). Washington, DC: Author.

Baranek, G. T. (2002). Efficacy of sensory and motor interventions in children with autism. *Journal of Autism and Developmental Disorders, 32*, 397–422.

Case-Smith, J., & Bryan, T. (1999). The effects of occupational therapy with sensory integration emphasis on preschool-age children with autism. *American Journal of Occupational Therapy, 53*, 489–497.

Case-Smith, J., & Miller, H. (1999). Occupational therapy with children with pervasive developmental disorders. *American Journal of Occupational Therapy, 53*, 506–513.

Dawson, G., & Osterling, J. (1997). *The effectiveness of early intervention*. Baltimore: P. H. Brookes.

Dawson, G., & Watling, R. (2000). Interventions to facilitate auditory, visual, and motor integration in autism: A review of the evidence. *Journal of Autism and Developmental Disorders, 30*, 415–421.

Dunlap, G. (1999). Consensus, engagement, and family involvement for young children with autism. *Journal of the Association for Persons with Severe Handicaps, 24*(3), 222–225.

Filipek, P. A., Accardo, P. J., Ashwal, S., Baranek, G. T., Cook, E. H., Jr., Dawson, G., et al. (2000). Practice parameter: Screening and diagnosis of autism: Report of the Quality Standards Subcommittee of the American Academy of Neurology and the Child Neurology Society. *Neurology, 55*, 468–479.

Fombonne, E. (2003). The prevalence of autism. *Journal of the American Medical Association, 289*(1), 87–89.

Frolek Clark, G., Miller-Kuhaneck, H., & Watling, R. (2004). Evaluation of the child with an autism spectrum disorder. In H. Miller-Kuhaneck (Ed.), *Autism: A comprehensive occupational therapy approach* (2nd ed., pp. 107–153). Bethesda, MD: AOTA Press.

Hurth, J., Shaw, E., Izeman, S., Whaley, K., & Rogers, S. (1999). Areas of agreement about effective practices among programs serving young children with autism spectrum disorders. *Infants and Young Children, 12*, 17–26.

Individuals with Disabilities Education Act Amendments of 1997, P. L. 105–17, 34 C.F.R., Part 300.

Individuals with Disabilities Education Improvement Act (IDEA) of 2004, P. L. 108–446, 20 U.S.C.

Kientz, M. A., & Dunn, W. (1997). A comparison of the performance of children with and without autism on the Sensory Profile. *American Journal of Occupational Therapy, 51*, 530–537.

Law, M., Polatajko, H., Baptiste, S., & Townsend, E. (1997). Core concepts of occupational therapy. In E. Townsend (Ed.), *Enabling occupation: An occupational therapy perspective* (pp. 29–56). Ottawa, ON: Canadian Association of Occupational Therapists.

Libby, S., Powell, S., Messer, D., & Jordan, R. (1998). Spontaneous play in children with autism: A reappraisal. *Journal of Autism and Developmental Disorders, 28*, 487–497.

National Research Council. (2001). *Educating children with autism.* Washington, DC: National Academy Press.

Rutherford, M. D., & Rogers, S. J. (2003). Cognitive underpinnings of pretend play in autism. *Journal of Autism and Developmental Disorders, 33,* 289–302.

Strain, P., Wolery, M., & Izeman, S. (1998). Considerations for administrators in the design of service options for young children with autism and their families. *Young Exceptional Children, Winter,* 8–16.

Tomchek, S. D. (2001). Sensorimotor assessment of individuals with autism spectrum disorders. In R. Huebner (Ed.), *Autism and related disorders: A sensorimotor approach to management* (pp. 103–133). Gaithersburg, MD: Aspen.

Watling, R., Deitz, J., Kanny, E. M., & McLaughlin, J. F. (1999). Current practice of occupational therapy for children with autism. *American Journal of Occupational Therapy, 53,* 498–505.

Watson, L. R., Baranek, G. T., & DiLavore, P. C. (2003). Toddlers with autism: Developmental perspectives. *Infants and Young Children, 16,* 201–214.

World Health Organization. (1993). *International Classification of Diseases: Diagnostic Criteria for Research* (10th Ed.). Geneva: World Health Organization.

World Health Organization. (2001). *International classification of functioning, disability and health (ICF).* Geneva, Switzerland: Author.

Authors

Renee Watling, PhD, OTR/L
Scott Tomchek, MS, OTR/L
Patti LaVesser, PhD, OTR/L

for

The Commission on Practice
Sara Jane Brayman, PhD, OTR/L, FAOTA, *Chairperson*

Adopted by the Representative Assembly 2005C220

PART II

Societal Statements

AOTA's Societal Statement on Autism Spectrum Disorders

The American Occupational Therapy Association (AOTA) asserts that occupational therapy services are grounded in the belief that persons with autism spectrum disorder (ASD) are integral members of their families and communities and have the right to fully participate in the educational, social, cultural, political, and economic life of society (AOTA, 2008).

ASD is a lifelong condition currently diagnosed in an estimated 1 in 150 children, and the rate of diagnosis is rapidly increasing (Centers for Disease Control and Prevention [CDC], 2007). Individuals with ASD experience significant challenges in communication, social interaction, sensory processing, play, and regulation of emotions and behavior as compared with peers (CDC, 2007). These differences affect the ability of individuals with ASD to make sense of the world around them and to participate in everyday activities such as interacting with others, performing educationally related tasks, obtaining and maintaining employment, and being involved in community events (AOTA, 2005). Although intellectual functioning among persons with ASD ranges from "profound mental retardation–extreme giftedness" (Sternberg, Lautrey & Lubart, 2002), fewer than 20% attend post-secondary education, and only 15% achieve independence as adults (Lawer, Brusilovskiy, Salzer, & Mandell, 2008).

Occupational therapy practitioners work collaboratively with individuals on the autism spectrum, their families, other professionals, and community members in multiple contexts to advocate for and provide a range of needed resources and services that support the individual's ability to participate fully in life (Case-Smith & Arbesman, 2008).

References

American Occupational Therapy Association. (2005). The scope of occupational therapy services for individuals with autism spectrum disorders across the lifespan. *American Journal of Occupational Therapy, 59*, 680–683.

American Occupational Therapy Association. (2008). Occupational therapy practice framework: Domain and process (2nd ed.). *American Journal of Occupational Therapy, 62*, 625–683.

Case-Smith, J. & Arbesman, M. (2008). Evidence-based review of interventions for autism used in or of relevance to occupational therapy. *American Journal of Occupational Therapy, 62*, 416–429.

Centers for Disease Control and Prevention. (2007, February 9). *Prevalence of autism spectrum disorders: Autism and developmental disabilities monitoring network, 14 sites, United States, 2002.* Retrieved February 5, 2009, from http://www.cdc.gov/mmwr/preview/mmwrhtml/ss5601a2.htm

Lawer, L., Brusilovskiy, E., Salzer, M. S., & Mandell, D. S. (2008). Use of vocational rehabilitative services among adults with autism. *Journal of Autism and Developmental Disorders.* Retrieved February 5, 2009, from www.springerlink.com/content/x4j736467lng8v36/?p=c616d9b82ea04d9bb34175afcdcf1d7d&pi=1

Sternberg, R. Lautrey, J., & Lubart, T. (2002) *Models of intelligence: International perspectives.* Washington, DC: American Psychological Association.

Authors

Renee Watling, PhD, OTR/L

Asha Asher, MA, (OTR), MEd, (Special Ed.)

Barbara Chandler, PhD, OTR/L, FAOTA

Lisa Mahaffey, MS, OTR/L

for

The Representative Assembly Coordinating Council (RACC):

Deborah Murphy-Fischer, MBA, OTR, IMT, *Chairperson*

Brent Braveman, PhD, OTR/L, FAOTA

Janet V. DeLany, DEd, OTR/L, FAOTA

René Padilla, PhD, OTR/L, FAOTA

Kathlyn Reed, PhD, OTR, FAOTA, MLIS

Barbara Schell, PhD, OTR/L, FAOTA

Pam Toto, MS, OTR/L, BCG, FAOTA

Carol H. Gwin, OT/L, *AOTA Staff Liaison*

Adopted by the Representative Assembly 2009AprCO140

Copyright © 2009, by the American Occupational Therapy Association. To be published in the *American Journal of Occupational Therapy, 63*(November/December).

AOTA's Societal Statement on Combat-Related Posttraumatic Stress

Self-report of symptoms of post-traumatic stress disorder (PTSD) have tripled among combat-exposed military personnel, compared to those who have not deployed, since 2001 (Smith et al., 2008). Tanielian and Jaycox (2008) have estimated that approximately 300,000 military personnel previously deployed to Iraq or Afghanistan currently experience PTSD or major depression. Military personnel are returning home and demonstrating signs and symptoms of combat-related PTSD, such as nightmares, flashbacks, memory loss, insomnia, depression, avoidance of social interaction, fear, decreased energy, drug and alcohol use, and the inability to concentrate. These signs and symptoms could affect these individuals' ability to effectively negotiate their personal lives and work roles. Specifically during work, the avoidance of social interactions and avoidance of situations that resemble the traumatic event may interfere with coworker relationships or may be perceived as the lack of motivation or ability to be successful in a work setting (Penk, Drebing, & Schutt, 2002).

Combat-related PTSD not only affects military personnel but also the family and the community in which military personnel interact. If unidentified and untreated, the effects of combat-related PTSD may have a delayed onset and cause problems such as depression, social alienation, marital communication problems, difficulty with parenting, and alcohol and drug abuse, and each can cause a disruption in military personnel's personal lives, professional abilities, and overall physical and mental health (Baum, 2008). It is vital for military personnel and health care providers to be educated on these signs and symptoms and detect them early to ensure that military personnel receive adequate opportunities for prompt intervention services and to access support. This is something that occupational therapists and occupational therapy assistants can do.

The overarching goal of occupational therapy for military personnel coping with combat-related PTSD is to use strategies to help them recover, compensate, or adapt so they can reengage with activities that are necessary for their daily life. Occupational therapists and occupational therapy assistants also help military personnel coping with combated-related PTSD to develop strategies to self-manage the long-term consequences of the condition. These strategies are important to promote their health and participation in family, community, and military life because these strategies support their ability to engage or re-engage in daily life activities and occupations that are necessary and meaningful to them. Because of their knowledge and skills in addressing the physical, cognitive, and psychosocial factors associated with combat-related PTSD, occupational therapists and occupational therapy assistants bring broad expertise to help personnel identify the barriers that are limiting their recovery and participation in meaningful activities (American Occupational Therapy Association [AOTA], 2005). AOTA supports recognition of and intervention services for military personnel coping with combat-related PTSD, including research, advocacy, education, and resource allocation consistent with professional standards and ethics.

References

American Occupational Therapy Association. (2005). Occupational therapy code of ethics (2005). *American Journal of Occupational Therapy, 59,* 639–642.

Baum, C. M. (2008, April 1). *Post traumatic stress disorder treatment and research: Moving ahead toward recovery.* Statement of Carolyn M. Baum, PhD, OTR/L, FAOTA, before the House Committee on Veterans' Affairs. Available online at http://veterans.house.gov/hearings/Testimony.aspx?TID=26235& Newsid=188 &Name=%20Carolyn%20M.%20Baum,%20Ph.D,%20OTR/L,%20FAOTA

Penk, W., Drebing, C., & Schutt, R. (2002). PTSD in the workplace. In J. C. Thomas & M. Hersen (Eds.), *Handbook of mental health in the workplace* (pp. 215–248). Thousand Oaks, CA: Sage.

Smith, T. C., Ryan, M. A., Wingard, D. L., Slymen, D. J., Sallis, J. F., & Kritz-Sivlerstein, D. (2008). New onset and persistent symptoms of post-traumatic stress disorder self-reported after deployment and combat exposures: prospective population-based US military cohort study. *British Medical Journal, 336,* 336–371.

Tanielian, T. L., & Jaycox, L. H. (Eds. 2008). *Invisible wounds of war: Psychological and cognitive injuries, their consequences, and services to assist recovery.* Santa Monica, CA: Rand Corporation. Available online at http://www.rand.org/pubs/monographs/2008/RAND_MG720.pdf

Authors

Robinette J., Amaker, PhD, OTR/L, CHT, FAOTA
Yvette Woods, PhD, OTR/L
Steven M. Gerardi, MS, OTR/L, CHT

The views expressed in this article are those of the authors and do not reflect the official policy or position of the Department of the Army, Department of Defense, or the U.S. Government.

for

The Representative Assembly Coordinating Council (RACC):
Deborah Murphy-Fischer, MBA, OTR, BCP, IMT, *Chairperson*
Brent Braveman, PhD, OTR/L, FAOTA
Coralie Glantz, OTR/L, BCG, FAOTA
René Padilla, PhD, OTR/L, FAOTA
Kathlyn Reed, PhD, OTR, FAOTA, MLIS
Barbara Schell, PhD, OTR/L, FAOTA
Pam Toto, MS, OTR/L, BCG, FAOTA
Carol H. Gwin, OT/L, *AOTA Staff Liaison*

Adopted by the Representative Assembly 2008CS84

AOTA's Societal Statement on Family Caregivers

Caregiving is often a desired and rewarding occupation. Sometimes caregiving needs occur unexpectedly. Whether planned or unexpected, the extent and need for caregiving for others changes over time, affecting the structure and priorities of engagement in daily occupations. Depending on individual circumstances, these life changes may be associated with health risks for the caregivers themselves.

It has been well documented that family caregivers (unpaid family and friends who are assisting loved ones) often experience negative health effects as a result of their efforts (Centers for Disease Control, 2005; Evercare & National Alliance for Caregiving, 2006). This not only affects their own well-being but can affect their ability to continue to provide care. Many areas of caregiver concern have been identified, including issues of life imbalance, stress, depression, and the need for training in task performance (National Alliance for Caregiving & AARP, 2004). Occupational therapy practitioners can help ensure a healthy balance and support caregivers who experience sudden or long-term changes in their lifestyle and priorities and assist caregivers who may be at risk for negative health consequences.

Occupational therapists and occupational therapy assistants bring broad expertise to intervene with family caregivers to facilitate caregiving and promote better health because of their knowledge and skills in addressing the physical, psychosocial, cognitive, sensory, and contextual elements that affect participation and engagement in everyday life activities (American Occupational Therapy Association [AOTA], 2005). AOTA supports recognition of families and caregivers across the life span, including research, education, advocacy, and resource allocation, consistent with the *Core Values* (AOTA, 1993) and the *Code of Ethics* (AOTA, 2005) for the profession of occupational therapy.

References

American Occupational Therapy Association. (1993). Core values and attitudes of occupational therapy practice. *American Journal of Occupational Therapy, 47,* 1085–1086.

American Occupational Therapy Association. (2005). Occupational therapy code of ethics (2005). *American Journal of Occupational Therapy, 59,* 639–642.

Centers for Disease Control and Prevention. (2005). *Summary health statistics for U.S. children: National health interview survey, 2003* (March 2005, Series 10, Number 223). Retrieved September 23, 2005, from http://www.cdc.gov/nchs/data/series/sr_10/sr10_223.pdf

Evercare, & National Alliance for Caregiving. (2006). *Study of caregivers in decline: Findings from a national survey.* Retrieved October 13, 2006, from http://www.caregiving.org/data/Caregivers%20in%20 Decline%20Study-FINAL-lowres.pdf

National Alliance for Caregiving, & AARP. (2004). *Family caregiving in the U.S.: Findings from a national survey.* Bethesda, MD: Authors.

Author

Ann O'Sullivan, OTR/L, LSW

for

The Representative Assembly Coordinating Council (RACC):
Deborah Murphy-Fischer, MBA, OTR, BCP, IMT, *Chairperson*
Brent Braveman, PhD, OTR/L, FAOTA
Linda Fazio, PhD, OTR/L, LPC, FAOTA
Coralie Glantz, OTR/L, BCG, FAOTA
Wendy C. Hildenbrand, MPH, OTR/L, FAOTA
Kathlyn L. Reed, PhD, OTR, FAOTA, MLIS
S. Maggie Reitz, PhD, OTR/L, FAOTA
Susanne Smith Roley, MS, OTR/L, FAOTA
Carol H. Gwin, OT/L, *AOTA Staff Liaison*

Adopted by the Representative Assembly 2007C81

AOTA's Societal Statement on Health Disparities

It is widely recognized that disparities in health status and the availability of health and social services exist in the United States. The Trans-National Institutes of Health (NIH) Work Group on Health Disparities defined the term *health disparities* as "the difference in the incidence, prevalence, morbidity, mortality, and burden of diseases and other adverse health conditions that exist among specific population groups" (NIH, 1999).

As noted by the NIH Work Group, experts assert that "health disparities arise from a complex combination of social and economic factors, the physical environments, cultural beliefs and values, educational level, personal behaviors, and genetic susceptibilities" (NIH, 1999). Occupational therapy is well positioned to intervene with individuals and communities to limit the effects of health disparities on participation in meaningful occupations because of practitioners' knowledge and skills in evaluating and intervening with persons who face physical, social, emotional, or cultural challenges to participation. Further, the American Occupational Therapy Association (AOTA) supports advocacy to increase access to health services for persons in need, and efforts to lessen or eliminate health disparities are consistent with the Core Values and the Code of Ethics for the profession of occupational therapy (AOTA, 1993, 2005).

References

American Occupational Therapy Association. (1993). Core values and attitudes of occupational therapy practice. *American Journal of Occupational Therapy, 47*, 1085–1086.

American Occupational Therapy Association. (2005). Occupational therapy code of ethics (2005). *American Journal of Occupational Therapy, 59*, 639–642.

National Institutes of Health. (1999). *Trans-NIH Work Group on Health Disparities.* Retrieved January 30, 2006, from http://www.nidcr.nih.gov/Research/HealthDisparities/TransWorkGroup.htm

Author
Brent Braveman, PhD, OTR/L, FAOTA

for

The Representative Assembly Coordinating Council (RACC):
Janet Raisor, OTR, *Chairperson*
Brent Braveman, PhD, OTR/L, FAOTA
Linda Fazio, PhD, OTR/L, LPC, FAOTA
Wendy C. Hildenbrand, MPH, OTR/L, FAOTA
Penelope Moyers, EdD, OTR, FAOTA
S. Maggie Reitz, PhD, OTR/L, FAOTA
Susanne Smith Roley, MS, OTR/L, FAOTA
Carol H. Gwin, OT/L, *AOTA Staff Liaison*

Adopted by the Representative Assembly 2006C360

AOTA's Societal Statement on Livable Communities

The demographic profile of the United States is rapidly changing, with an increasing number of older adults and persons with disabilities who desire to remain in their homes and communities as they grow older, a concept referred to as *aging-in-place*. According to the United Nations (2007), persons with disabilities have the same right as all other members of society to live in the community with opportunities to choose their place of residence and to have equal access to support services that promote full participation in all aspects of community living. To support these rights, society must create communities that enable all residents to live, work, play, and participate in locations of their choice (AARP, 2005; National Council on Disability, 2004). "A livable community is one that has affordable and appropriate housing, supportive community features and services, and adequate mobility options, which together facilitate personal independence and engagement of the residents in civic and social life" (AARP, 2005, p. 4).

The American Occupational Therapy Association's (AOTA's) *Core Values and Attitudes of Occupational Therapy Practice* (AOTA, 1993) and *Occupational Therapy Code of Ethics* (AOTA, 2005) support equality for all individuals, and are congruent with the goals of livable communities. Occupational therapy practitioners plan and implement strategies that promote their client's participation in community life by creating opportunities to establish, restore, or maintain the skills used in activities of daily living and other meaningful occupations and by supporting clients' who are advocating for their own and others' rights. Further, occupational therapy practitioners advocate for universal design and environmental modifications that remove barriers in homes and communities to ensure access to supportive community services, including transportation, personal care, health care, education, employment, and other services, and to facilitate engagement in social and civic activities. Occupational therapy promotes public health and civic engagement by advocating for and assisting in the creation of more livable communities through effective partnerships with individuals, private organizations, and government agencies. Supporting health and participation through active engagement in meaningful activities in the home and community contributes to health, wellness, and quality of life for all individuals (AOTA, 2006).

References

AARP Public Policy Institute. (2005). *Beyond 50.05—A report to the nation on livable communities: Creating environments for successful aging.* Washington, DC: Author.

American Occupational Therapy Association. (1993). Core values and attitudes of occupational therapy practice. *American Journal of Occupational Therapy, 47,* 1085–1086.

American Occupational Therapy Association. (2005). Occupational therapy code of ethics (2005). *American Journal of Occupational Therapy, 59,* 639–642.

American Occupational Therapy Association. (2006). *AOTA Board Task Force on Health and Wellness: Report to the Executive Board.* Retrieved February 4, 2008, from www.atoa.org/News/Centennial/AdHoc/2006/40407.aspx

National Council on Disability. (2004, December). *Livable communities for adults with disabilities: The 2004 report, executive summary.* Available online at http://www.ncd.gov/newsroom/publications/2004/pdf/livablecommunities.pdf

United Nations. (2007). *Rights and dignity of persons with disabilities, Article 19.* Retrieved May 11, 2008, from http://www.un.org/disabilities/documents/convention/convoptprot-e.pdf

Authors
Lisa Ann Fagan, MS, OTR/L
Cheri Cabrera, OTR

for

The Representative Assembly Coordinating Council (RACC):
Deborah Murphy-Fischer, MBA, OTR, BCP, IMT, *Chairperson*
Brent Braveman, PhD, OTR/L, FAOTA
René Padilla, PhD, OTR/L, FAOTA
Kathlyn Reed, PhD, OTR, FAOTA, MLIS
Janet V. DeLany, DEd, OTR/L, FAOTA
Pam Toto, MS, OTR/L, BCG, FAOTA
Barbara Schell, PhD, OTR/L, FAOTA
Carol H. Gwin, OT/L, *AOTA Staff Liaison*

Adopted by the Representative Assembly 2008CS85

AOTA's Societal Statement on Obesity

Obesity is the result of complex social, behavioral, cultural, environmental, physiological, and genetic factors. In the United States, 65% of adults and one-third of the children and adolescents are overweight secondary to diet and sedentary lifestyle (U.S. Department of Health and Human Services [DHHS], 2006c). Obesity is the leading modifiable risk factor contributing to early mortality; type 2 diabetes; cardiovascular disease; metabolic syndrome; breast, prostate, and colon cancer; gallbladder disease; sleep apnea; musculoskeletal disorders; and associated limitations in physical activity (Bungum, Satterwhite, Jackson, & Morrow, 2003; Manson, Skerrett, Greenland, & VanItallie, 2004). Within the United States, millions of people struggle and fail to achieve a healthy weight using current methods (Manson et al., 2004). Occupational therapy's holistic and unique focus on occupation and daily life activities offers structured intervention and support for the management of obesity across the life span regardless of ability. Consistent with the first goal of *Healthy People 2010* (DHHS, 2000, 2001, 2006a, 2006b, 2006c), The American Occupational Therapy Association (AOTA) supports primary, secondary, and tertiary prevention for the management of obesity. The AOTA is firmly dedicated to serving the needs for community health, increasing life expectancy, and improving the quality of life for all people.

References

Bungum, T., Satterwhite, M., Jackson, A. W., & Morrow, J. R. (2003). The relationship of body mass index, medical costs, and job absenteeism. *American Journal of Health Behavior, 27,* 456–462.

Manson, J. E., Skerrett, P. J., Greenland, P., & VanItallie, T. B. (2004). The escalating pandemics of obesity and sedentary lifestyle: A call to action for clinicians. *Archives of Internal Medicine, 164,* 249–258.

U.S. Department of Health and Human Services. (2000). *Healthy People 2000: Understanding and improving health.* Conference edition. Washington, DC: Government Printing Office.

U.S. Department of Health and Human Services. (2001, June). *Healthy People 2010: A systematic approach to health improvement.* Retrieved June 4, 2002, from http://www.health.gov/healthypeople/document/html/uih/uih_2.htm

U.S. Department of Health and Human Services. (2006a, February). *Healthy People 2010: Leading health indicators.* Retrieved February 26, 2006, from http://www.healthypeople.gov/document/html/uih/uih4.htm

U.S. Department of Health and Human Services. (2006b, February). *Nutrition and overweight.* Retrieved February 26, 2006, from http://www.healthypeople.gov/Document/HTML/Volume2/19Nutrition.htm

U.S. Department of Health and Human Services. (2006c, February). *Physical activity and fitness.* Retrieved February 26, 2006, from http://www.healthypeople.gov/Document/HTML/Volume2/22Ph

Author

Shirley A. Blanchard, PhD, ABDA, OTR/L

for

The Representative Assembly Coordinating Council (RACC):
Janet Raisor, OTR, *Chairperson*
Brent Braveman, PhD, OTR/L, FAOTA
Linda Fazio, PhD, OTR/L, LPC, FAOTA
Wendy C. Hildenbrand, MPH, OTR/L, FAOTA
Penelope Moyers, EdD, OTR, FAOTA
S. Maggie Reitz, PhD, OTR/L, FAOTA
Susanne Smith Roley, MS, OTR/L, FAOTA
Carol H. Gwin, OT/L, *AOTA Staff Liaison*

Adopted by the Representative Assembly 2006C359

AOTA's Societal Statement on Play

Every child has the right to play (Office of the United Nations High Commissioner for Human Rights, 1989). Childhood play is the context for children's development and is fundamental to their growth and learning from infancy through adolescence, contributing to their physical, cognitive, social, and emotional development (Isenberg & Quisenberry, 2002). The right of every child to play is challenged worldwide by child labor, commercial exploitation, war, exposure to violence in homes and communities, changes in family structure, and living in poverty (American Association for the Child's Right to Play [AACRP], 2007; Ginsburg, 2007). Time and spaces for play in children's lives have been reduced by pressured lifestyles that rush children into adult roles; emphasis on academic preparation, organized activities, and sports; elimination of recess in the school day; proliferation of electronic media and passive entertainment; and inadequate and unsafe outdoor play environments due to urban growth, neighborhood violence, high levels of traffic, and lack of green spaces and access to nature (AACRP, 2007; Ginsburg, 2007; National Association of Early Childhood Specialists in State Departments of Education, 2007).

The absence of childhood play, or reduced opportunities for it, deprives children of an essential context for their optimal development and learning. The American Occupational Therapy Association (AOTA) recognizes play as a domain of occupational therapy practice applicable to people throughout the life span (AOTA, 2002). Occupational therapy practitioners support, enhance, and defend children's right to play as individuals and as members of their families, peer groups, and communities by promoting recognition of play's crucial role in children's development, health, and well-being; establishing and restoring children's skills needed to engage in play; adapting play materials, objects, and environments to facilitate optimal play experiences; and advocating for safe, inclusive play environments that are accessible to all.

References

American Association for the Child's Right to Play. (2007). *IPA declaration of a child's right to play*. Retrieved August 19, 2007, from http://www.ipausa.org/declare/htm

American Occupational Therapy Association. (2002). Occupational therapy practice framework: Domain and process. *American Journal of Occupational Therapy, 56*, 609–639.

Ginsburg, K. R. (with the Committee on Communications and the Committee on Psychosocial Aspects of Child and Family Health). (2007). The importance of play in promoting healthy child development and maintaining strong parent–child bonds. *Pediatrics, 119*, 182–191.

Isenberg, J. P., & Quisenberry, N. (2002). *Play: Essential for all children—A position paper of the Association for Childhood Education International*. Retrieved August 19, 2007, from http://www.acei.org/playpaper.htm

National Association of Early Childhood Specialists in State Departments of Education. (2007). *Recess and the importance of play: A position statement on young children and recess*. Retrieved August 19, 2007, from http://naecs.crc.uiuc.edu/position/recessplay.html

Office of the United Nations High Commissioner for Human Rights. (1989). *Convention on the rights of the child: General Assembly Resolution 44/25 of 20 November 1989.* Retrieved August 19, 2007, from http://www.unhchr.ch/html/menu3/b/k2crc.htm

Author

Loree A. Primeau, PhD, OTR, FAOTA

for

The Representative Assembly Coordinating Council (RACC):
Deborah Murphy-Fischer, MBA, OTR, BCP, IMT, *Chairperson*
Brent Braveman, PhD, OTR/L, FAOTA
Janet V. Delany, DEd, OTR/L, FAOTA
Coralie Glantz, OTR/L, BCG, FAOTA
René Padilla, PhD, OTR/L, FAOTA
Kathlyn L. Reed, PhD, OTR, FAOTA, MLIS
Barbara Schell, PhD, OTR/L, FAOTA
Susanne Smith Roley, MS, OTR/L, FAOTA
Carol H. Gwin, OT/L, *AOTA Staff Liaison*

Adopted by the Representative Assembly 2007CO143

AOTA'S Societal Statement on Stress and Stress Disorders

Stress is a pervasive societal challenge that affects the social participation of people of varying ages, ethnicity, gender, and socioeconomic status (U.S. Department of Health and Human Services [USDHHS], 2000). It is a significant risk factor in a number of health problems, including mental illness, cognitive decline, cardiovascular disease, musculoskeletal disorders, and workplace injuries. Individuals with disabilities are disproportionately affected, with 49 percent of these people reporting adverse health effects from stress, compared with 34 percent of the general population (USDHHS, 2000).

Individuals, families, organizations, and communities differ significantly in their perceptions of and vulnerability to stressful events, as well as in their coping strategies. Organizational stressors, such as relocation or restructuring, may result in financial strain and loss of personnel. Community or population catastrophes, such as natural disasters or wars, result in stress from overwhelming personal loss, forced displacement, and a disruption of massive proportions in familiar daily routines and occupations (Wein, 2000).

The occupational therapy profession promotes the establishment of healthy habit patterns; familiar, predictable routines; and increased engagement in meaningful occupations that serve both as protective and healing factors in combating the negative effects of stress. Occupational therapy practitioners[1] develop evidence-based interventions based on this philosophy, and conduct research to establish their efficacy for coping with stress (Jackson, Carlson, Mandel, Zemke, & Clark, 1998; Nelson, 1996; Oaten & Chen, 2006; Wein, 2000).

References

American Occupational Therapy Association. (2006). Policy 1.44: Categories of occupational therapy personnel. *American Journal of Occupational Therapy, 60,* 683–684.

Hinojosa, J., & Kramer, P. (1997). Statement—Fundamental concepts of occupational therapy: Occupation, purposeful activity, and function. *American Journal of Occupational Therapy, 51,* 864–866.

Jackson, J., Carlson, M., Mandel, D., Zemke, R., & Clark, F. (1998). Occupation in lifestyle redesign: The Well Elderly Study Occupational Therapy Program. *American Journal of Occupational Therapy, 52,* 326–336.

Nelson, D. L. (1996). Therapeutic occupation: A definition. *American Journal of Occupational Therapy, 50,* 775–782.

Oaten, M., & Chen, K. (2006). Longitudinal gains in self-regulation from regular physical exercise. *British Journal of Health Psychology, 11,* 717–733.

U.S. Department of Health and Human Services. (2000). *Healthy people 2010: Understanding and improving health* (2nd ed.). Washington, DC: U.S. Government Printing Office.

---

[1]When the term *occupational therapy practitioner* is used in this document, it refers to both occupational therapists and occupational therapy assistants (AOTA, 2006).

Wein, H. (2000). *Stress and disease: New perspectives* [NIH Word on Health]. Retrieved October 20, 2006, from http://www.nih.gov/news/WordonHealth/oct2000/story01.htm

Related Reading

Selye, H. (1975). Stress and distress. *Comprehensive Therapy, 1*(8), 9–13.

Author
Susan Stallings-Sahler, PhD, OTR/L, FAOTA

for

The Representative Assembly Coordinating Council (RACC):
Deborah Murphy-Fischer, MBA, OTR, BCP, IMT, *Chairperson*
Brent Braveman, PhD, OTR/L, FAOTA
Linda Fazio, PhD, OTR/L, LPC, FAOTA
Coralie Glantz, OTR/L, BCG, FAOTA
Wendy C. Hildenbrand, MPH, OTR/L, FAOTA
Kathlyn L. Reed, PhD, OTR, FAOTA, MLIS
S. Maggie Reitz, PhD, OTR/L, FAOTA
Susanne Smith Roley, MS, OTR/L, FAOTA
Carol H. Gwin, OT/L, *AOTA Staff Liaison*

Adopted by the Representative Assembly 2007C82

AOTA'S Societal Statement on Youth Violence

A nationwide crisis related to youth violence has resulted in this being the second-leading cause of death among all youth aged 15 to 24 years and the leading cause of death among African American youth of the same age (U.S. Department of Health and Human Services, 2000). Acts of violence include bullying, verbal threats, physical assault, domestic abuse, and gunfire. Premature death, disability, and academic failure occur due to violent activity that surrounds youth. Risk factors that lead to youth violence include history of being abused or abusing others, school truancy, poor time use, exposure to crime, mental illness, drug and alcohol use, gang involvement, access to guns, and absence of familial and social support structures. Rising health care costs, decreased property values, and social services disruption are indicators of the impact that violence has on the health of communities, as well as on individual participation in society (Centers for Disease Control & Prevention, 2006). Individual participation can be limited by reduced access to services, fear of harm to self or others, and the inability to perform valued roles. The severity of this issue has forced policymakers, health care providers, teachers, parents, and students to recognize, examine, and alter social conditions, cultural influences, and relationships.

The profession of occupational therapy has the societal duty and expertise to respond to youth violence by promoting overall health and well-being among youth (American Occupational Therapy Association, 2006). Occupational therapy practitioners work toward understanding the occupational nature of violence, researching effective interventions, creating collaborations, and advocating for public health and social services for youth. Violence and its antecedents can deprive this growing segment of youth of necessary and meaningful occupations (Whiteford, 2000), leaving them insufficiently prepared for their future. Positive change can occur by providing youth with opportunities to replace poor occupational choices with healthy, safe, productive, and socially acceptable activities (Snyder, Clark, Masunaka-Noriego, & Young, 1998). Ultimately, occupational therapy practitioners provide services that support a vision of social justice, dignity, and social action throughout the life span by addressing the engagement patterns and lifestyle choices of at-risk youth through methods such as effective transition services and life skills remediation.

References

American Occupational Therapy Association. (2006). *Centennial Vision: Ad hoc report on children and youth.* Retrieved August 7, 2007, from http://www.aota.org/News/Centennial/Updates/AdHoc.aspx

Centers for Disease Control and Prevention. (2006). *Understanding youth violence* [Fact Sheet]. Retrieved August 9, 2007, from http://www.cdc.gov/ncipc/pub-res/YVFactSheet.pdf

Snyder, C., Clark, F., Masunaka-Noriega, M., & Young, B. (1998). Los Angeles street kids: New occupations for life program. *Journal of Occupational Science, 5,* 133–139.

U.S. Department of Health and Human Services. (2000). *Healthy People 2010: Injury and violence prevention.* Retrieved November 17, 2006, from http://www.healthypeople.gov/docuament/html/volume1/07ed.htm

Whiteford, G. (2000). Occupational deprivation: Global challenge in the new millennium. *British Journal of Occupational Therapy, 63,* 200–204.

Author
Heather D. Goertz, OTD, OTR/L

Author
Creighton University Class of 2007 occupational therapy doctoral students:
  Bryan Benedict, Oanh Bui, Stacy Peitz, Rose Ryba
Susan Cahill, MAEA, OTR/L, Clinical Instructor, University of Illinois at Chicago

for

The Representative Assembly Coordinating Council (RACC):
Deborah Murphy-Fischer, MBA, OTR, BCP, IMT, *Chairperson*
Brent Braveman, PhD, OTR/L, FAOTA
Janet V. Delany, DEd, OTR/L, FAOTA
Coralie Glantz, OTR/L, BCG, FAOTA
René Padilla, PhD, OTR/L, FAOTA
Kathlyn L. Reed, PhD, OTR, FAOTA, MLIS
Barbara Schell, PhD, OTR/L, FAOTA
Susanne Smith Roley, MS, OTR/L, FAOTA
Carol H. Gwin, OT/L, *AOTA Staff Liaison*

Adopted by the Representative Assembly 2007CO144

Copyright © 2008, by the American Occupational Therapy Association. Previously published in the *American Journal of Occupational Therapy, 62,* 709–710.

PART III

The American Occupational Therapy Foundation, Inc.

Bylaws: The American Occupational Therapy Foundation, Inc. (Delaware)

Revised March 26, 1998
Amended March 25, 2006
Amended June 27, 2006
Amended September 4, 2006

ARTICLE I: NAME

The name of this corporation shall be The American Occupational Therapy Foundation, Inc. (hereinafter called the Foundation).

ARTICLE II: PURPOSE

The Foundation is organized exclusively for the charitable, scientific, literary, or educational purposes within the meaning of Section 501(C)(3) of the Internal Revenue Service Code of 1954, or corresponding Section of any future federal tax code as stated in its Certificate of Incorporation.

The particular business and objects of the corporation shall be to advance the science of occupational therapy and increase the public knowledge and understanding thereof by the encouragement of the study of occupational therapy (1) through the provision of scholarships and fellowships, (2) by engaging in studies, surveys and research, and (3) by all other proper means.

ARTICLE III: OFFICES

Section 1. Principal Office. The principal office of the Foundation in the State of Delaware shall be at No. 1209 Orange Street, City of Wilmington, County of New Castle, and the resident agent in charge thereof shall be The Corporation Trust Company.

Section 2. Other Offices. The Foundation may have offices either within or without the State of Delaware and at such place or places as may from time to time be designated by the Board of Directors. Until further action by the Board of Directors, the principal office of the Foundation shall be designated by the Board of Directors.

ARTICLE IV: MEMBERSHIP

The members of the Foundation shall be the voting members of the Board of Directors, including officers and directors.

ARTICLE V: BOARD OF DIRECTORS

Section 1. Responsibilities and Powers.

A. The Board of Directors may exercise all such powers of the corporation required to govern the organization with prudence and ethics within the laws of the State of Delaware, including but not limited to: consent to the appointment of members of all committees and their chairmen; elect individuals to fill vacancies on the Board of Directors including officers; adopt standing rules consistent with the Bylaws to regulate matters; and select a certified public accountant to audit the financial statements and accounts.

B. The Board of Directors shall operate with integrity. The Board of Directors shall assure that there is no discrimination on the basis of creed, religion, race, age, gender, sexual orientation, disability or national origin.

C. Notwithstanding any other provision of these articles, the Foundation shall not conduct any activities not permitted by (I) an organization exempt from federal income tax under the IRS Code, (ii) an organization whose contributions are deductible under Section 170. (C). (2) of the IRS Code (or corresponding provision of any future United States Internal Revenue

Law), and (iii) an organization recognized as tax-exempt under the laws of the State of Delaware.

D. The Board of Directors shall employ, monitor and remove an Executive Director upon such terms and conditions as shall be determined by the Board to carry out the operations of the organization. The policies of the Board will be communicated to the Executive Director on a regular basis.

Section 2. Composition. The organization will be governed by a Board of eleven voting members, including officers and directors who shall be elected at the annual meeting. A majority of the voting members of the Board of Directors shall be occupational therapy practitioners and members of the American Occupational Therapy Association.

Non-voting members shall be the Honorary President Emerita of the Foundation who shall serve in perpetuity, the Chair of the Research Advisory Council, the Executive Director of the Foundation and a liaison from the American Occupational Therapy Association (AOTA) to be appointed annually by the AOTA President.

Honorary life members of the Board of Directors may be elected from time to time, at the discretion of the Board of Directors, in recognition of exemplary service as defined in Board policies. Honorary life members of the Board of Directors shall serve without vote, may speak, but may not make motions.

Section 3. Election and Term of Office. The directors shall be elected to serve for three years or until their successors are elected, and their term of office shall begin at the close of the meeting at which they are elected. No director shall be eligible to serve more than two consecutive terms in office unless the term of office is extended one year, for purposes of continuity, by a two-thirds vote of the members of the board.

Section 4. Resignation. Any director may resign at any time by written notice to the President. Any resignation shall take effect at the time specified, or if not specified, shall take effect immediately upon its receipt by the President.

Section 5. Removal. For cause outlined in Board policies, the Board of Directors may by a two-thirds vote remove a director and declare the office vacant.

Section 6. Vacancies. Any vacancy on the Board of Directors caused by death, resignation or removal of a director shall be filled by a majority vote of the remaining members of the Board.

A person elected to a vacancy shall serve the unexpired term of the director. If a director whose office has become vacant has served more than half of a three-year term, his successor shall be eligible to be re-elected to two successive three-year terms. If the director whose office has become vacant has served less than one half of his term, then the replacement director shall be eligible to be re-elected to one three-year term and thereafter, may not serve an additional successive term.

Section 7. Compensation. Members of the Board of Directors shall not be entitled to any compensation for their services, but voting members of the Board of Directors shall be reimbursed for expenses related to Board service. No salaried staff member of the Foundation shall serve as a director of the Foundation.

ARTICLE VI: MEETINGS

Section 1. Regular Meetings. There shall be at least one regular meeting each year, held in conjunction with the Annual Meeting of the Board of Directors, for the purpose of conducting business. Additional regular meetings may be held at any time and place on the direction of the President with written notice.

Section 2. Annual Meeting. The Annual Meeting for the purpose of electing officers and directors and for any other business that may arise shall be held on the first Sunday in November. The President, upon thirty days prior notice in writing, may change the time, date and place for this meeting.

Section 3. Special Meetings. Special meetings of the Board of Directors, for the purpose of considering one or more items of business specified in the call for the meeting, can be called by the President or by the Executive Committee and shall be called upon the written request of five of the members of the Board. Except in an emergency, written notice of such meetings of the Board of Directors shall be sent to each director and officer at least two days before the day upon which the meeting is to be held. Each such notice shall state the time, place, and purpose(s) of the meeting being called.

Section 4. Quorum. A majority of the voting members of the Board of Directors, including directors and officers present shall constitute a quorum for the transaction of business at any meeting of the Board of Directors. The act of a majority of such members of the Board of Directors present at any meeting, at which a quorum is present, shall be the act of the Board of Directors, except as may be otherwise specifically provided by statute, or by the Certificate of Incorporation, or by these Bylaws.

Section 5. Members of the Board of Directors, or any committee of the Board of Directors, may participate in and act at any meeting of such Board or committee through the use of a conference telephone or other communications equipment by means of which all persons participating in the meeting can communicate with each other. Participation in such a meeting shall constitute attendance and presence in person at the meeting of the person or persons so participating.

Section 6. Any action required to be taken at a meeting of the Board of Directors, or of any committee thereof, may be taken without a meeting if a consent in writing, setting forth the action so taken, shall be signed by all members of the Board of Directors entitled to vote with respect to the subject matter thereof, or by all the members of such committee, as the case may be. Any such consent signed by all voting members of the Board of Directors, or all the members of the committee shall have the same effect as a unanimous vote at a meeting of the Board of Directors at which a quorum was present, and may be stated as such in any document to be filed with the Secretary of State, or with anyone else.

ARTICLE VII: OFFICERS

Section 1. The President and Vice President of the American Occupational Therapy Foundation shall be occupational therapists and a current or previous member of the Board of Directors of the Foundation. The Secretary and Treasurer shall also be a current or previous member of the Board of Directors of the Foundation. Officers shall be voting members of the Board of Directors and shall have all powers and duties generally assigned their respective positions by Roberts Rules of Order Newly Revised and as specifically stated in Board Policies. The President is an ex-officio member of all committees except the Nominating Committee. The President shall vote only when his or her vote is required to break a tie vote of the members of the Board of Directors.

Honorary officers may be elected from time to time, at the discretion of the Board of Directors, in recognition of exemplary service as defined in Board policies. Honorary officers shall serve without vote, may speak but may not make motions.

Section 2. Election, Term of Office. The officers shall be elected to serve for three years or until their successors are elected, and their term of office shall begin at the close of the meeting at which they are elected. No officer shall be eligible to serve more than two consecutive terms in the same office or more than twelve successive years on the board without a three-year leave of absence unless the term of office is extended one year, for purposes of continuity, by a two-thirds vote of the members of the board.

Section 3. Resignation. Any officer may resign at any time by written notice to the President. Any resignation shall take effect at the time specified, or if not specified, shall take effect immediately upon its receipt by the President. In the event of the resignation of the President, such shall be submitted in writing to the Secretary, acting as the representative of the Board of Directors.

Section 4. Removal. For cause, outlined in Board Policies, the Board of Directors by a two-thirds vote shall remove any officer and declare the office vacant.

Section 5. Vacancies. Any vacancy in any office caused by death, resignation or removal of an officer shall be filled by majority vote of the remaining members of the Board at the Annual Meeting or a special meeting held for that purpose.

A person elected to a vacant office shall serve the unexpired term of the officer. If the officer whose office has become vacant has served more than one half of a three-year term, his successor shall be eligible to be re-elected to serve two three-year terms. If the officer whose office has become vacant has served less than one half of a three-year term, then the replacement officer shall be eligible to be re-elected to one three-year term and thereafter, may not serve an additional successive term.

Section 6. Compensation of Officers. Officers shall not be entitled to any compensation for their services as officers, but may be reimbursed for expenses related to their service as officers. No salaried staff member of the Foundation shall serve as an officer of the Foundation.

ARTICLE VIII: COUNCILS

Research Advisory Council. The purpose of the Research Advisory Council shall be to promote research in occupational therapy, anticipate the research needs for the profession and coordinate research activities within the profession. The Chairman of the Council shall be appointed by the President of the Foundation in consultation with the President of AOTA, and shall be accountable to the President of the Foundation. The Chairman shall serve on the Foundation Board of Directors without vote for a term of three years, and may be appointed to serve an additional three-year term. The membership of the Council shall be defined by the Standard Operating Procedures for this group.

ARTICLE IX: COMMITTEES

Section 1. Nominating Committee. Annually, at least sixty days in advance of the scheduled Annual Meeting, the President shall appoint a Chairman of the Nominating Committee who must be a voting member of the Board of Directors. The Chairman shall appoint two committee members who must also be voting members of the Board of Directors. The Board of Directors shall confirm the Chairman and the members of the Nominating Committee. The Nominating Committee shall prepare a slate of candidates for the election of officers and directors to be mailed to members of the Board of Directors at least thirty days prior to the Annual Meeting and elected by ballot by a quorum of the members of the Board of Directors present at the Annual Meeting.

Section 2. The Executive Committee. The Executive Committee shall consist of elected officers of the Board including the President, Vice-President, Secretary, and Treasurer. Meetings of the Executive Committee may be called by the President at such times as are necessary to take action on items of business which shall be binding until ratified by the Board of Directors at its next meeting.

Section 3. Standing Committees.

    A. The Standing Committees of the Foundation shall be the Bylaws, Policies and Procedures, the Awards of Recognition Committee, and the Investment Committee.

    B. The President shall nominate, and the Board of Directors shall confirm the appointment of all committee chairmen and the President shall serve as ex-officio member of all standing committees.

C. Chairmen of Standing Committees must be voting members or previous members of the Board of Directors. The membership of these Committees need not be restricted to members of the Board of Directors.

D. Committees shall report to the Board of Directors and shall assume such duties as shall be assigned by the Board of Directors.

E. A committee chairman shall appoint the members of the committee with the advice and consent of the President acting on behalf of the Board of Directors. A majority of the members of any committee shall constitute a quorum.

Section 4. Special Committees. If the Board of Directors shall create committees for special purposes, the chairs and membership need not be restricted to members of the Board of Directors. Committees shall report to the Board of Directors and shall assume such duties as shall be assigned by the Board of Directors. A committee chairman shall appoint the members of the committee with the advice and consent of the President acting on behalf of the Board of Directors. A majority of the members of any committee shall constitute a quorum.

ARTICLE X: INDEMNIFICATION

The Foundation shall indemnify (a) any person who was or is a party or is threatened to be made a party to any threatened, pending or completed action or suit by or in the right of the Foundation to procure a judgment in its favor by reason of the fact that such person is or was a director, officer, employee or agent of the Foundation or is or was serving at the request of the Foundation as a director, officer, employee or agent of another corporation, partnership, joint venture, trust or other enterprise, against expenses (including attorney's fees) actually and reasonably incurred by such person in connection with the defense or settlement of such action or suit, and by any person who was or is a party or is threatened to be made a party to any threatened, pending, or completed action, suit or proceeding, whether civil, criminal, administrative or investigative (other than an action by or in the right of the Foundation) by reason of the fact that he is or was a director, officer, employee or agent of the Foundation, or who was serving at the request of the Foundation as a director, officer, employee, or agent of another corporation, partnership, joint venture, trust or other enterprise, against expenses (including attorney's fees), judgements, fines and amounts paid in settlement actually and reasonably incurred by him in connection with any such action, suit or proceeding, in each case to the fullest extent permissible under applicable laws, as amended from time to time, or in the indemnification provision of any successor statute.

ARTICLE XI: DISSOLUTION CLAUSE

In the event the Foundation should be dissolved for any reason, any remaining assets shall be distributed for purposes within the scope of the Internal Revenue Service Code 501(c) 3, or any amendment thereto and according to the Eleventh Article of the Certificate of Incorporation of the American Occupational Therapy Foundation, Inc.

ARTICLE XII: SEAL

The corporate seal shall bear the name of the Foundation, the year of its organization and the words "Corporate Seal, Delaware".

ARTICLE XIII: PARLIAMENTARY AUTHORITY

The rules contained in Robert's Rules of Order Newly Revised shall govern the Foundation in all cases to which they are applicable and in which they are not inconsistent with these Bylaws and/or the Foundation's Articles of Incorporation.

ARTICLE XIV: AMENDMENTS

The Foundation shall make and from time to time alter and amend these Bylaws as may be necessary to carry into effect any of the purposes of the Foundation, or which may be needful in its governance, or in the conduct of its business. Such Bylaws may be made or amended at any regular or special meeting of the Foundation, provided, however, that any proposed Bylaw change shall be made available to all voting members of the Board of Directors no less than twenty days prior to the meeting at which such proposed Bylaw change shall be considered for adoption.

Certificate of Incorporation

CERTIFICATE OF INCORPORATION

OF

THE AMERICAN OCCUPATIONAL THERAPY FOUNDATION, INC.

FIRST. The name of the corporation is The American Occupational Therapy Foundation, Inc.

SECOND. Its principal office in the State of Delaware is located at No. 100 West Tenth Street, in the City of Wilmington, County of New Castle. The name and address of its resident agent is The Corporation Trust Company, No. 100 West Tenth Street, Wilmington 99, Delaware.

THIRD. The corporation is organized exclusively for charitable, scientific, literary, and educational purposes, including, for such purposes, the making of distributions to organizations that qualify as exempt organizations under Section 501(c)(3) of the Internal Revenue Code of 1954. The particular business and objects of the corporation shall be to advance the science of occupational therapy and increase the public knowledge and understanding thereof by the encouragement of the study of occupational therapy (1) through the provision of scholarships and fellowships, (2) by engaging in studies, surveys and research, and (3) by all other proper means. No

REC C 85 PAGE 692

activities shall be pursued by the corporation for a profit, to such an extent as to constitute such activities a trade or business, but solely for the purposes hereinabove set forth; and no part of the net earnings of the corporation shall inure to the benefit of any member, director, officer or employee of the corporation or any other individual, except reasonable compensation for services actually rendered in effecting one or more of the corporation's purposes set forth hereinabove. The corporation shall not in any way, directly or indirectly, carry on propaganda, or otherwise attempt to influence legislation, or participate in, or intervene in (including the publishing or distributing of statements), any political campaign on behalf of any candidate for public office; nor shall any of its funds, property or income be used for such purpose.

In pursuance of and not in limitation of the general powers conferred by law, and the objects and purposes herein set forth, it is expressly provided that the corporation shall also have the following powers:

To do all such acts as are necessary or convenient to attain the objects and purposes herein set forth, to the same extent and as fully as any natural person could or might do, and as are not forbidden by law or by this certificate of incorporation or by the by-laws of this corporation;

To purchase, lease, receive by gift, devise or bequest, or otherwise acquire, either absolutely or in trust,

2

REC C 85 PAGE 693

hold, sell, mortgage, or otherwise dispose of real, personal or mixed property; and to invest the principal thereof, to accumulate, administer, expend and distribute any such property or the income therefrom in the form of gifts, grants, and endowments for and to institutions and organizations primarily engaged in charitable, scientific, literary or educational purposes, or gifts, grants and endowments to individuals for educational or scientific purposes or research;

To enter into, make, perform and carry out contracts of every kind with any person, firm, corporation, or association; to do any acts necessary or expedient for carrying on any and all of the activities and pursuing any and all of the objects and purposes set forth in this certificate of incorporation and not forbidden by the laws of the State of Delaware.

To have offices and promote and carry on its objects and purposes within or without the State of Delaware, in other states, the District of Columbia, the territories or colonies of the United States.

In general, to have all powers conferred upon a corporation by the laws of the State of Delaware, except as herein prohibited, or forbidden by the by-laws of this corporation.

3

REC C 85 PAGE 694

FOURTH: The corporation shall not have authority to issue capital stock. The conditions of membership of the corporation shall be stated in the by-laws.

FIFTH: The names and places of residence of the incorporators are as follows:

NAMES	RESIDENCES
Ruth W. Brunyate, OTR	306 South Wind Road Ruxton 4, Maryland
Alice C. Jantzen, OTR	2711 N.W. 2nd Avenue Gainesville, Florida
Mary Frances Keermans, OTR	429 West Prospect Appleton, Wisconsin
Ethel E. Huebner, OTR	13 Pennwood Drive Trenton, New Jersey 08638
Marion W. Crampton, OTR	109 Bartlett Avenue Arlington, Massachusetts 02174
Janet C. Stone, OTR	4435 East Ocean Blvd., Apt. 12, Long Beach, California 90803
Sister Miriam Joseph, OTR	Chairman, Dept. of OT, College of St. Catherine 2004 Randolph St. Paul, Minn. 55116
Florence Cromwell, OTR	1179 Yocum Street Pasadena, California
Dean R. Tyndall, OTR	444 Campbell Avenue Kalamazoo, Michigan
Mary Van Gorden, OTR	401 East 2nd Street Duluth, Minnesota 55805

4

REC C 85 PAGE 695

SIXTH. The corporation shall have perpetual existence.

SEVENTH. The private property of the members shall not be subject to the payment of corporate debts to any extent whatever.

EIGHTH. The activities and affairs of the corporation shall be managed by a board of directors. The number of directors which shall constitute the whole board shall be such as from time to time shall be fixed by or in the manner provided in the by-laws, but in no case shall the number be less than three. The incorporators shall act as the members and first Board of Directors until the adoption of by-laws and the first election of directors.

The corporation may in its by-laws confer powers upon the Board of Directors in addition to the foregoing, and in addition to the powers and authority expressly conferred upon them by statute, provided that the Board of Directors shall not exercise any power or authority reserved herein or by statute to the members.

NINTH. Meetings of members may be held without the State of Delaware, if the by-laws so provide. The books of the corporation may be kept (subject to any provision contained in the statutes), outside of the State of Delaware at such place or places as may be from time to time

5

REC C 85 PAGE 696

designated by the Board of Directors. Election of directors need not be by ballot unless the by-laws of the corporation shall so provide.

TENTH. The corporation reserves the right to amend, alter, change or repeal any provision contained in this certificate of incorporation, in the manner now or hereafter prescribed by statute, and all rights conferred upon members herein are granted subject to this reservation.

ELEVENTH. No dividends of any nature whatsoever nor any other distribution of earnings or surplus shall be declared or paid to the members of the corporation; and no part of the net earnings of the corporation shall enure to the benefit of any member or individual. All profits or surplus shall be used by the corporation to further its purposes. Upon any dissolution of the corporation no member or any other private individual shall be entitled to any distribution or division of its remaining assets, but the net assets of the corporation, after the payment of debts and necessary expenses, shall be distributed to or among one or more other organizations organized and operated exclusively for charitable, religious, scientific, literary and/or educational purposes.

WE, THE UNDERSIGNED, being each of the incorporators hereinbefore named, for the purpose of forming a corporation pursuant to the General Corporation Law of the State of

6

REC C 85 PAGE 697

Delaware, do make this certificate, hereby declaring and certifying that the facts herein stated are true, and accordingly have hereunto set our hands and seals this 5th day of April, A. D. 1965.

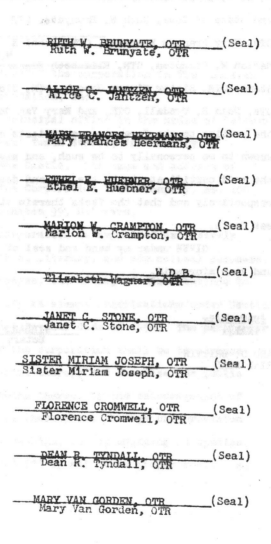

RUTH W. BRUNYATE, OTR _____ (Seal)
Ruth W. Brunyate, OTR

ALICE C. JANTZEN, OTR _____ (Seal)
Alice C. Jantzen, OTR

MARY FRANCES HEERMANS, OTR (Seal)
Mary Frances Heermans, OTR

ETHEL E. HUEBNER, OTR _____ (Seal)
Ethel E. Huebner, OTR

MARION W. CRAMPTON, OTR _____ (Seal)
Marion W. Crampton, OTR

W.D.B. _____ (Seal)
Elizabeth Wagner, OTR

JANET C. STONE, OTR _____ (Seal)
Janet C. Stone, OTR

SISTER MIRIAM JOSEPH, OTR _____ (Seal)
Sister Miriam Joseph, OTR

FLORENCE CROMWELL, OTR _____ (Seal)
Florence Cromwell, OTR

DEAN R. TYNDALL, OTR _____ (Seal)
Dean R. Tyndall, OTR

MARY VAN GORDEN, OTR _____ (Seal)
Mary Van Gorden, OTR

REC C 85 PAGE 698

STATE OF IOWA   )
                    : ss.:
COUNTY OF POLK)

              BE IT REMEMBERED that on this 5 day of April A. D. 1965, personally came before me, a Notary Public for the State of Iowa, Ruth W. Brunyate, OTR, Alice C. Jantzen, OTR, Mary Frances Heermans, OTR, Ethel E. Huebner, OTR, Marion W. Crampton, OTR, Elizabeth Wagner, OTR, W.D.B. Janet C. Stone, OTR, Sister Miriam Joseph, OTR, Florence Cromwell, OTR, Dean R. Tyndall, OTR, and Mary Van Gorden, OTR, all of the parties to the foregoing certificate of incorporation, known to me personally to be such, and severally acknowledged the said certificate to be the act and deed of the signers respectively and that the facts therein stated are truly set forth.

              GIVEN under my hand and seal of office the day and year aforesaid.

[NOTARIAL
SEAL]

                                 WILLARD D. BRITTIN
                                  Notary Public

WILLARD D. BRITTIN
NOTARIAL SEAL
IOWA

8

PART IV

Recisions, Revisions, and Changes

Recisions, Revisions, and Changes

The following recisions, revisions, and changes have been made since the publication of previous editions of the *Reference Manual of the Official Documents of the American Occupational Therapy Association, Inc.*

Bylaws

Incorporation Papers and Bylaws (1991, 1996, 1999, 2002, 2003, 2005). Bylaws and Glossary Sections **revised** and **replaced** 2007.

Accreditation

Essentials and Guidelines for an Accredited Educational Program for the Occupational Therapist (1935, 1943, 1949, 1965, 1973, 1983, 1991, 1995, 1998). **Rescinded** 2007. **Replaced** by Accreditation Standards for a Doctoral-Degree-Level Educational Program for the Occupational Therapist (2007) and Accreditation Standards for a Master's-Degree-Level Educational Program for the Occupational Therapist (2007).

Essentials and Guidelines for an Accredited Educational Program for the Occupational Therapy Assistant (1958, 1962, 1967, 1970, 1975, 1983, 1991, 1995, 1998). **Rescinded** 2007. **Replaced** by Accreditation Standards for an Educational Program for the Occupational Therapy Assistant (2007).

Concept Papers

Cross-Training Concept Paper (1997). **Rescinded** 2002.

Scholorship and Occupational Therapy (2003). **Revised** 2009.

Service Delivery in Occupational Therapy (1995). **Rescinded** 2004.

Education

Academic Terminal Degree (2003). **Replaced** by Academic Terminal Degree (2008).

Philosophy of Professional Education (1997, 2003). **Replaced** by Philosophy of Occupational Therapy Education (2007).

Purpose and Value of Occupational Therapy Fieldwork Education (1996). **Replaced** by The Purpose and Value of Occupational Therapy Fieldwork Education (2003). **Replaced** by Occupational Therapy Fieldwork Value and Purpose (2009).

Standards and Guidelines for an Occupational Therapy Affiliation Program (1970). **Rescinded** 1983.

The Viability of Occupational Therapy Assistant Education (2002). **Replaced** by the Importance of Occupational Therapy Assistant Education (2008).

Ethics

Occupational Therapy Code of Ethics (1988, 1994, 2000). **Replaced** by Occupational Therapy Code of Ethics (2005, **edited** 2006).

Enforcement Procedures for Occupational Therapy Code of Ethics (1994, 1996, 1998, 2000, 2002, 2004, 2005, **edited** 2006). **Replaced** by Enforcement Procedures for Occupational Therapy Code of Ethics (2007).

Guidelines to the Occupational Therapy Code of Ethics (1998). **Replaced** by the Guidelines to the Occupational Therapy Code of Ethics (2006).

Guidelines

Elements of Clinical Documentation (1994). **Rescinded** 2003. **Replaced** by Guidelines for Documentation of Occupational Therapy (2003, **edited** 2007).

Guide for Supervision of Occupational Therapy Personnel (1994). **Rescinded** 1999. **Replaced** by Guide for Supervision of Occupational Therapy Personnel in the Delivery of Occupational Therapy Services (1999, *AJOT*, *53*(6):592–594 [correction, *54*(2):235]).

Guide for Supervision of Occupational Therapy Personnel in the Delivery of Occupational Therapy Services (1994, 1999). **Rescinded** 2004. **Replaced** by Guidelines for Supervision, Roles, and Responsibilities During the Delivery of Occupational Therapy Services (2004, **edited** 2009).

Guide to Classification of Occupational Therapy Personnel (1987). **Rescinded** 1991. **Replaced** by Occupational Therapy Roles (1993) and Companion Guide (1994).

Guidelines for an Occupational Therapist Providing Services as a Supervisor (1974). **Replaced** by Guide for Supervision of Occupational Therapy Personnel (1981, 1994).

Guidelines for Occupational Therapy Documentation (1986). **Replaced** by Elements of Clinical Documentation (1994).

Guidelines for the Use of Aides in Occupational Therapy Practice (1996, 1999). **Rescinded** 2004. **Replaced** by Guidelines for Supervision, Roles, and Responsibilities During the Delivery of Occupational Therapy Services (2004, **edited** 2009).

Hierarchy of Competencies Relating to the Use of Standardized Instruments and Evaluation Techniques by Occupational Therapists (1984). **Rescinded** 1992.

Minimal Occupational Therapy Classification Standards (1971). **Revised** 1997. Replaced by Guide to Classification of Occupational Therapy Personnel (1985, **edited** 1987). **Replaced** by Occupational Therapy Roles (1993) and Companion Guide (1994).

Occupational Therapy Practice Framework. **Replaced** by Occupational Therapy Practice Framework: Domain and Process, 2nd Edition (2008).

Occupational Therapy Product Output Reporting System (1979). **Rescinded** 1994.

Supervision Guidelines (1986). **Rescinded** 1992. **Replaced** by Guidelines for Supervision, Roles, and Responsibilities during the Delivery of Occupational Therapy Services (2004, **edited** 2009).

Supervision Guidelines for Certified Occupational Therapy Assistants (1990). **Rescinded** 1993.

Uniform Occupational Therapy Evaluation Checklist (1981). **Rescinded** 1994.

Uniform Terminology for Reporting Occupational Therapy Services—First Edition (1979). **Replaced** by Uniform Terminology for Occupational Therapy (Second Edition) and the Application of Uniform Terminology to Practice (1989). **Replaced** by Uniform Terminology for Occupational Therapy (Third Edition) and Application to Practice (1994). **Rescinded** 2002.

Work Hardening Guidelines (1986). **Replaced** by Statement: Occupational Therapy Services in Work Practice (1992).

Specialized Knowledge and Skills Papers

Specialized Knowledge and Skills for Occupational Therapy Practice in the Neonatal Intensive Care Unit (1993, 2000). **Replaced** by Specialized Knowledge and Skills for Occupational Therapy Practice in the Neonatal Intensive Care Unit (2006).

Specialized Knowledge and Skills in Adult Vestibular Rehabilitation for Occupational Therapy Practice (2000). **Replaced** by Specialized Knowledge and Skills in Adult Vestibular Rehabilitation for Occupational Therapy Practice (2006).

Specialized Knowledge and Skills in Eating and Feeding in Occupational Therapy Practice (2000). **Replaced** by Specialized Knowledge and Skills in Feeding, Eating, and Swallowing for Occupational Therapy Practice (2007).

Position Papers

AOTA Position Paper on Early Childhood Intervention (1986). **Replaced** by Occupational Therapy Services in Early Intervention and Preschool Services (1988). **Rescinded** 2002.

Broadening the Construct of Independence (1995, 2002). **Rescinded** 2007.

Human Immunodeficiency Virus (1984). **Replaced** by Providing Services for Persons with HIV/AIDS and Their Caregivers (1996). **Rescinded** 2002.

Occupation: A Position Paper (1995). **Rescinded** 2004.

Occupational Performance: Occupational Therapy's Definition of Function (1995). **Rescinded** 2002.

Occupational Therapy: A Profession in Support of Full Inclusion (1995) with White Paper: The Role of the Occupational Therapy Practitioner in the Implementation of Full Inclusion (1996). Position Paper and White Paper **rescinded** 1999. **Replaced** by Position Paper, Occupational Therapy's Commitment to Non-discrimination and Inclusion (1999, *AJOT*, 53(6):598 [correction, 54(2):235]).

Occupational Therapy and Assistive Technology (1991). **Replaced** by The Use of General Information and Assistive Technology Within Occupational Therapy Practice (1998).

Occupational Therapy and Eating Dysfunction (1989). **Replaced** by Eating Dysfunction Position Paper (1996). **Replaced** by Specialized Knowledge and Skills for Eating and Feeding in Occupational Therapy Practice (2000).

Occupational Therapy and Hospice (1986,1991). **Replaced** by Statement, Occupational Therapy and Hospice (1998).

Occupational Therapy and Long-Term Services and Supports (1994). **Rescinded** 2002.

Occupational Therapy and The Americans With Disabilities Act (ADA) (1993, 2000). **Rescinded** 2005.

Occupational Therapy as an Education-Related Service (1981). **Rescinded** 1987.

Occupational Therapy for Sensory Integrative Dysfunction (1982). **Rescinded** 1991.

Occupational Therapy in Adult Day-Care (1986). **Rescinded** 1992.

Occupational Therapy in the Promotion of Health and the Prevention of Disease and Disability (1989). **Rescinded** 2000. **Replaced** by Statement: Occupational Therapy in the Promotion of Health and the Prevention of Disease and Disability (2000).

Occupational Therapy Services for Alzheimer's Disease and Related Disorders Position Paper (1986). **Replaced** by Occupational Therapy Services for Persons with Alzheimer's Disease and Other Dementias (Statement [1994]). **Rescinded** 2000.

Occupational Therapy's Commitment to Nondiscrimination and Inclusion (1999). **Replaced** by Occupational Therapy's Commitment to Nondiscrimination and Inclusion (2004, **edited** 2009).

Physical Agent Modalities: A Position Paper (1992). **Replaced** by Physical Agent Modalities Position Paper (**edited** 1997). **Rescinded** 2003. **Replaced** by Physical Agent Modalities: A Position Paper (2003, **edited** 2007).

Purposeful Activities (1983). **Replaced** by Position Paper: Purposeful Activity (1993). **Rescinded** 2002.

The Psychosocial Core of Occupational Therapy (1995, **edited** 1997). **Rescinded** 2004. **Replaced** by Psychosocial Aspects of Occupational Therapy (2004).

Scope of Practice (2005). **Replaced** by Scope of Practice (2009).

Use of Occupational Therapy Aides in Occupational Therapy Practice (1995, **edited** 1996). **Rescinded** 1999. **Replaced** by Guidelines for the Use of Aides in Occupational Therapy Practice—Guidelines (1999, *AJOT, 53*(6):595–597 [correction, *54*(2):235]).

The Use of General Information and Assistive Technology Within Occupational Therapy Practice (1991, 1998). **Rescinded** 2004. **Replaced** by Assistive Technology Within Occupational Therapy Practice (2004, **Rescinded** 2009).

Roles Papers

Entry-Level Role Delineation for OTRs and COTAs (1981). **Revised** 1990. **Rescinded** 1994. **Replaced** by Occupational Therapy Roles (1993) and Companion Guide (1994).

Occupational Therapy: Its Definitions and Functions (1972). **Replaced** by Definitions (1981). **Rescinded** 1992.

Occupational Therapy Roles (1993) and Career Exploration and Development: A Companion Guide to the Occupational Therapy Roles Document (1994). **Rescinded** 2004. **Replaced** by Guidelines for Supervision, Roles, and Responsibilities During the Delivery of Occupational Therapy Services (2004, **edited** 2009) and Scope of Practice (2004, **edited** 2009).

Occupational Therapy's Role in Independent or Alternative Living Situations (1981). **Rescinded** 1991. **Replaced** by The Role of Occupational Therapy in the Independent Living Movement (Statement [1993]). **Rescinded** 1999.

Role Competencies for An Academic Fieldwork Coordinator (2003). **Rescinded** 2009. **Replaced** by Specialized Knowledge and Skills of Occupational Therapy Educators of the Future (2009).

Role Competencies for a Faculty Member in an OTA Academic Setting (2005). **Rescinded** 2009. **Replaced** by Specialized Knowledge and Skills of Occupational Therapy Educators of the Future (2009).

Role Competencies for a Fieldwork Educator (2005). **Rescinded** 2009. **Replaced** by Specialized Knowledge and Skills of Occupational Therapy Educators of the Future (2009).

Role Competencies for a Professional-Level OT Faculty memeber in an Academic Setting (2005). **Rescinded** 2009. **Replaced** by Specialized Knowledge and Skills of Occupational Therapy Educators of the Future (2009).

Role Competencies for a Professional-Level Program Director in an Academic Setting (2009). **Rescinded** 2009. **Replaced** by Specialized Knowledge and Skills of Occupational Therapy Educators of the Future (2009).

Role Competencies for a Program Director in an OTA Academic Setting (2003). **Rescinded** 2009. **Replaced** by Specialized Knowledge and Skills of Occupational Therapy Educators of the Future (2009).

Roles and Functions of Occupational Therapy in Adult Day-Care (1986). **Rescinded** 1992.

Roles and Functions of Occupational Therapy in Burn Care Delivery (1985). **Rescinded** 1991.

Roles and Functions of Occupational Therapy in Hand Rehabilitation (1985). **Rescinded** 1991.

Roles and Functions of Occupational Therapy in Long-Term Care: Occupational Therapy and Activity Programs (1983). **Rescinded** 1992. **Replaced** by Occupational Therapy and Long-Term Services and Supports (Position Paper [1994]).

Roles and Functions of Occupational Therapy in the Management of Patients with Rheumatic Diseases (1986). **Rescinded** 1992.

Roles and Functions of Occupational Therapy in Mental Health (1986). **Rescinded** 1991.

Roles and Functions of Occupational Therapy Services for the Severely Disabled (1983). **Rescinded** 1992.

Roles and Functions of the Occupational Therapist in the Treatment of Sensory Integrative Dysfunction (1982). **Rescinded** 1991.

Roles of Occupational Therapists and Occupational Therapy Assistants in Schools (1987). **Rescinded** 1997.

The Role of the Occupational Therapist in Home Health Care (1981). **Rescinded** 1991.

The Role of the Occupational Therapist in the Promotion of Health and Prevention of Disabilities (1976). **Replaced** by Occupational Therapy in the Promotion of Health and the Prevention of Disease and Disabilities (1976). **Replaced** by Occupational Therapy in the Promotion of Health and the Prevention of Disease and Disability (Position Paper [1989]).

The Role of Occupational Therapy in the Vocational Rehabilitation Process (1980). **Rescinded** 1991.

Standards

Glossary of Terms Used in the Standards of Practice (1985). **Rescinded** 1991.

Standards for Continuing Competence (1999). **Replaced** by Standards for Continuing Competence (2005).

Standards of Practice for Occupational Therapy (1983, 1992, 1994, 1998). **Replaced** by Standards of Practice for Occupational Therapy (2005).

Standards of Practice: Developmental Disabilities (1979, 1988). **Rescinded** 1991.

Standards of Practice: Home Health (1979, 1988). **Rescinded** 1991.

Standards of Practice: Mental Health (1979, 1988). **Rescinded** 1991.

Standards of Practice: Physical Disabilities (1979, 1988). **Rescinded** 1991.

Standards of Practice for Occupational Therapy Services in Schools (1987). **Rescinded** 1994.

Statements

Applying Sensory Integration Framework in Educationally Related Occupational Therapy Practice (2003). **Rescinded** 2009. **Replaced** by *Providing Occupational Therapy Using Sensory Integration Therapy and Methods in School-Based Practice* (2009).

Assistive Technology Within Occupational Therapy Practice (2004). **Rescinded** 2009. **Replaced** by *Specialized Knowledge and Skills in Technology and Environmental Interventions for Occupational Therapy Practice* (2009).

AOTA Statement of Physical Agent Modalities (1991). **Rescinded** 1997.

Fundamental Concepts of Occupational Therapy: Occupation, Purposeful Activity, Function (1997). **Rescinded** 2005.

Management of Occupational Therapy Services for Persons with Cognitive Impairments (1999). **Rescinded** 2003.

Nondiscrimination and Inclusion Regarding Members of the Occupational Therapy Professional Community (1995). **Rescinded** 2005.

Ocupational Therapy and Hospice (1998). **Replaced** by Occupational Therapy and Hospice (2004).

Occupational Therapy for Individuals with Learning Disabilities (1991, 1998). **Rescinded** 2004. **Replaced** by Occupational Therapy Services in Early Intervention and School-Based Programs (2004).

Occupational Therapy in the Promotion of Health and the Prevention of Disease and Disability (2000). **Replaced** by Occupational Therapy in the Promotion of Health and the Prevention of Disease and Disability 2007).

Occupational Therapy Provision for Children with Learning Disabilities and/or Mild to Moderate Perceptual and Motor Deficits (1991). **Replaced** by Occupational Therapy for Individuals with Learning Disabilities (1998).

Occupational Therapy Services for Persons with Alzheimer's Disease and Other Dementias (1994). **Rescinded** 2000.

Occupational Therapy Services in Work Practice (1992). **Replaced** by Statement, Occupational Therapy Services in Facilitating Work Performance (2000). **Replaced** by Occupational Therapy Services in Facilitating Work Performance (2005).

Occupational Therapy Services Management of Persons With Cognitive Impairments (1991). **Rescinded** 1999. **Replaced** by Management of Occupational Therapy Services for Persons With Cognitive Impairments (1999).

Psychosocial Concerns Within Occupational Therapy Practice (1995). **Rescinded** 2004.

The Occupational Therapist as Case Manager (1991). **Rescinded** 2002.

The Role of Occupational Therapy in the Independent Living Movement (1993). **Rescinded** 1999.

Sensory Integration Evaluation and Intervention in School-Based Occupational Therapy (1997). **Rescinded** 2003. **Replaced** by Applying Sensory Integration Framework in Educationally Related Occupational Therapy Practice (2003).

Statement of Occupational Therapy Referral (1969, 1980, 1994). **Rescinded** 2004. **Replaced** by the Guidelines for Supervision, Roles, and Responsibilities During the Delivery of Occupational Therapy Services (2004, **edited** 2009) and Scope of Practice (2004, **edited** 2005).

Certification Document Changes

The following certification documents have been removed from earlier editions of this manual:

AOTA Certification Requirements. **Rendered moot** by the formation of the American Occupational Therapy Certification Board.

Requirements for Graduates from Foreign Schools to Become OTRs. **Rendered moot** by the formation of the American Occupational Therapy Certification Board.

Policy Governing Lapsed Certification of Occupational Therapists and Occupational Therapy Assistants. **Rescinded** 1986.

Index

Note: Page references in *italic* refer to figures and tables.